# An Introduction to Intermediate and Advanced Statistical Analyses for Sport and Exercise Scientists

# An Introduction to Intermediate and Advanced Statistical Analyses for Sport and Exercise Scientists

Edited by

**Nikos Ntoumanis**

*School of Psychology & Speech Pathology,
Curtin University, Perth, Australia*

**Nicholas D. Myers**

*School of Education and Human Development,
University of Miami, Florida, USA*

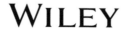

*Registered Office*
John Wiley & Sons, Ltd, The Atrium, Southern Gate, Chichester, West Sussex, PO19 8SQ, United Kingdom

For details of our global editorial offices, for customer services and for information about how to apply for permission to reuse the copyright material in this book please see our website at www.wiley.com.

*Library of Congress Cataloging-in-Publication Data*

Names: Ntoumanis, Nikos, 1971– , editor. | Myers, Nicholas D., editor.
Title: An Introduction to Intermediate and Advanced Statistical Analyses for Sport and Exercise Scientists / edited by Nikos Ntoumanis, Nicholas D. Myers.
Description: Chichester, West Sussex ; Hoboken : John Wiley & Sons Inc., 2016. | Includes bibliographical references and index.
Identifiers: LCCN 2015036901 | ISBN 9781118962053 (cloth)
Subjects: | MESH: Sports Medicine–methods. | Athletic Performance–statistics & numerical data. | Statistics as Topic–methods.
Classification: LCC RC1210 | NLM QT 261 | DDC 617.1–dc23 LC record available at http://lccn.loc.gov/2015036901

A catalogue record for this book is available from the British Library.

Set in 10/12pt Times by SPi Global, Pondicherry, India
Printed and bound in Singapore by Markono Print Media Pte Ltd

1   2016

*To Anna Maria, Zoe, and Cecilie: thank you for your love,*
*support, and companionship!*
*(Nikos Ntoumanis)*

*My work on this book is dedicated to my lovely partner, Ahnalee,*
*and our wonderful children, Benjamin and Amelia.*
*(Nicholas D. Myers)*

# Contents

# About the editors

**Nikos Ntoumanis** is currently a Professor of Psychology at Curtin University, in Perth, Australia. He earned his PhD at the University of Exeter (United Kingdom) in 1999. In 2001, he joined the University of Birmingham (United Kingdom) where he worked until 2014. In 2001, Nikos authored a step-by-step guide to SPSS for sport and exercise sciences; the book was published by Routledge. Nikos taught statistics for many years at the University of Birmingham. His research examines personal and contextual factors that optimize motivation and promote performance, psychological well-being, and health-conducive behaviors in various physical activity settings 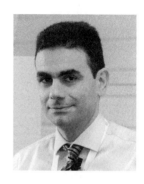 (exercise, sport, physical education). Nikos is a fellow of the UK's Academy of Social Sciences and coeditor-in-chief of the journal *Psychology of Sport and Exercise*. Nikos' research has received funding from major research councils in the United Kingdom, charities, health authorities, private companies, and the European Union. His research has been published in various journals, such as *Perspectives on Psychological Science*, *Developmental Psychology*, *Personality and Social Psychology Bulletin*, *Annals of Behavioral Medicine*, and *Sports Medicine*. Nikos often engages with the media (e.g., *The Times*, *Le Figaro*, *Men's Health*) in an effort to disseminate his research. He is the proud father of two girls, Anna Maria and Zoe.

**Nicholas D. Myers** is currently an Associate Professor of Research, Measurement, and Evaluation at the University of Miami School of Education and Human Development. He earned a dual discipline (i.e., psychosocial aspects of sport and physical activity, measurement and quantitative methods) PhD at Michigan State University in 2005. Nick currently serves as editor-in-chief of the journal *Measurement in Physical Education and Exercise Science*.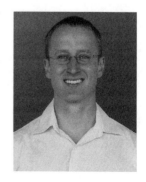

# List of contributors

**Soyeon Ahn**, School of Education and Human Development, University of Miami, Coral Gables, FL, USA

**Paul R. Appleton**, School of Sport, Exercise and Rehabilitation Sciences, University of Birmingham, Birmingham, UK

**Seniz Celimli**, School of Education and Human Development, University of Miami, Coral Gables, FL, USA

**David E. Conroy**, College of Health & Human Development, The Pennsylvania State University, University Park, PA USA

**Michael J. Duncan**, Faculty of Health and Life Sciences, Coventry University, Coventry, UK

**Alicia L. Fedewa**, Department of Educational, School, and Counseling Psychology, University of Kentucky, Lexington, KY, USA

**Alexandre Gareau**, École de Psychologie/School of Psychology, Université d'Ottawa/University of Ottawa, Ottawa, ON, Canada

**Patrick Gaudreau**, École de Psychologie/School of Psychology, Université d'Ottawa/University of Ottawa, Ottawa, ON, Canada

**Daniel F. Gucciardi**, School of Physiotherapy and Exercise Science, Curtin University, Perth, WA, Australia

**Katie E. Gunnell**, Healthy Active Living and Obesity (HALO) Research Group, the Children's Hospital of Eastern Ontario Research Institute, Ottawa, ON, Canada

**Gregory R. Hancock**, Department of Human Development and Quantitative Methodology, University of Maryland, College Park, MD, USA

**Andreas Ivarsson**, Center of Research on Welfare, Health and Sport, Halmstad University, Halmstad, Sweden

**Ying Jin**, Assistant Professor, Quantitative Psychology, Middle Tennessee State University, Murfreesboro, TN, USA

**Minsoo Kang**, Professor, Health and Human Performance, Middle Tennessee State University, Murfreesboro, TN, USA

**Andrew M. Lane**, Faculty of Education, Health and Wellbeing, University of Wolverhampton, Walsall, UK

**Magnus Lindwall**, Department of Food and Nutrition, and Sport Science, Department of Psychology, University of Gothenburg, Gothenburg, Sweden

**Min Lu**, School of Education and Human Development, University of Miami, Coral Gables, FL, USA

**Herbert W. Marsh**, Institute for Positive Psychology and Education, Australian Catholic University, Strathfield, NSW, Australia

**Jeffrey J. Martin**, Division of Kinesiology, Health and Sport Studies, Wayne State University, Detroit, MI, USA

**Alexandre J. S. Morin**, Institute for Positive Psychology and Education, Australian Catholic University, Strathfield, NSW, Australia

**Nicholas D. Myers**, School of Education and Human Development, University of Miami, Coral Gables, FL, USA

**Alan M. Nevill**, Faculty of Education, Health and Wellbeing, University of Wolverhampton, Walsall, UK

**Nikos Ntoumanis**, School of Psychology & Speech Pathology, Curtin University, Perth, WA, Australia

**Philip D. Parker**, Institute for Positive Psychology and Education, Australian Catholic University, Strathfield, NSW, Australia

**Andreas Stenling**, Department of Psychology, Umeå University, Umeå, Sweden

**Marietta Suarez**, School of Education and Human Development, University of Miami, Coral Gables, FL, USA

**G. Tyler Lefevor**, School of Education and Human Development, University of Miami, Coral Gables, FL, USA

**John C. K. Wang**, Physical Education and Sports Science, National Institute of Education, Nanyang Technological University, Singapore

**Yan Yang**, Department of Kinesiology & Community Health, University of Illinois at Urbana-Champaign, Urbana, IL, USA

**Weimo Zhu**, Department of Kinesiology & Community Health, University of Illinois at Urbana-Champaign, Urbana, IL, USA

**Michael J. Zyphur**, Department of Management and Marketing, The University of Melbourne, Parkville, VIC, Australia

# Foreword

Many years ago, when I taught basic statistics to undergraduate sport and exercise science students, I thought that statistics were analogous to the study and teaching of anatomy—it would never change! How naïve was that? Maybe it was due to the difficulty of calculating statistical procedures at the time that led me to that conclusion. For example, I started learning SPSS using punch cards whereby I would submit my cards to the computer center on the way into work, collect them on the way out, and then repeat it the next day because I had made an error on the first card! Three days later, I had my correlation coefficient. I was also in awe of my PhD supervisor being able to calculate a factor analysis—by hand!

So these early experiences made me think that statistics did not really exist beyond correlations, ANOVAs, and factor analysis. How wrong could I be? With the advent of fast computers and associated software and, of course, developments in methods themselves, such as meta-analysis and structural equation modeling, the era of accessible sophisticated statistics crept up on me and my colleagues in the sport and exercise sciences.

It seems to me that there are many good books on more basic statistical procedures that are applied to sport and exercise science. Indeed, Nikos authored the excellent *A Step-by-Step Guide to SPSS for Sport and Exercise Science Studies* in 2001. However, that market is now quite crowded, and indeed, some general statistics books are highly popular and have probably "cornered the market." That said, students do like to see stats related to their field of interest and with examples that resonate.

Where there is clearly a gap is in the presentation of more sophisticated procedures, especially applied to sport and exercise science. This is where Nikos and Nick have done such a great job. In short, this is not just another stats book. With each chapter written by experts in a particular method and technique and with experience of application to sport and exercise science, readers of this book have the "go-to" text for intermediate and advanced statistics for our field. Chapters range from factorial and repeated (M)ANOVA to structural equation modeling (SEM). In addition, topics include sample size estimation for SEM, change statistics (e.g., latent growth curve modeling), psychometric issues (e.g., item response theory), intervention-relevant statistics (e.g., mediation analysis), and review-level statistics (i.e., meta-analysis).

While there is no substitute for actually doing statistical calculations, not everyone will have this opportunity. Indeed, I recall being told when studying for my MSc degree that even if we may not be research "producers," many are research "consumers." For example, students may learn and perform one or two of the methods described in this book. But they and others are likely to need to understand—as consumers of research—many more.

I look forward to "consuming" the contents of this excellent text myself for many years to come, including any updates that may follow. I expect there will be updates as I now realize statistics is not all at like anatomy!

**Stuart Biddle,**
Professor of Active Living and Public Health
Institute of Sport, Exercise and Active Living,
Victoria University, Melbourne, Australia

# Preface

*"Anyone who stops learning is old, whether at twenty or eighty. Anyone who keeps learning stays young"*
*(Henry Ford).*

A challenge that most (if not all!) researchers are facing is to keep up with developments (conceptual, methodological, policy and practice, etc.) in the areas of their research interests. Given that time is a precious and limited resource nowadays, we (Nikos and Nick) realized that there is a need for a book that will attempt to summarize and present in a simple manner some recent developments in the statistics literature which have implications for quantitative data analysis in sport and exercise sciences (kinesiology). To this end, we were fortunate to secure the collaboration of a large and diverse group of experts in quantitative methodology in sport and exercise sciences (and beyond) to write chapters for our book. These experts, from various continents, have the methodological training, teaching background, and publication experience that were required for this project.

With this book, we aim to introduce the reader to a variety of intermediate and advanced statistical tests that are utilized, or should be utilized more, by the sport and exercise scientists. We hope to lay the foundations for understanding these tests and guide readers to more specialized resources for additional information on those statistical tests. Currently, there is no book in the market covering a wide variety of intermediate to advanced statistical tests with examples from sport and exercise sciences. Hence, readers with a sport and exercise science background either (a) are not using these tests (but would have liked to, if provided appropriate mentoring) or (b) are using texts from other substantive fields (e.g., business, psychology, sociology) to understand these tests. However, students, particularly those with limited formal training, often have difficulties to relate the examples from these fields to their own research. Our book attempts to address some of these problems by using examples from sport and exercise sciences only. Further, this book is pioneer in that it offers to the readers electronic supplemental material with data sets, screenshots, program code, and outputs, so that the reader can replicate the examples presented in the book or adapt them to their own research questions.

The structure of each chapter was determined by the authors. We offered some general expectations and guidelines to all authors, but at the same time, we respected their autonomy to present their chapter in the way they deemed as best. Our general expectations were that all chapters should include a description of a research question(s) from sport and exercise sciences, a justification of why the described statistical technique(s) is (are) suitable to address the research question(s), a step-by-step illustration of the different procedures required to carry out the analysis, an explanation of the results, how they relate back to the research question(s), and their implications for sport and exercise sciences. By and large, we think that this structure has been followed by all authors. The electronic supplementary material illustrates program code and outputs from a number of different software. Some readers might have preferred examples from only a very small number of software; however, this was not always practically possible (given the large number of contributors to this book) or desirable.

The statistical tests presented in the book are increasingly used in publications in prestigious journals; hence, the reader should welcome a book that explains how to utilize such tests and how to interpret their results. Given that many postgraduate courses in sport and exercise sciences, particularly outside North America, do not offer systematic training in using the statistical tests covered in the book, we hope that this book will serve as a valuable resource for many postgraduate students and faculty members worldwide. The book can also be a useful resource for postgraduate students and faculty members in other subject areas. There are not many books available that cover the variety of intermediate to advanced statistical tests we present (particularly accompanied with program code, screenshots, and data files).

The tests we describe in the book do not represent an exhaustive list of available intermediate and advanced tests that are utilized or could be utilized by sport and exercise scientists. However, the 13 chapters represented a good compromise for a timely completion of the project and the publication of a resource that will be affordable to students and faculty around the world. We are confident that we have covered a large percentage of the intermediate and advanced statistical tests taught in graduate classes and published in peer-reviewed journals in the sport and exercise science field.

Chapters 1–3 cover "traditional" techniques (factorial ANOVA/MANOVA, repeated measures ANOVA/MANOVA, mediation and moderation via regression analysis) which are widely employed within sport and exercise sciences. Advances in these techniques are illustrated where appropriate. These chapters aim to serve as a "bridge" between what many readers will view as "traditional" techniques and the "newer," more sophisticated techniques described in the subsequent chapters. Chapter 4 presents item response theory, which is important for the design, testing, and scoring of questionnaires, but it is rarely used in scale construction (despite the abundance of questionnaire development studies, particularly in the sport and exercise psychology field). Chapter 5 presents an introduction to confirmatory factory analysis and structural equation modeling. Both techniques are widely utilized but not always correctly; appropriate guidelines and suggestions are offered to readers. This chapter serves as the stepping stone to more advanced analyses such as invariance of models across groups and time (Chapter 6), analysis of longitudinal data via structural equation modeling (Chapter 7), new factor models which serve as alternative to confirmatory factor models (exploratory structural equation modeling and Bayes modeling; Chapter 8), and person-based approaches (mixture modeling; Chapter 9). Chapter 10 explains how multilevel modeling can be used to analyze data with a nested structure; such nesting can be due to group effects (e.g., athletes nested within a team) or due to the longitudinal nature of the data. Meta-analysis is a relatively common statistical technique in sport and exercise sciences. Chapter 11 presents some of the latest approaches to meta-analysis. Chapter 12 presents tests that have been developed to assess the reliability and stability of physiological/biological and psychological data. Chapter 13 illustrates contemporary approaches for power calculations and effect sizes via the use of structural equation modeling.

This book is an example of our motivation to keep learning and improving our statistical knowledge and skills. To paraphrase Henry Ford, we think that by continuously learning about new developments in statistics, researchers will retain their vitality and be creative in their efforts to answer important research questions, with the assistance of the most appropriate analytical tools available at the time.

This project is a collective effort. We thank all contributing authors for sharing their expert advice, our publisher for their trust in us, our universities for giving us the time to carry out this project, and our family and friends for their support and patience throughout this project. We hope and anticipate that the readers will e-mail us their comments and suggestions about this book.

April 2015
Nikos Ntoumanis and Nicholas D. Myers

# 1

# Factorial ANOVA and MANOVA

## Minsoo Kang[1] and Ying Jin[2]

[1] Health and Human Performance, Middle Tennessee State University, Murfreesboro, TN, USA
[2] Quantitative Psychology, Middle Tennessee State University, Murfreesboro, TN, USA

## General Introduction

The ANOVA is a statistical method used to test mean differences among groups. In its simplest form, a one-way ANOVA with two groups functions the same as a *t*-test for independent samples. Unlike the *t*-test, however, more elaborate forms of ANOVA have the ability to test for mean differences among three or more groups of a single variable. The independent variable or variables in an ANOVA, also called factors or predictors, are categorical variables. Nominal and ordinal variables are common independent variables. The dependent variables are continuous (i.e., interval and ratio) variables.

The true advantage of the ANOVA, compared to *t*-test, comes from its ability to test for mean differences between two or more groups across multiple independent variables. When an ANOVA model has two independent variables, it is called a two-way ANOVA; when there are three independent variables, the ANOVA is called a three-way ANOVA; and so on. However, any ANOVA with two or more independent variables falls under the label of a factorial ANOVA. The multivariate analysis of variance (MANOVA) is an extension of the ANOVA that allows for multiple

*An Introduction to Intermediate and Advanced Statistical Analyses for Sport and Exercise Scientists*, First Edition.
Edited by Nikos Ntoumanis and Nicholas D. Myers.
© 2016 John Wiley & Sons, Ltd. Published 2016 by John Wiley & Sons, Ltd.
Companion website: www.wiley.com/go/ntoumanis/sport

dependent variables. The following sections will discuss the hypotheses and assumptions of a factorial ANOVA analysis with one dependent variable and also with multiple dependent variables (i.e., factorial MANOVA).

## Hypothesis Testing

The factorial ANOVA and MANOVA test the main effects for each independent variable on a dependent variable, as well as any possible interactions between independent variables. A hypothesis test is required for each main effect and interaction effect.

A significant main effect indicates that the independent variable is a significant predictor of the dependent variable(s). A significant main effect in a factorial ANOVA indicates that at least one group in the independent variable differs on the dependent variable. In a factorial ANOVA, there is only one dependent variable for the independent variables to differ on. The null hypothesis for each main effect in a factorial MANOVA is that the dependent variables are the same across all conditions of that independent variable. The alternative hypothesis is that at least one group in the independent variable differs on at least one dependent variable.

For an interaction, the null hypothesis is that the effect of one independent variable on the dependent variable(s) is the same across each level of another independent variable. The alternative hypothesis is that the effect of an independent variable on the dependent variable(s) differs for the levels of another independent variable. For example, the benefits associated with being physically active (low, medium, and high) on health outcomes are likely to be different depending on an individual's body mass index (underweight, normal, overweight, and obese). To test this hypothesis, an interaction term between physical activity and body mass index groups is introduced and tested along with the main effects of these variables.

## Alpha Level

Alpha level is related to the type I error rate, the chance that a researcher infers that there is a significant difference when the groups do not differ. The nominal alpha level is what the researcher sets as the chance of a type I error rate, usually 0.05 (or 5% chance). The empirical alpha level is the actual chance that a type I error occurs. Various approaches have been proposed to control the empirical alpha level in post hoc procedures. In a two-way factorial ANOVA, each main effects and interaction are considered a family and are compared to an alpha of 0.05. When the interaction is nonsignificant, the pairwise comparisons of the main effects are performed with a nominal alpha level of 0.05/comparison in order to control the familywise empirical alpha level close to 0.05. With a significant interaction, the nominal alpha level is split for each follow-up ANOVA (0.05/levels of other factor) and again for the number of pairwise comparisons ([0.05/levels of other factor]/comparison). When dealing with factorial MANOVAs, the same approach of splitting the alpha level is used until the analyses become univariate (one dependent variable) in nature. All univariate analyses retain the alpha level of the preceding multivariate analysis. This is called a protected F procedure. Even when the nominal alpha is controlled at a familywise alpha of 0.05, the empirical alpha can differ drastically from the nominal alpha level if the following assumptions are not met.

# Assumptions

## Independence Assumption

The independence assumption means that the dependent variable scores of one participant are not affected by the dependent variable scores of another participant. ANOVAs are sensitive to violations of the independence assumption. Therefore, it is important to adhere to this assumption in two ways. First, each participant contributes only one score to the data; repeated assessments of the same participant require repeated measures ANOVA/MANOVA (see Chapter 2). Second, no outside influence can systematically affect the groups. For example, if two coaches are keeping track of the number of push-ups attainable by their players, and coach A accepts push-ups from the knees and coach B does not, the coaches have systematically influenced the measurements of their groups.

## Normality Assumption

Normality refers to the distribution of the participants' scores on the dependent variable(s). The bell curve is the common conceptual image of univariate normality. Dealing with multiple dependent variables requires multivariate normality. Data that are multivariate normal are univariate normal as well. However, variables can be univariate normal without the data possessing a multivariate normal distribution. The effect of nonnormality on the ANOVA/MANOVA results is influenced by two main factors:

1. The extent of departure from normality (i.e., skewness and kurtosis)

2. Sample size ($n$)

The extent of the departure from normality diminishes in influence on test results with larger sample sizes. The influence due to departures from univariate normality on the ANOVA results is almost nonexistent when the sample size is above 30 participants per group (Myers, Well, & Lorch, 2010). The number of participants needed to reduce the effects of multivariate nonnormality relates to the number of dependent variables in the model. However, Seo, Kanda, and Fujikoshi (1995) demonstrated that the MANOVA is actually fairly robust to departures from multivariate normality with 10 participants per group. While there are statistical tests for normality (i.e., Kolmogorov–Smirnov test), these tests are more likely to indicate normality as sample size increases. As mentioned previously, the ANOVA and MANOVA are more robust to nonnormality as sample size increases. Often, a visual inspection of a histogram, Q–Q plot, or the skewness and kurtosis statistics can provide sufficient evidence for or against normality. Histograms can be produced with an added bell-shaped overlay to help assess normality. On a Q–Q plot, nonnormality is indicated by the dots straying from the diagonal line. Deviations from a bell shape are expected due to random error. Skewness and kurtosis can help describe just how far the data actually stray from normality. Skewness and kurtosis ratios can be calculated by dividing the respective statistic by its standard error. Ratios greater than two or less than negative two are indicative of potential nonnormality.

### Univariate: Homogeneity of Variance

The variance of the dependent variable should be the same for each group. The ANOVA is fairly robust to differences in variances as long as groups are of equal sample size (Maxwell & Delaney, 2004). In situations with small (<10 per group) or unequal sample sizes, it is best to utilize the Welch ANOVA (Myers et al., 2010) instead of the usual one-way ANOVA. The Welch ANOVA does not rely on the assumption of equal variance because it weights each group mean by its sample size. Levene's test provides a statistical test of the homogeneity of variance assumption. SPSS makes Levene's test (T2) available, but Nordstokke and Zumbo (2007) have shown that the empirical alpha level of Levene's test (T2) can be two to four times the nominal alpha level, resulting in a high chance of a type I error. Therefore, in situations with small or unequal sample sizes, it is recommended to not assume equal variance (Maxwell & Delaney, 2004).

### Multivariate: Homogeneity of Variance–Covariance Matrix

Each group created by a unique combination of factor levels contains its own variance–covariance matrix for the dependent variables. The multivariate homogeneity of variance– covariance matrix assumption requires that this matrix is the same for each group. Box's M is available from SPSS for testing multivariate homogeneity of variance–covariance. With equal sample sizes, robustness can be expected regardless of Box's M significance (Tabachnick & Fidell, 2013).

### Multicollinearity

When dealing with multiple dependent variables, each of these variables should be highly correlated with the independent variables but not highly correlated with the other dependent variables. If dependent variables are highly correlated with each other, multicollinearity can occur. This can drastically reduce the power of the MANOVA and potentially result in unstable solutions. In such cases, consider deleting one or more of the redundant dependent variables or use a principal component analysis (PCA) as a dimensionality reduction technique. The factors that are extracted by a PCA (assuming they are conceptually plausible) are completely uncorrelated and therefore address the issue of multicollinearity.

## Further Considerations

### A Priori Power Calculations

Power calculation should be done prior to data collection in order to identify the minimum number of participants required in order to achieve sufficient power. Without theory dictating an expected effect size, it is recommended to use a medium effect size (Maxwell & Delaney, 2004) with an alpha of 0.05 and an expected power of 0.80 (Tabachnick & Fidell, 2013). G*Power is a freeware program able to perform a priori power calculation.

## Post Hoc Analyses Following a Significant Interaction

Significant interactions supersede main effects in a factorial ANOVA because comparisons of marginal means may no longer be appropriate. Significant interactions must be further analyzed in order to better understand the effects of the independent variables on the dependent variable(s). One approach to further analyze an interaction in any ANOVA with two or more factors is to perform simple effects ANOVAs. Simple effects tests analyze the effect of one or more factors at each level of another factor. The following SPSS syntax can be altered to fit any factorial ANOVA:

UNIANOVA **Yvar**
BY **Afactor Bfactor**
/CRITERIA ALPHA(**.05/#LevelsBfactor**)
/EMMEANS = TABLES (**Afactor\* Bfactor**) compare (**Afactor**) adj (SIDAK).

UNIANOVA **Yvar**
BY **Afactor Bfactor**
/CRITERIA ALPHA(**.05/#LevelsAfactor**)
/EMMEANS = TABLES (**Afactor\* Bfactor**) compare (**Bfactor**) adj (SIDAK).

where **Yvar** is the dependent variable and **Afactor** and **Bfactor** are the two independent variables. This syntax pools error terms and is therefore not appropriate in situations with unequal variance (Maxwell & Delaney, 2004). With unequal variance, the data must be manually split in order to calculate separate error terms for the simple effects ANOVAs and pairwise comparisons. The following SPSS syntax command will split the data by **Bfactor**:

SPLIT FILE SEPARATE BY **Bfactor**.

A Welch ANOVA may then be performed looking at the effect of **Afactor** for each level of **Bfactor**. Splitting the data again by **Afactor** allows for the effect of **Bfactor** to be analyzed for each level of **Afactor**.

## Multivariate F Statistics

Four statistics are available for determining the significance of an independent variable's main or interaction effect in the MANOVA. Roy's largest root and Hotelling's trace are both liberal statistics and therefore overestimate actual significance. Wilks' lambda and Pillai's trace are much more conservative and less biased estimates of the significance. The values reported are the approximate $F$ values associated with the multivariate statistic. Wilks' $F$ is commonly reported. However, Pillai's $F$, being the most conservative, can help control the type I error rate with small or unequal sample sizes (Tabachnick & Fidell, 2013).

## Univariate/Multivariate Effect Size

Effect sizes are important to report because as sample size increases, so does statistical power. With very large sample sizes, ANOVA will eventually produce a significant $F$ test even though the differences between the groups are practically insignificant. Several effect sizes are available for the factorial ANOVA. Eta squared

$(\eta^2)$ is easily calculated by hand as $[SS_{Effect}/SS_{Total}]$. Partial $\eta^2$ $\left(\eta_p^2\right)$ is readily available from SPSS and is calculated as $[SS_{Effect}/(SS_{Effect}+SS_{Error})]$. In a one-way ANOVA, $\eta^2$ and $\eta_p^2$ are identical. Partial $\eta^2$ allows the effect size to only measure the unique variance accountable for by that independent variable. However, $\eta^2$ and $\eta_p^2$ are known to be overestimates, but $\eta_p^2$ is less biased than $\eta^2$ (Grissom & Kim, 2005). A more accurate and nearly unbiased measure of effect size is omega squared $(\omega^2)$ (Grissom & Kim, 2005). Partial $\eta^2$ and $\omega^2$ are both considered appropriate. The formula for $\omega^2$ is

$$\omega^2 = \frac{\left[SS_{Effect} - \left(df_{Effect} \times MS_{Within}\right)\right]}{\left(SS_{Total} + MS_{Within}\right)}$$

There is not a multivariate equivalent to $\omega^2$, but partial $\eta_p^2$ for multivariate effects is provided by SPSS.

# Utility in Sport and Exercise Sciences

This section provides a discussion of the usefulness of the ANOVA model in the field of sport and exercise sciences. Examples of different types of independent variables are discussed briefly.

## Treatment Conditions

Developing a new workout routine, contrasting coaching techniques, and comparing the health benefits of various types of physical activity all require the use of different treatment conditions. For example, in the development of a new workout routine, it may useful to include commonly accepted workout routines similar to the one in development in order to compare and contrast the potential of the new routine. Not every group requires an actual treatment. The control group is a common addition to the treatment group(s). The control group allows the comparison to a comparable group of matched individuals who received no treatment.

Sisson et al. (2009) performed a study looking at fitness gains in women (45–75 years of age). In their study, they randomly assign women to one of three different exercise treatment conditions (4, 8, and 12 kcal/kg) with a fourth control group. The exercise routines were maintained for 6 months. While the control group was not of interest, it allowed Sisson et al. to have a comparable group of participants to control for other confounding effects (i.e., yearly weight fluctuations) that could influence the results of the treatment conditions.

## Existing Conditions

It is not always possible for researchers to assign participants to certain groups. For instance, when analyzing injury rates between sports, sport membership is a preexisting condition. Working in schools also requires that researchers work with existing groups of students already assigned to different classes.

Beighle, Morgan, Le Masurier, and Pangrazi (2006) provide an example of an existing condition (grade level) in their study of children's physical activity in and out of school. Third, fourth, and fifth graders were monitored for step counts and amount of time spent being physically active during recess and outside of school. Beighle et al. (2006) found no significant difference between grade levels and no significant interaction between grade levels and gender. Boys were significantly more active than girls.

## Individual Characteristics

Gender, ethnicity, and age groups are commonly included in ANOVAs in order to test for differences across individual characteristics. An interaction between new treatment condition (e.g., different workout routines) and an individual characteristic such as gender could indicate that a particular workout routine is more effective with men, while a different workout routine is more effective with women.

Seabra et al. (2013) used gender as an individual characteristic variable to study difference in the perception of physical activity and its enjoyment between boys and girls (8–10 years of age). Boys reported greater enjoyment of physical activity than girls.

Nyberg, Nordenfelt, Ekelund, and Marcus (2009) studied the differences between 6-, 7-, 8-, and 9-year-olds' physical activity levels for both boys and girls. Their study concluded that 9-year-olds are less physically active than 6-year-olds and boys are more physically active than girls.

## Recent Usage

From 2010 through 2014, 12 peer-reviewed journals in the field of sport and exercise sciences were used to assess the frequency of the factorial ANOVA and MANOVA reporting. Appendix 1.5 provides the frequency of factorial ANOVA and MANOVA usage. The 12 peer-reviewed journals published a total of 8027 articles. Some form of a factorial ANOVA or MANOVA appeared in 519 of these articles. A one-way ANOVA or MANOVA was reported in 864 of these articles.

# The Substantive Example

Kang and Brinthaupt (2009) developed a school-based pedometer intervention program. Previous studies have suggested the use of group goals (every student is attempting to reach the same step count) or individual goals (5% of baseline increase) to increase walking. Extant research provided little direction on which goal one to choose and when. Kang and Brinthaupt performed a 6-week study to analyze the effects of individual- and group-based step count goals. Groups differing in baseline physical activity level were included in the analysis as an independent variable to see if goal types were more effective for different physical activity levels. This section will use goal type and physical activity level as independent variables to analyze the differences in step goal attainment and postintervention (PI) step count.

Physical activity level for each participant was defined as their average step counts per day at baseline, broken down into low (<4800), medium, and high (>6300). Goal type was either individual- or group-based step count goal. The factorial ANOVA analysis will test if the number of days of goal attainment over the 6-week period differs by baseline physical activity level, goal type, or their interaction. The factorial MANOVA will keep the same model (for comparative purposes) and will introduce a second dependent variable, PI step counts.

# Univariate: Factorial ANOVA

*Dependent variable*:
Number of days of goal attainment (hereafter referred to as goal attainment (days)): ratio data.
*Independent variables and main effect hypotheses*:
Baseline physical activity level: ordinal data with three levels [low ($n=31$), medium ($n=38$), and high ($n=30$)].
Null hypothesis: Physical activity level is not a significant predictor of goal attainment (days), *or* goal attainment (days) does not differ across physical activity levels.
Goal type: nominal data with two groups [(group-based ($n=57$) and individual-based ($n=42$)] step count goals.
Null hypothesis: Goal type is not a significant predictor of goal attainment (days), *or* goal attainment(days) does not differ across goal type.
*Interaction effect hypothesis*:
Physical activity level X goal type.
Null hypothesis: The effect of physical activity level on goal attainment (days) is the same across conditions of goal type.

# Univariate Assumptions

*Independence*:
The data were collected from individual students who only contributed once to step count and goal attainment (days). Each wore his/her own pedometer, and no sharing of pedometers was reported. There is no evidence to suggest that the independence assumption was violated.
*Normality*:
Analysis of descriptive statistics indicates very low skewness or kurtosis in all the groups.
*Homogeneity of variance*:
Due to small and unequal sample sizes, the homogeneity of variance assumption is likely to have been violated. To maintain empirical alpha levels close to nominal alpha levels, the error terms will not be pooled. The data will be manually split in SPSS, and simple effects Welch ANOVAs and Games–Howell pairwise comparisons will be subsequently performed.

*A priori power*:
A priori power calculations were conducted using G*Power with the following parameters:

Effect size *f*: 0.25 (medium; Cohen, 1988)

$\alpha$: 0.05

Power: 0.8

Numerator *df*: 2 ([3 levels of physical activity level − 1] * [2 levels of goal types − 1])

Number of groups: 6 (3 levels of physical activity level * 2 levels of goal type)

The resulting recommendation is a sample size of 158 that is not met by our sample size of 99 students. The example below is given for illustrative purposes. Adequate power is strongly advised for all studies.

## Multivariate: Factorial MANOVA

*Dependent variables*:
Number of days of goal attainment (hereafter referred to as goal attainment (days)): ratio data.
Postintervention step count (hereafter referred to as PI step count): ratio data.
*Independent variables and main effect hypotheses*:
Physical activity level: same as before.
Null hypothesis: Physical activity level is not a significant predictor of goal attainment (days) and PI step count, *or* goal attainment (days) and PI step count do not differ across physical activity levels.
Goal type: same as before.
Null hypothesis: Goal type is not a significant predictor of goal attainment (days) and PI step count, *or* goal attainment (days) and PI step count do not differ across goal type.
*Interaction effect hypothesis*:
Physical activity level X goal type.
Null hypothesis: The effect of physical activity level on goal attainment (days) and PI step count is the same across conditions of goal type.

## Multivariate Assumptions

*Independence*:
See univariate assumption.
*Multivariate normality*:
With more than 10 participants per group, the factorial MANOVA is fairly robust to any divergence from multivariate normality. In addition, no indication of univariate nonnormality, while not sufficient to demonstrate multivariate normality, also suggests that the normality assumption is valid for all post hoc analyses.
*Homogeneity of variance–covariance*:
Due to small and unequal sample sizes, the homogeneity of variance–covariance assumption is likely to have been violated. To maintain empirical alpha levels close

to nominal alpha levels, the error terms will not be pooled. The data will be manually split in SPSS, and subsequently simple effects Welch ANOVAs and Games–Howell pairwise comparisons will be performed. Pillai's $F$ will be reported in order to keep in control type I error rate.

*A priori power*:

A priori power calculations were conducted using G*Power with the following parameters:

Effect size $f^2$(V): 0.15 (medium; Cohen, 1988)
α err prob: 0.05
Power (1-β err prob): 0.8
Number of groups: 6 (3 levels of physical activity level * 2 levels of goal type)
Number of predictors: 2 (# of independent variables)
Response Variables: 2 (# of dependent variables)

The resulting recommendation is a sample size of 43 that is met by our sample of 99 students.

# The Synergy

This section will illustrate the analysis plan for a factorial ANOVA and a factorial MANOVA and the reporting of the output in a way that is compatible with the American Psychological Association (APA) publication manual. We will also highlight what is most important and necessary to report. The SPSS syntax and data can be found in the Appendices 1.1 and 1.3.

## Factorial ANOVA Analysis Plan

The full model was analyzed for the main effects and any possible interactions (see Figure 1.1 for the ANOVA analysis plan). In this example, the main effects of physical activity and goal type and the interaction of the two independent variables were explored (see Appendix 1.2 for the abbreviated output).

This example contains a significant interaction. With equal variance, the EMMEANS command could have been used in order to produce the necessary post hoc analyses. Given a significant interaction with unequal variance, the data were split by one of the variables involved in the interaction, analyzed, split by the other variable, and analyzed again. For this example, the data were split first by goal type, and the effect of physical activity level was analyzed and reported for each goal type (alpha = 0.05/2 goal types = 0.025). Physical activity level is comprised of three levels and thus requires follow-up comparisons. Given the small and unequal sample sizes, Games–Howell pairwise comparisons were analyzed. The Games–Howell procedure is commonly used for situations where equal variance cannot be assumed, as it is the same as Tukey's HSD adjusted for each pairwise comparison.

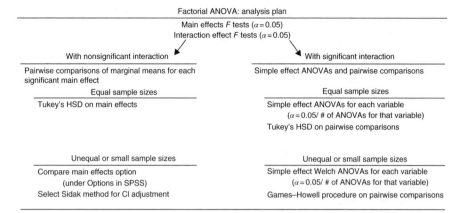

<figure>
Factorial ANOVA: analysis plan

Main effects $F$ tests ($\alpha = 0.05$)
Interaction effect $F$ tests ($\alpha = 0.05$)

| With nonsignificant interaction | With significant interaction |
|---|---|
| Pairwise comparisons of marginal means for each significant main effect | Simple effect ANOVAs and pairwise comparisons |
| Equal sample sizes | Equal sample sizes |
| Tukey's HSD on main effects | Simple effect ANOVAs for each variable ($\alpha = 0.05$/ # of ANOVAs for that variable) Tukey's HSD on pairwise comparisons |
| Unequal or small sample sizes | Unequal or small sample sizes |
| Compare main effects option (under Options in SPSS) Select Sidak method for CI adjustment | Simple effect Welch ANOVAs for each variable ($\alpha = 0.05$/ # of ANOVAs for that variable) Games–Howell procedure on pairwise comparisons |
</figure>

*Figure 1.1    Factorial ANOVA analysis plan.*

Next, the data were split by physical activity level, and the effect of goal type was analyzed and reported for each level of physical activity level (alpha = 0.05/3 levels of physical activity = 0.0167). Given that goal type is a dichotomous variable, a follow-up pairwise comparison is redundant with the simple effects ANOVA.

If the interaction was not significant, comparisons of the marginal means would be reported for each significant main effect with Tukey's HSD or the Sidak adjustment for small or unequal sample (Games–Howell is unavailable for comparisons of marginal means). Tukey's HSD and Sidak assume equal variance, while the Sidak is slightly more conservative.

# Example of a Write-Up Compatible with the APA Publication Manual

A two-way ANOVA was used to evaluate the number of days that each student attained their goal based on their goal type and physical activity level (see Table 1.1 for descriptive statistics). Physical activity level and goal type were significant predictors of the number of days of goal attainment, $F(2, 93) = 17.67$, mean square error (MSE) = 33.33, $p < 0.001$, $\eta_p^2 = 0.275$, and $F(1, 93) = 6.85$, $p = 0.010$, $\eta_p^2 = 0.069$, respectively. There was a significant interaction between goal type and physical activity level, $F(2, 93) = 10.25$, $p < 0.001$, $\eta_p^2 = 0.181$ (Figure 1.3). As a result, simple effects ANOVAs were conducted to probe the interaction effect.

Welch ANOVAs and Games–Howell pairwise comparisons were used to conduct simple effects tests for predicting goal attainment based on physical activity level for each goal type (see Table 1.2 for pairwise comparisons). The alpha for each ANOVA was 0.025 because there were two different groups in goal type. The results indicated that physical activity level was a significant predictor of goal attainment for students in the group goal program, $F(2, 35.04) = 38.17$, MSE = 34.37, $p < 0.001$, $\eta_p^2 = 0.529$. High activity level student attained significantly more goals than middle activity level students who also attained significantly more goals than low activity level students.

Table 1.1    Descriptive statistics for goal attainment (days) and postintervention (PI) step count.

| | Goal attainment (days) | | PI step count | | $n$ |
|---|---|---|---|---|---|
| | $M$ | SD | $M$ | SD | |
| *Group goal* | | | | | |
| Physical activity level | | | | | |
| Low | 6.22 | 4.88 | 5467.06 | 1029.44 | 18 |
| Middle | 15.57 | 6.74 | 6121.00 | 1363.23 | 23 |
| High | 21.69 | 5.49 | 7883.25 | 2084.39 | 16 |
| *Individual goal* | | | | | |
| Physical activity level | | | | | |
| Low | 16.38 | 3.10 | 4493.77 | 1402.98 | 13 |
| Middle | 17.93 | 7.23 | 7065.33 | 2486.28 | 15 |
| High | 18.43 | 5.53 | 7970.71 | 1720.71 | 14 |

Table 1.2    Factorial ANOVA: Games–Howell comparisons of days of goal attainment (days).

| (I) | (J) | Mean difference | 97.5% CI | |
|---|---|---|---|---|
| | | (I–J) | Lower limit | Upper limit |
| *Comparisons for physical activity level* | | | | |
| Subgroup = group goal | | | | |
| Physical activity level | | | | |
| Low | Middle | −9.34* | −14.31 | −4.38 |
| Low | High | −15.47* | −20.42 | −10.51 |
| Middle | High | −6.12* | −11.51 | −0.74 |
| Subgroup = individual goal | | | | |
| Physical activity level | | | | |
| Low | Middle | −1.55 | −7.44 | 4.34 |
| Low | High | −2.04 | −6.92 | 2.83 |
| Middle | High | −0.50 | −7.16 | 6.16 |

*Significant at a familywise alpha of 0.05 (0.025 per simple effects).

Physical activity level was not a significant predictor of goal attainment for students in the individual goal program, $F(2, 24.08) = 0.82$, MSE $= 31.88$, $p = 0.450$, $\eta_p^2 = 0.024$. The pairwise comparisons were nonsignificant.

Simple effects Welch ANOVAs were used to predict the number of days of goal attainment based on the goal type for each level of physical activity. An alpha of 0.0167 was used to determine significance for the simple effects ANOVAs. No pairwise comparisons were used as there are only two groups within goal type. Low physical activity students in the individual goal program attained their goal more often than the group goal program, $F(1, 28.63) = 50.10$, MSE $= 17.94$, $p < 0.001$, $\eta_p^2 = 0.600$. However, goal type was not a significant predictor of goal attainment for middle and high physical activity level students, $F(1, 28.55) = 1.03$, MSE $= 48.07$, $p = 0.319$, $\eta_p^2 = 0.029$, and $F(1, 27.41) = 2.613$, MSE $= 30.32$, $p = 0.117$, $\eta_p^2 = 0.085$, respectively.

## Factorial MANOVA Analysis Plan

As with the ANOVA analysis plan, the full model was analyzed in order to inform the direction of the post hoc analyses. Wilks' lambda is commonly reported and considered to be sufficient at controlling type I error rates. Pillai's is the most conservative and should be used with small or unequal sample sizes in order to control for type I error rate. In this example, Pillai's F statistic will be reported for the main effects of physical activity level and goal type and their interaction.

Post hoc analyses will be conducted using the protected F procedure. The protected $F$ test is a commonly used procedure to further analyze the effects of the independent variables on the dependent variables.

The same variables from the factorial ANOVA example are included and will provide the same significant interaction. This is intentional in order to highlight the process of simple effects MANOVAs with a protected F procedure. The data are split first by goal type, and the effect of physical activity level is analyzed in simple effects MANOVAs for each goal type (alpha $= 0.05/2$ goal types $= 0.025$). Where physical activity is a significant predictor, follow-up Welch ANOVAs will be reported for physical activity level predicting goal attainment (days) and PI step count (alpha $= 0.025$). Games–Howell pairwise comparisons will be used because physical activity level is comprised of three levels.

Next, the data are split by physical activity level, and the effect of goal type is analyzed in simple effects MANOVAs for each level of physical activity level (alpha $= 0.05/3$ level of physical activity $= 0.0167$). Where goal type is a significant predictor, follow-up Welch ANOVAs, due to unequal variance, will be reported for goal type predicting goal attainment (days) and PI step count (alpha $= 0.0167$).

With a nonsignificant interaction, the independent variables are analyzed in a factorial ANOVA plan for each dependent variable (see Figure 1.2 for the MANOVA analysis plan). This reduces the MANOVA down to a series of factorial ANOVAs, each with its own analysis plan.

## Example of a Write-Up Compatible with the APA Publication Manual

A two-way MANOVA was used to evaluate the number of days that each student attained their goals and their PI step count based on their physical activity level and goal type. An alpha of 0.05 was used. Physical activity level and goal type were both significant predictors, *Pillai's* $F(4, 186) = 9.49$, $p < 0.001$, $\eta_p^2 = 0.169$, and *Pillai's* $F(2, 92) = 8.05$, $p = 0.001$, $\eta_p^2 = 0.149$. There was a significant interaction between physical activity level and goal type, *Pillai's* $F(4, 186) = 15.39$, $p < 0.001$, $\eta_p^2 = 0.249$ (see Figures 1.3 and 1.4). As a result, simple effects MANOVAs were conducted.

Simple effects MANOVAs were conducted to predict the number of days that each student attained their goal and their PI step count based on the physical

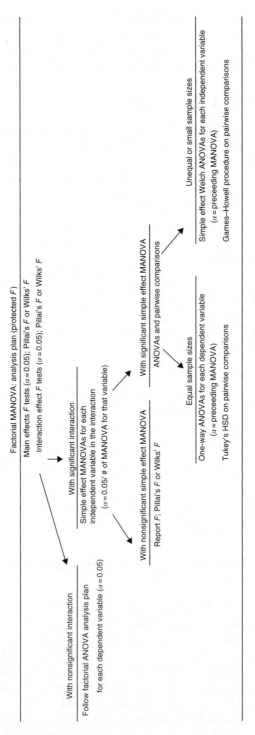

*Figure 1.2  Factorial MANOVA analysis plan (protected F).*

Estimated marginal means of number of days goal attained

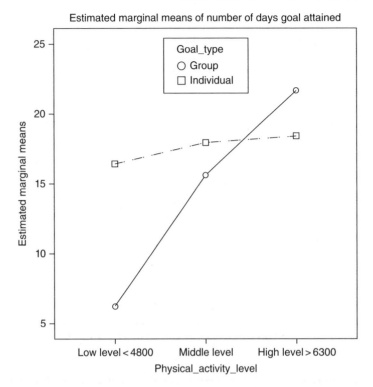

*Figure 1.3    Marginal means plot of goal attainment (days) (a clear interaction can be visualized by the differences in slopes between individual and group goal types).*

activity level for each goal type. An alpha of 0.025 was used to determine significance. For the group goal program, physical activity level was a significant predictor, Pillai's $F(4, 108) = 13.81$, $p < 0.001$, $\eta_p^2 = 0.338$. Follow-up Welch ANOVAs, with an alpha of 0.025, and Games–Howell pairwise comparisons were conducted (see Table 1.3 for pairwise comparisons). Physical activity level was a significant predictor of goal attainment, $F(2, 35.04) = 38.17$, $p < 0.001$, $\eta_p^2 = 0.529$. High activity level student attained more goals than middle activity level students who also attained significantly more goals than low activity level students. Physical activity level was also a significant predictor of PI step count, $F(2, 31.63) = 8.84$, $p = 0.001$, $\eta_p^2 = 0.298$. High activity level students had significantly higher PI step count than middle and low activity level students; the latter two groups did not differ significantly from each other. For the individual goal program, physical activity level was a significant predictor, *Pillai's* $F(4, 78) = 7.41$, $p < 0.001$, $\eta_p^2 = 0.275$. Follow-up Welch ANOVAs, with an alpha of 0.025, indicated that physical activity level was not a significant predictor of goal attainment, $F(2, 24.08) = 0.82$, $p = 0.450$, $\eta_p^2 = 0.024$, but was a significant predictor of PI step count, $F(2, 25.61) = 17.46$, $p < 0.001$, $\eta_p^2 = 0.370$. Low activity level students maintained lower step count compared to middle and high activity level students who did not differ in step count.

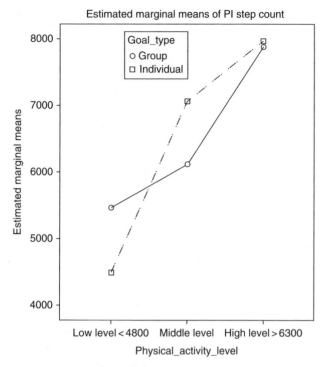

*Figure 1.4    Marginal means plot of postintervention step count (a clear interaction can be seen between low- and middle-level physical activity and goal type).*

Simple effects MANOVAs were conducted to predict the number of days that each student attained their goal and their PI step count based on the goal type for each physical activity level. An alpha of 0.0167 was used to determine significance for the simple effects MANOVAs. Goal type was a significant predictor for low activity level students, *Pillai's* $F(2, 28)=55.24$, $p<0.001$, $\eta_p^2=0.798$. Follow-up Welch ANOVAs, alpha$=0.0167$, indicated that low activity level students in the individual goal program attained their goal more often than those in the group goal program, but no difference was found in PI step count, $F(1, 28.63)=50.10$, $p<0.001$, $\eta_p^2=0.600$, and $F(1, 20.91)=4.51$, $p=0.046$, $\eta_p^2=0.147$ (recall that an alpha of 0.167 was used to establish significance). Goal type was not a significant predictor for middle and high activity level students, *Pillai's* $F(2, 35)=1.19$, $p=0.317$, $\eta_p^2=0.064$, and *Pillai's* $F(2, 27)=3.33$, $p=0.051$, $\eta_p^2=0.198$, respectively.

# Summary

The factorial ANOVA and MANOVA are natural extensions of the one-way ANOVA. The strength of these tests is that multiple independent variables can be analyzed simultaneously, testing their main and interaction effects. The example in this chapter reported an interaction within the data and demonstrated how to further probe it.

Table 1.3    Factorial MANOVA: Games–Howell comparisons of days of goal attainment (days) and PI step count.

| (I) | (J) | Mean difference | 97.5% CI | |
|---|---|---|---|---|
| | | (I–J) | Lower limit | Upper limit |
| *Comparisons for physical activity level on goal attainment (days)* | | | | |
| Subgroup = group goal | | | | |
| Physical activity level | | | | |
| Low | Middle | −9.34* | −14.31 | −4.38 |
| Low | High | −15.47* | −20.42 | −10.51 |
| Middle | High | −6.12* | −11.51 | −0.74 |
| Subgroup = individual goal | | | | |
| Physical activity level | | | | |
| Low | Middle | −1.55 | −7.44 | 4.34 |
| Low | High | −2.04 | −6.92 | 2.83 |
| Middle | High | −0.50 | −7.16 | 6.16 |
| *Comparisons for physical activity level on PI step count* | | | | |
| Subgroup = group goal | | | | |
| Physical activity level | | | | |
| Low | Middle | −653.94 | −1674.70 | 366.81 |
| Low | High | −2416.19* | −4051.36 | −781.03 |
| Middle | High | −1762.25* | −3434.84 | −89.66 |
| Subgroup = individual goal | | | | |
| Physical activity level | | | | |
| Low | Middle | −2571.56* | −4695.94 | −447.19 |
| Low | High | −3476.95* | −5169.98 | −1783.91 |
| Middle | High | −905.38 | −3122.20 | 1311.44 |

*Significant at a familywise alpha of 0.05 (0.025 per simple effects).

This chapter covered the theoretical framework of the factorial analyses starting with hypothesis testing. The hypotheses are laid out prior to analysis and help to drive the interpretation of the results. The assumptions of the ANOVA are necessary in order to maintain the power of the analysis. Keeping high numbers in terms of group membership (where possible) and minimizing attrition rates can help to keep sample sizes large and equal. Large and equal sample sizes guard against unequal variance and ensure that researchers have enough degrees of freedom for adequate power. The independence assumption should be considered during the design of the study. If the independence assumption is violated, it can have a detrimental effect on the type I error rate within the analysis procedures.

The analysis plan laid out within this chapter is easy to generalize and adapt to factorial ANOVAs with more than 2 predictors. Significant interactions can occur with three- and four-way interactions. The highest interactions term should be analyzed first through splitting the data by each variable involved. The simple effects tests provide a strong and easily interpreted approach to isolating the way that independent variables differ in their effect on the dependent variable across levels of other independent variables. Descriptive statistics ($M$, SD, $n$) are best presented in a table. However, if only a few variables are analyzed, the descriptive statistics can be presented in the write-up when the variables are first mentioned. If model summary statistics ($F$, MSE, $R^2$, and $p$) are not presented within the Results section, they should be included in a model summary table. Pairwise comparisons of either the marginal means or the simple effects pairwise comparisons (e.g., Tukey's or Games–Howell) should be presented in a table but still discussed in the write-up.

# Acknowledgment

The authors would like to thank Hershel Eason from Middle Tennessee State University for his contribution in the preparation of this chapter.

# References

Beighle, A., Morgan, C. F., Le Masurier, G., & Pangrazi, R. P. (2006). Children's physical activity during recess and outside of school. *Journal of School Health, 76*(10), 516–520.

Cohen, J. (1988). *Statistical power analysis for the behavioral sciences* (2nd ed.). Hillsdale, NJ: Lawrence Erlbaum Associates.

Grissom, R. J., & Kim, J. J. (2005). *Effect sizes for research: A broad practical approach.* Mahwah, NJ: Lawrence Erlbaum Associates.

Kang, M., & Brinthaupt, T. (2009). Effects of group- and individual-based step goals on children's physical activity levels in school. *Pediatric Exercise Science, 21*, 148–158.

Maxwell, S. E., & Delaney, H. D. (2004). *Designing experiments and analyzing data: A model comparison perspective* (2nd ed.). Mahwah, NJ: Lawrence Erlbaum Associates.

Myers, J. L., Well, A. D., & Lorch, R. F., Jr. (2010). *Research design and statistical analysis* (3rd ed.). New York, NY: Routledge.

Nordstokke, D. W., & Zumbo, B. D. (2007). A cautionary tale about Levene's tests for equal variances. *Journal of Educational Research and Policy Studies, 7*, 1–14.

Nyberg, G. A., Nordenfelt, A. M., Ekelund, U., & Marcus, C. (2009). Physical activity patterns measured by accelerometry in 6- to 10-yr-old children. *Medicine and Science in Sports and Exercise, 41*(10), 1842–1848.

Seabra, A., Mendonça, D., Maia, J., Welk, G., Brustad, R., Fonseca, A. M., & Seabra, A. F. (2013). Gender, weight status and socioeconomic differences in psychosocial correlates of physical activity in schoolchildren. *Journal of Science and Medicine in Sport, 16*(4), 320–326.

Seo, T., Kanda, T., & Fujikoshi, Y. (1995). The effects of nonnormality on tests for dimensionality in canonical correlation and MANOVA models. *Journal of Multivariate Analysis, 52*, 325–337.

Sisson, S. B., Katzmarzyk, P. T., Earnest, C. P., Bouchard, C., Blair, S. N., & Church, T. S. (2009). Volume of exercise and fitness nonresponse in sedentary, postmenopausal women. *Medicine and Science in Sports and Exercise, 41*(3), 539–545.

Tabachnick, B. C., & Fidell, L. S. (2013). *Using multivariate statistics* (6th ed.). Boston, MA: Pearson.

# 2

# Repeated measures ANOVA and MANOVA

## Minsoo Kang[1] and Ying Jin[2]

[1] *Health and Human Performance, Middle Tennessee State University, Murfreesboro, TN, USA*
[2] *Quantitative Psychology, Middle Tennessee State University, Murfreesboro, TN, USA*

## General Introduction

The repeated measures analysis of variance (ANOVA) is a natural extension of the one-way and factorial ANOVAs (see Chapter 1) and is designed for the analysis of longitudinal studies, that is, when participants are measured multiple times on one or more dependent variables. In its simplest form, a pre- and posttest repeated measures ANOVA design functions just as a paired samples *t*-test. As with the factorial ANOVA, the repeated measures ANOVA can accommodate multiple independent variables. The repeated measures multivariate analysis of variance (MANOVA) procedure can also be used to accommodate research designs with multiple dependent variables. Repeated measures ANOVA and MANOVA require the distinction between two kinds of independent variables.

### Between- versus Within-Subjects Variables

Between-subjects variables distinguish between participants in each group and can only accommodate one score per participant. In a one-way or factorial ANOVA, all

*An Introduction to Intermediate and Advanced Statistical Analyses for Sport and Exercise Scientists*, First Edition.
Edited by Nikos Ntoumanis and Nicholas D. Myers.
© 2016 John Wiley & Sons, Ltd. Published 2016 by John Wiley & Sons, Ltd.
Companion website: www.wiley.com/go/ntoumanis/sport

independent variables are between-subjects variables. For example, gender is a between-subjects variable because each participant is only male or female.

Within-subjects variables distinguish between an individual's multiple assessments. The full independence assumption is not applicable here because each individual is included in every assessment of a dependent variable (e.g., measures of daily physical activity over a 1-week period). Repeated measures ANOVAs and MANOVAs are used whenever one or more within-subjects independent variables are in the ANOVA model. Repeated measures ANOVAs and MANOVAs can also include one or more between-subjects factors (in such cases, they are often called mixed-design ANOVAs and MANOVAs). The independent variables of a repeated measures ANOVA or MANOVA are categorical (i.e., nominal or ordinal), whereas the dependent variables are continuous (i.e., interval or ratio).

# Hypothesis Testing

The general null hypothesis for each within-subjects main effect in a repeated measures ANOVA/MANOVA is that the participants' scores on the dependent variable(s) are the same across all conditions and/or times that the dependent variables were measured (i.e., baseline, 6 weeks, 12 weeks). The alternative hypothesis is that participants differ on at least one dependent variable between the conditions or times of measurement (i.e., baseline scores were smaller than 6 weeks' scores). In essence, a significant main effect indicates that the conditions are (or time is) a significant predictor of at least one dependent variable. The null and alternative hypotheses for a between-subjects main effect are the same as in a factorial ANOVA/MANOVA (see Chapter 1).

With regard to the interaction of a between-subjects variable and a within-subjects variable, the null hypothesis is that the effects of one independent variable (either a between-subjects or a within-subjects variable) on the dependent variable(s) do not differ across the conditions of the other independent variable. The alternative hypothesis is that the effects of one independent variable on at least one dependent variable differ across the conditions of the other independent variable.

# Assumptions

The assumptions of the repeated measures ANOVA and MANOVA are similar to the assumptions of the factorial ANOVA and MANOVA (see Chapter 1). The following sections discuss some changes in the independence assumption and the homogeneity of variance assumption.

## Independence Assumption

The full independence assumption is required for between-subjects variables. Participants can only contribute one score to each dependent variable. Within-subjects variables do not adhere to the requirement of one score per participant per dependent variable. The independence assumption still requires that no outside influence can systematically affect the measurement of dependent variables between conditions or times. An example of this is if a coach wanted to measure push-ups pre- and postseason but allowed some players to perform modified push-ups in the postseason.

This would most likely show an increase in average push-ups, but it is unclear whether the training affected strength or the modified push-ups allowed the players to perform a greater number of push-ups. If an outside influence is present, empirical alpha (actual potential for type I error) will be greater than nominal alpha (the potential for type I error that is set by the researcher; see Chapter 1 for more information about the alpha level), leading to an increase in the type I error rate.

### Univariate: Homogeneity of Variance and Sphericity

The repeated measures ANOVA requires that the difference scores across the levels of the within-subjects variable are equal (e.g., Time1 – Time2 = Time1 – Time3 = Time2 – Time3). Additionally, the repeated measures ANOVA requires all covariances between the difference scores to be equal. The combination of equal variances and equal covariances is referred to as the sphericity assumption. Sphericity is achieved with only two groups in a within-subjects variable because there is only one set of difference scores. However, with three or more groups, the sphericity assumption is rarely met, even with equal sample sizes.

### Multivariate: Homogeneity of Variance–Covariance Matrix

Each group created by a unique combination of factor levels (e.g., when factors are gender and time of the day, a unique combination could be females and morning) contains its own variance–covariance matrix for the dependent variables. The multivariate homogeneity of variance–covariance matrix assumption requires that this matrix is the same for each group. The repeated measures MANOVA makes no assumption about sphericity and does not require adjustments similar to the repeated measures ANOVA (Tabachnick & Fidell, 2013).

## Further Considerations

### Repeated Measures Univariate $F$

Substantial departures from sphericity can drastically reduce the power and increase the type I error rate of the univariate $F$. One solution is to use the repeated measures MANOVA which does not assume sphericity (Myers, Well, & Lorch, 2010). The second solution is to use an adjusted $F$ value. Most statistical software will report four adjusted $F$ statistics: sphericity assumed, Greenhouse–Geisser, Huynh–Feldt, and lower bound. Greenhouse–Geisser is slightly more conservative than the Huynh–Feldt adjustment, but both are considered to adequately control type I error rates (Myers et al., 2010). The correction only affects the degrees of freedom and the $p$ value. When the sphericity assumption is met (i.e., 2 within-subjects groups), the corrected degrees of freedom and associated $p$ value will be the same as the sphericity-assumed $F$ statistic.

### A Priori Power Calculations

Power calculation should be done prior to data collection in order to identify the minimum number of participants required in order to achieve sufficient power. Without theory dictating an expected effect size, it is recommended to use a medium effect size (Maxwell & Delaney, 2004), with an alpha of 0.05 and an expected power of 0.80 (Tabachnick & Fidell, 2013). G*Power is a freeware program able to perform a priori power calculations.

Between-subjects effects will always require more participants than the within-subjects effects. This is due to within-subjects variables measuring the same people multiple times, whereas the between-subjects variables measure separate people each time. It is recommended to assess sample size needed for detecting a between-subjects effect, a within-subjects effect, and also the interaction effect between the between-subjects and the within-subjects variables for a full view prior to data collection.

**Post Hoc Analyses Following a Significant Interaction**

One approach to further analyze an interaction effect in any repeated measures ANOVA with two or more factors is to perform simple effects ANOVAs. The idea is to analyze the effect of one or more factors at each level of another factor. The following SPSS syntax can be altered to fit any repeated measures ANOVA:

GLM  **Yvar_pre Yvar_post** BY **Afactor**
/WSFACTOR = **Time** 2 Polynomial
/MEASURE = **Yvar**
/CRITERIA ALPHA(.05/#Levels**Time**)
/EMMEANS = TABLES (**Afactor*** **Time**) compare (**Afactor**) adj (SIDAK).

GLM  **Yvar_pre Yvar_post** BY **Afactor**
/WSFACTOR = **Time** 2 Polynomial
/MEASURE = **Yvar**
/CRITERIA ALPHA(.05/#Levels**Afactor**)
/EMMEANS = TABLES (**Afactor*** **Time**) compare (**Time**) adj (SIDAK).

where **Yvar** is the dependent variable and **Afactor** and **Time** are the two independent variables.

As with the factorial ANOVA, if homogeneity of variance cannot be assumed, then the syntax approach is inappropriate due to pooled error terms. The error terms must be calculated separately in order to maintain type I error rates. In situations where separate error terms are needed, the data must be manually split and analyzed separately.

# Utility in Sport and Exercise Sciences

Within-subjects variables are relevant in three situations: multiple treatment conditions, multiple measures, and longitudinal studies. This section discusses these three situations and the current usage of the repeated measures ANOVA (or MANOVA if several dependent variables are tested simultaneously) in the field of sport and exercise sciences.

## Multiple Treatment Conditions

When the available participants are scarce, it may be advisable to consider using all the participants in every treatment condition. One drawback to this approach is that it takes much longer to run participants through each condition and baseline phases. A positive aspect of this procedure is that individuals are compared against themselves. This provides a natural protection against confounds that are associated with selection techniques for between-subjects factors.

As an example, Clemes and Deans (2012) conducted a multiple treatment step count study to examine reactivity to pedometers in adults. The participants wore a sealed pedometer for the first week of the study with no knowledge that the device was a pedometer. For the second and third week of the study, the participants were aware that the device was a pedometer. The three weeks were compared in a repeated measures ANOVA design; results showed that after the first week of aware wear (week 2), the participants returned to normal walking activity levels (i.e., week 1 step count = week 3 step count).

## Multiple Assessments

This is commonly referred to as a profile analysis (Tabachnick & Fidell, 2013). Each test must have the same scale in order to establish meaningful interpretations. A profile analysis involves using the subtests of a scale rather than the total score. One example of this would be the use of various components of fitness rather than an overall fitness score. The benefit of profile analysis is that differences between groups (e.g., sports teams) may not be evident on an overall score, but when broken down to various fitness components, differences may be detected. This analysis can also provide clarity in situations where mean differences between groups on an overall score are widely different. The profile analysis can help shed light on exactly which subscales are differing and by how much.

As an example, Demarini, Koo, and Hockman (2006) used profile analyses to compare twins and singletons on body composition. Each newborn's bone, lean tissue, and fat composition were recorded and used as variables in the profile analysis. No differences in overall body composition were found between twins and singletons when controlling for birth weight. However, profile analyses did show a lower absolute amount of lean tissue in twins whose birth weights were less than the 10th percentile.

## Longitudinal Studies

Longitudinal studies are the most common application of the repeated measures approach. A longitudinal study involves the measurement of a dependent variable (or variables) at multiple times (usually with consistent intervals) throughout a treatment phase. More samplings of the dependent variables can lead to trend analyses that may provide useful information about the dependent variables over time. A trend analysis relays significance about linear, quadratic, and cubic (or even more complex) trends in the relationship between the dependent variable and time.

As an example, Till, Jones, Darrall-Jones, Emmonds, and Cooke (2015) tracked anthropometric (height, body mass, etc.) and physical (10 m sprint, 20 m sprint, max squat, max bench press, vertical jump, etc.) assessments of rugby league players (16–20 years). Over the course of 4 years, Till et al. (2015) found statistically significant increases in these variables, both year over year and from the beginning to the end of the study. Some assessments did not show significant year over year increases, but did show long-term improvement (i.e., vertical jump). Other assessments showed greater improvement in earlier assessments than later assessments (i.e., max squat).

## Recent Usage

From 2010 to 2014, 12 peer-reviewed journals in the field of sports and exercise science were used to assess the frequency of the repeated measures ANOVA and MANOVA reporting. Appendix 2.5 provides the frequency of the ANOVA and MANOVA usage. The 12 peer-reviewed journals published a total of 8027 articles. Some form of a repeated measures ANOVA or MANOVA was reported for 2069 of these articles.

# The Substantive Example

Anshel, Brinthaupt, and Kang (2010) studied the effects of a 10-week wellness intervention that focused on improving physical and mental well-being for full-time university employees. The intervention was centered on the disconnected values model (Anshel, 2008) and involved discussing with individuals about their core values about physical health and how/whether their daily routines were aligned with their values. From the variables measured, upper body strength from the physical fitness tasks and anxiety from the Psychological Mental Well-Being Inventory (Dupuy, 1984) were selected as the dependent variables for the examples in this chapter. Assessment period was an independent variable (a within-subjects factor with two levels: pretest and post-test). Gender, a between-subjects variable, was the second independent variable.

Upper body strength was determined by a one repetition max bench press. Anxiety was reverse coded so that higher scores indicated lower levels of experienced anxiety. The repeated measures ANOVA will assess whether anxiety levels differ between pre- and postintervention assessments and between males and females. The multivariate analysis will maintain the same variables (for comparative purposes) and introduce a second dependent variable, upper body strength, as a miniature full health (mind and body) analysis of a participant's well-being.

## Univariate: Repeated Measures ANOVA

*Dependent variable*:
    Anxiety level: interval data
    *Independent variables and main effect hypotheses*:
    Gender: nominal data with two groups [male ($n=25$), female ($n=46$)]
    Null hypothesis: Gender is not a significant predictor of anxiety level, *or* anxiety levels do not differ between males and females.

Assessment: nominal data with two groups [preintervention ($n=71$), postintervention ($n=71$)]

Null hypothesis: Assessment is not a significant predictor of anxiety level, *or* anxiety levels do not differ between pre- and postintervention assessments.

*Interaction effect hypothesis*:

Gender X assessment

Null hypothesis: The effect of gender on anxiety level is the same between pre- and postintervention assessments.

## Univariate Assumptions

*Independence*:

The data were collected from individual employees who only contributed one score to each dependent variable for each assessment. There is no evidence to suggest that the data were systematically influenced and that the independence assumption has been violated.

*Normality*:

Analysis of descriptive statistics indicates no concern for issues with skewness or kurtosis associated with males or females at either assessment.

*Homogeneity of variance*:

Due to small and unequal sample sizes, the homogeneity of variance assumption is likely to have been violated. To maintain empirical alpha levels close to nominal alpha levels, the error terms will not be pooled. The data will need to be manually split in SPSS, with simple effects Welch ANOVAs and Games–Howell pairwise comparisons conducted, if the $F$ values are significant. Because the within-subjects variable is dichotomous (pre and postassessment), there is only one difference score. The Greenhouse–Geisser and Huynh–Feldt adjustments will be the same as the sphericity-assumed $F$ statistics, but in order to illustrate the reporting of a corrected $F$ test, the following examples will report the Greenhouse–Geisser corrected statistics (denoted by G–G p). It is advised to report a corrected $F$ statistic even when sphericity is met as the two statistics will be the same.

*A Priori Power*:

A priori power calculations were conducted using G*Power with the following parameters looking at the between-subjects effects:

Effect size $f$: 0.25 (medium; Cohen, 1988)

$\alpha$ err prob: 0.05

Power ($1 - \beta$ err prob): 0.8

Number of groups: 2

Number of measurements: 2

Corr among rep measures: 0.5 (standard assumption if no prior theory is available)

The resulting recommended sample size of 98 is higher than our sample size of 71 participants. The same parameters for the within- and between-subjects interaction effect (nonsphericity correction $\varepsilon = 1$) indicate a total sample size of 34 (36 for within-subjects main effect). The available sample size should provide ample power for the within-subjects effects but may be lacking in detecting between-subjects effects. The example below is given for illustrative purposes. Readers are strongly advised that their studies are adequately powered.

## Multivariate: Repeated Measures MANOVA

*Dependent variables*:
Anxiety level: interval data
Upper body strength: ratio data
*Independent variables and main effect hypotheses*:
Gender: nominal data with two groups [male ($n=25$), female ($n=46$)]
Null hypothesis: Gender is not a significant predictor of anxiety level and upper body strength, *or* anxiety level and upper body strength do not differ between males and females.
Assessment: nominal data with two groups [preintervention ($n=71$), postintervention ($n=71$)]
Null Hypothesis: Assessment is not a significant predictor of anxiety level and upper body strength, *or* anxiety level and upper body strength do not differ between pre- and postintervention assessments.
*Interaction effect hypothesis*:
Gender X assessment
Null hypothesis: The effect of gender on anxiety level and upper body strength is the same between pre- and postintervention assessments.

## Multivariate Assumptions

*Independence*:
See univariate assumption.
*Multivariate normality*:
With more than 10 participants per group, the repeated measures MANOVA is fairly robust to any divergence from multivariate normality (see Chapter 1 for a discussion of the robustness of the MANOVA). In addition, no indication of univariate nonnormality, while not sufficient to demonstrate multivariate normality, also suggests that the normality assumption may be valid for all post hoc analyses.
*Homogeneity of variance–covariance*:
Due to small and unequal sample sizes, the homogeneity of variance–covariance assumption is likely to have been violated. To maintain empirical alpha levels close to nominal alpha levels, the error terms will not be pooled. The data will need to be manually split in SPSS, with simple effects Welch ANOVAs and Games–Howell pairwise comparisons, conducted, if the $F$ values are significant. Pillai's $F$ will be reported in order to reduce the possibility for type 1 error.
*A priori power*:
A priori power calculations were conducted using G*Power with the following parameters looking at the interaction effect:
Effect size $f$: 0.25 (medium; Cohen, 1988)

$\alpha$ err prob: 0.05
Power $(1 - \beta$ err prob): 0.8
Number of groups: 2
Number of measurements: 2
The resulting recommended sample size of 128 (for the interaction effect) is higher than our sample size of 71 participants. The recommended sample for the between-subjects main effect (Corr among rep measures = 0.5) is 98 participants and 34 participants for the within-subjects main effect. The available sample size should provide ample power for the within-subjects effects but may be lacking in detecting between-subjects effects or the interaction.

# The Synergy

This section will focus on presenting the analysis plan for a repeated measures ANOVA and reporting the output in a way that is compatible with the American Psychological Association (APA) publication manual. A version of potential interpretation which is compatible with the APA publication manual will be provided after each example in order to highlight what is most important and necessary to report. The SPSS syntax and data can be found in the appendix.

## Repeated Measures ANOVA Analysis Plan

The SPSS output for the repeated measures ANOVA is drastically different in the layout compared to that for the factorial ANOVA (see Appendix 2.1 for the syntax and Appendix 2.2 for the abbreviated output). Most statistical programs provide the output for the repeated measures ANOVA and MANOVA together. The analysis plan is driven by the presence or not of a significant interaction. If the interaction is significant, the researcher should follow it up. If it is not significant, the researcher should follow up significant main effects (see Figure 2.1 for the analysis plan and Table 2.1 for the descriptive statistics).

The example provided here contains a significant interaction in order to demonstrate the analysis plan. To begin the analysis of the interaction, the simple effects Welch ANOVAs of gender predicting anxiety are analyzed for each assessment (alpha = 0.05/2 assessments = 0.025).

Next, the data are split by gender and simple effects repeated measures ANOVAs are analyzed to assess the effects of the intervention for males and females [alpha = 0.05/2 gender (male and female) = 0.025]. There is no need to report any pairwise comparisons because both gender and assessment are dichotomous variables. The following write-up example uses the Greenhouse–Geisser adjustment.

Following a nonsignificant interaction, Tukey's HSD or the Sidak adjustment for small or unequal sample (Games–Howell is unavailable for comparisons of marginal means) should be reported for each significant main effect with more than two groups. Tukey's HSD assumes equal variance, while the Sidak adjustment accounts for the actual variance of each comparison.

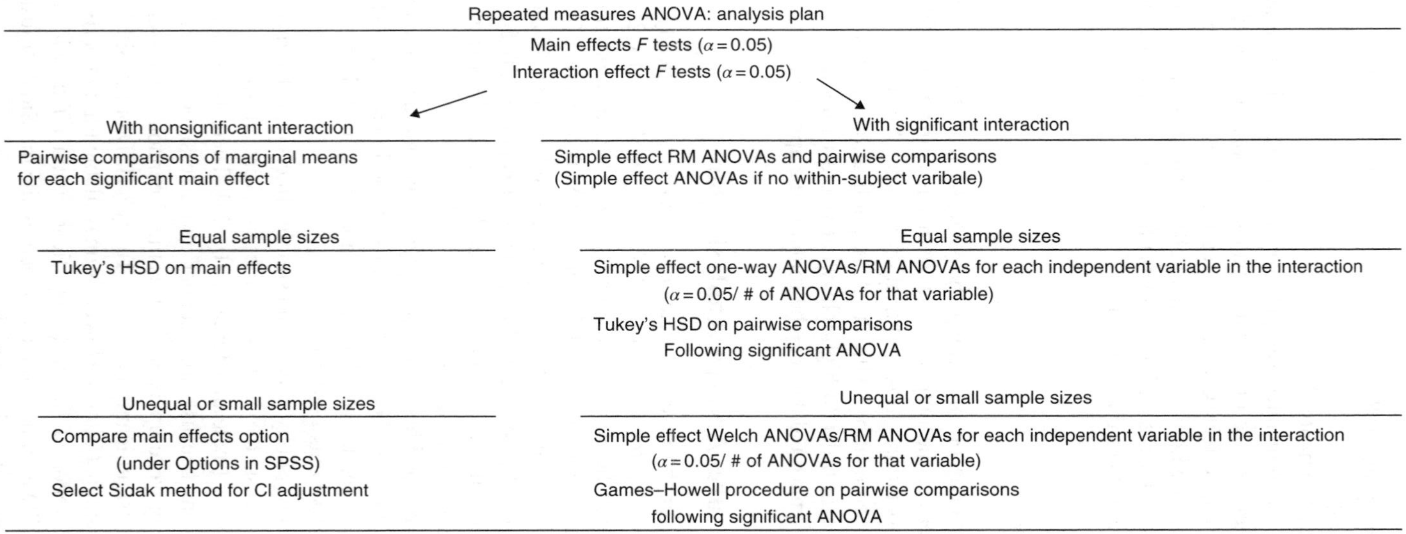

Repeated measures ANOVA: analysis plan

Main effects F tests ($\alpha = 0.05$)
Interaction effect F tests ($\alpha = 0.05$)

With nonsignificant interaction

Pairwise comparisons of marginal means
for each significant main effect

Equal sample sizes

Tukey's HSD on main effects

Unequal or small sample sizes

Compare main effects option
(under Options in SPSS)
Select Sidak method for CI adjustment

With significant interaction

Simple effect RM ANOVAs and pairwise comparisons
(Simple effect ANOVAs if no within-subject variable)

Equal sample sizes

Simple effect one-way ANOVAs/RM ANOVAs for each independent variable in the interaction
($\alpha = 0.05/$ # of ANOVAs for that variable)

Tukey's HSD on pairwise comparisons
Following significant ANOVA

Unequal or small sample sizes

Simple effect Welch ANOVAs/RM ANOVAs for each independent variable in the interaction
($\alpha = 0.05/$ # of ANOVAs for that variable)

Games–Howell procedure on pairwise comparisons
following significant ANOVA

*Figure 2.1  Repeated measures ANOVA analysis plan.*

Table 2.1    Descriptive statistics for anxiety and upper body strength.

| | Anxiety | | Upper body strength | | n |
|---|---|---|---|---|---|
| | M | SD | M | SD | |
| *Preintervention* | | | | | |
| Male | 20.28 | 4.03 | 99.66 | 35.92 | 25.00 |
| Female | 18.54 | 4.55 | 46.18 | 14.37 | 46.00 |
| *Postintervention* | | | | | |
| Male | 20.40 | 4.47 | 119.62 | 40.56 | 25.00 |
| Female | 20.46 | 4.76 | 60.30 | 14.42 | 46.00 |

# Example of a Write-Up Compatible with the APA Publication Manual

A two-way repeated measures ANOVA was used to predict anxiety scores based on gender as a between-subjects factor and assessment (pre- and postintervention) as a within-subjects factor. Anxiety was measured before and after the intervention using the Psychological General Well-Being Index (PGWBI). High scores represent lower anxiety. An alpha of 0.05 was used, and the Greenhouse–Geisser adjusted $F$ and degrees of freedom are reported. Anxiety differed between pre- and posttest assessment, $F(1, 69) = 6.93$, mean square error $(MSE) = 4.83$, G–G $p = 0.010$, $\eta_p^2 = 0.091$, but gender was not a significant predictor of anxiety level, $F(1, 69) = 0.63$, $MSE = 36.04$, $p = 0.429$, $\eta_p^2 = 0.009$. However, there was a significant interaction between gender and assessment, $F(1, 69) = 5.39$, G–G $p = 0.023$, $\eta_p^2 = 0.072$ (see Figure 2.3). As a result, simple effects ANOVAs were conducted as a result of this significant interaction.

Simple effects Welch ANOVAs were conducted to compare the average anxiety level of men and women for each assessment. An alpha of 0.025 was used to determine significance. Gender was not a significant predictor of anxiety for the pre- or posttest assessments, $F(1, 81.59) = 0.05$, $p = 0.818$, $\eta_p^2 = 0.001$, and $F(1, 55.59) < 0.001$, $p = 0.996$, $\eta_p^2 < 0.001$, respectively.

Simple effects repeated measures ANOVAs were conducted to compare the average anxiety level of pre- and postassessment for each gender. An alpha of 0.025 was used to determine significance. For men, the pre- and postintervention anxiety levels did not differ, $F(1, 24) = 0.06$, G–G $p = 0.808$, $\eta_p^2 = 0.003$. Women were significantly less anxious after the intervention, $F(1, 45) = 14.47$, G–G $p < 0.001$, $\eta_p^2 = 0.243$.

# Repeated Measures MANOVA Analysis Plan

The repeated measures MANOVA begins with reporting the main effects and interactions (alpha = 0.05) (see Figure 2.2 for the repeated measures MANOVA analysis plan). This MANOVA example intentionally contains an interaction in order to demonstrate the analysis plan when an interaction is present (see Appendix 2.3 for the syntax and Appendix 2.4 for the abbreviated output). Because our independent variables are dichotomous, pairwise comparisons are redundant.

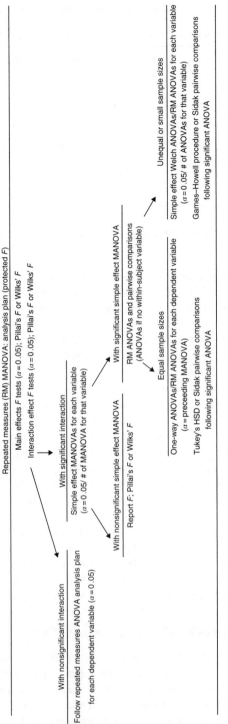

*Figure 2.2   Repeated measures MANOVA analysis plan (protected F).*

The protected $F$ procedure is utilized here. In other words, once an analysis is split into univariate ANOVAs, the alpha level of the preceding MANOVA is adopted for each dependent variable rather than split by each dependent variable. The effect of gender on the dependent variables is analyzed for each assessment (alpha=0.05/2, assessments=0.025). Because there is no longer a within-subjects variable, simple effects one-way MANOVAs will be used. Following a significant MANOVA, one-way ANOVAs are used to identify which dependent variables gender is a significant predictor of at each assessment (alpha of preceding MANOVA=0.025).

Next, the data are split by gender and simple effects repeated measures MANOVAs are used to determine if assessment is a significant predictor of the dependent variables for each gender (alpha=0.05/2, genders=0.025). Following a significant MANOVA, repeated measures ANOVAs are used to determine which dependent variables the pre- and postintervention assessment scores differ for each gender (alpha of preceding MANOVA=0.025).

If the interaction is not significant and at least one main effect is significant, the analysis can be divided up into multiple repeated measures ANOVAs predicting each significant dependent variable separately (alpha=0.05). The repeated measures ANOVA analysis plan would be followed from there.

# Example of a Write-Up Compatible with the APA Publication Manual

A two-way repeated measures MANOVA was used to predict anxiety scores and upper body strength, with gender as a between-subjects factor and assessment (pre- and postintervention) as a within-subjects factor. An alpha of 0.05 was used. Gender and assessment were both significant predictors, Pillai's $F(2, 68)=44.73$, $p<0.001$, $\eta_p^2=0.568$, and Pillai's $F(2, 68)=31.36$, $p<0.001$, $\eta_p^2=0.480$. The interaction of gender and assessment was significant, Pillai's $F(2, 68)=4.00$, $p=0.023$, $\eta_p^2=0.105$ (see Figures 2.3 and 2.4). Simple effects MANOVAs were conducted to further examine the interaction.

Simple effects MANOVAs were used to predict anxiety scores and upper body strength from gender for each assessment. Alpha of 0.025 was used to determine significance. For the preintervention assessment, gender was a significant predictor, Pillai's $F(2, 84)=51.39$, $p<0.001$, $\eta_p^2=0.550$. Welch ANOVAs (with an alpha of 0.025) indicated that preintervention anxiety was not different between males and females, $F(1, 81.59)=0.05$, $p=0.818$, $\eta_p^2=0.001$. Preintervention upper body strength was greater for males than females, $F(1, 71.94)=125.66$, $p<0.001$, $\eta_p^2=0.540$. For the postintervention assessment, gender was a significant predictor, Pillai's $F(2, 69)=40.74$, $p<0.001$, $\eta_p^2=0.541$. Welch ANOVAs, with an alpha of 0.025, indicated that postintervention anxiety was not different between males and females, $F(1, 55.59)<0.001$, $p=0.996$, $\eta_p^2<0.001$. Postintervention upper body strength was greater for males than females, $F(1, 66.89)=106.76$, $p<0.001$, $\eta_p^2=0.503$.

Simple effects repeated measures MANOVAs were used to predict anxiety scores and upper body strength for males and again for females. An alpha of 0.025 was used to determine significance, and the Greenhouse–Geisser adjusted $F$ and degrees of

Estimated marginal means of anxiety

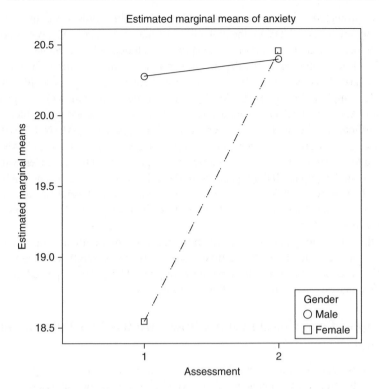

*Figure 2.3    Interaction plot for gender and assessment predicting anxiety.*

freedom are reported. For males, assessment was a significant predictor, Pillai's $F(2,23)=6.52, p=0.006, \eta_p^2=0.362$. Repeated measures ANOVAs, with an alpha of 0.025, indicated that male anxiety did not differ between pre- and postintervention, $F(1, 24)=0.06$, G–G $p=0.808$, $\eta_p^2=0.003$. However, males possessed more upper body strength in the postintervention assessment, $F(1, 50)=16.33$, G–G $p<0.001$, $\eta_p^2=0.246$. For females, assessment was a significant predictor, Pillai's $F(2, 44)=66.97$, $p<0.001$, $\eta_p^2=0.753$. Repeated measures ANOVAs, with an alpha of 0.025, indicated that females reported lower anxiety levels in the postintervention assessment, $F(1, 45)=14.47$, G–G $p<0.001, \eta_p^2=0.243$. Females possessed more upper body strength in the postintervention assessment $F(1, 45)=128.81$, G–G $p<0.001, \eta_p^2=0.741$.

## Summary

The repeated measures ANOVA and MANOVA are special cases of ANOVA and MANOVA in which a within-subjects variable (or variables) is included in the model (in addition to or without a between-subjects variable). Our examples included a between-subjects and a within-subjects variable.

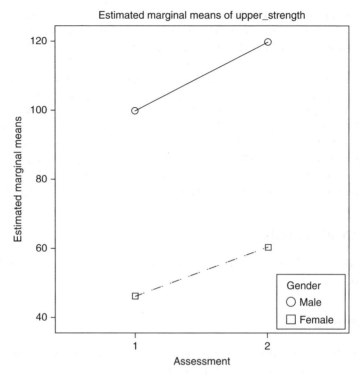

*Figure 2.4    Interaction plot for gender and assessment predicting upper body strength.*

The analytical frameworks of the repeated measures ANOVA and MANOVA are very similar to those for factorial ANOVA and MANOVA with minor differences. The most notable difference in the univariate assumptions is the sphericity assumption for the repeated measures. The univariate $F$ adjustments help address the violations of this assumption in order to preserve the alpha level. Both Greenhouse–Geisser and Huynh–Feldt are considered appropriate adjustments. Alternatively, the multivariate (i.e., MANOVA) approach is available in situations with substantial sphericity violations.

The usage of the repeated measures ANOVA and MANOVA is quite common. Nearly 1 out of every 4 of the 12 peer-reviewed journal articles in sport and exercise sciences over the past 5 years (refer to Appendix 2.5) included some form of a repeated measures ANOVA/MANOVA. The analytical power available from analyzing participants on multiple treatment conditions, profile analyses, or longitudinal studies warrants more use of these analytical procedures in situations with less than ideal numbers of participants or situations that may suffer from large variability between subjects. It should be noted, however, that lengthy data acquisition and attrition rates are a consideration in longitudinal studies and multiple treatment conditions.

The analysis plans laid out in this chapter for both the repeated measures ANOVA and MANOVA are easily adapted to situations with multiple between- and within-subjects variables. Descriptive statistics ($M$, SD, $n$) are best reported in a table.

The model statistics (G–G and H–F $F$ values, Pillai's $F$, Wilks' $F$) should be reported in the text. Pairwise comparisons of marginal means (Tukey's or Sidak's) or simple effects (Tukey's or Games–Howell) are commonly reported in a table. Tukey's assumes equal variance and is available for marginal means and simple effects tests. Games–Howell is the equal variance unassumed, equivalent of Tukey's, but Games–Howell is unavailable whenever comparisons of marginal means are performed. Pairwise comparisons are not required with dichotomous variables because such comparisons make sense when an independent variable has three or more levels.

Myers et al. (2010) provide a thorough presentation of the univariate repeated measures ANOVA. Hair, Black, Babin, and Anderson (2009) provide a thorough overview of the repeated measures MANOVA, and Tabachnick and Fidell (2013) cover multivariate techniques, including repeated measures MANOVA, in great length.

# Acknowledgment

The authors would like to thank Hershel Eason from Middle Tennessee State University for his contribution in the preparation of this chapter.

# References

Anshel, M. H. (2008). The disconnected values model: Intervention strategies for exercise behavior change. *Journal of Clinical Sports Psychology, 2*, 357–380.

Anshel, M. H., Brinthaupt, T. M., & Kang, M. (2010). The disconnected values model improves mental well-being and fitness in an employee wellness program. *Behavioral Medicine, 36*(4), 113–122.

Clemes, S. A., & Deans, N. K. (2012). Presence and duration of reactivity to pedometers in adults. *Medicine and Science in Sports and Exercise, 44*(6), 1097–1101.

Cohen, J. (1988). *Statistical power analysis for the behavioral sciences* (2nd ed.). Hillsdale, NJ: Lawrence Erlbaum Associates.

Demarini, S., Koo, W. W., & Hockman, E. M. (2006). Bone, lean and fat mass of newborn twins versus singletons. *Acta Paediatrica, 95*(5), 594–599.

Dupuy, H. J. (1984). The psychological general well-being (PGWB) index. In N. K. Wenger, M. E. Mattson, C. D. Furberg, & J. Elinson (Eds.), *Assessment of quality of life in clinical trials of cardiovascular therapies* (pp. 170–183). New York, NY: Le Jacq Publishing.

Hair, J. F., Jr., Black, W. C., Babin, B. J., & Anderson, R. E. (2009). *Multivariate data analysis* (7th ed.) Englewood Cliffs, NJ: Prentice Hall.

Maxwell, S. E., & Delaney, H. D. (2004). *Designing experiments and analyzing data: A model comparison perspective* (2nd ed.). Mahwah, NJ: Lawrence Erlbaum Associates, Inc.

Myers, J. L., Well, A. D., & Lorch, R. F., Jr. (2010). *Research design and statistical analysis* (3rd ed.). New York, NY: Routledge.

Tabachnick, B. C., & Fidell, L. S. (2013). *Using multivariate statistics* (6th ed.). Boston, MA: Pearson.

Till, K., Jones, B., Darrall-Jones, J., Emmonds, S., & Cooke, C. (2015). Longitudinal development of anthropometric and physical characteristics within academy rugby league players. *Journal of Strength and Conditioning Research, 29*(6), 1713–1722.

# 3

# Mediation and moderation via regression analysis

## Nikos Ntoumanis[1] and Paul R. Appleton[2]

[1] School of Psychology & Speech Pathology, Curtin University, Perth, WA, Australia
[2] School of Sport, Exercise and Rehabilitation Sciences, University of Birmingham, Birmingham, UK

## General Introduction

Mediation and moderation analyses are frequently used statistical techniques in sport and exercise science, primarily in the area of sport and exercise psychology. The classic 1986 paper by Baron and Kenny on the mediation versus moderator distinction had nearly 50 000 citations on Google Scholar in October 2014. Mediation analysis examines intermediary variables in a nomological network of variables, hence its popularity in various areas of social and health sciences which focus on mechanisms of change (e.g., in terms of health behavior). In its simplest form, mediation analysis tests whether the prediction of an outcome (criterion) variable ($Y$) by a predictor variable ($X$) is exerted via an intermediary variable, the mediator ($M$). For example, Thøgersen, Fox, and Ntoumanis (2002) showed that the positive relation between physical activity and global self-esteem was partially explained by physical satisfaction. Specifically, individuals with higher levels of physical activity were more satisfied with their physical self, which in turn predicted more positive global evaluations of one's self-worth. More complex versions of this scenario are possible, for example, having multiple $X$, $Y$, and/or $M$ variables, repeated measures of these variables, or measures of these variables at different levels of analysis (e.g., individual and group).

*An Introduction to Intermediate and Advanced Statistical Analyses for Sport and Exercise Scientists*, First Edition.
Edited by Nikos Ntoumanis and Nicholas D. Myers.
© 2016 John Wiley & Sons, Ltd. Published 2016 by John Wiley & Sons, Ltd.
Companion website: www.wiley.com/go/ntoumanis/sport

Moderator analysis, in its simplest form, tests whether the prediction of an outcome (criterion) variable $(Y)$ by a predictor variable $(X)$ varies, in strength and/or direction, as a function of the scores of a third variable $(Z)$. For example, Amireault, Godin, Vohl, and Pérusse (2008) showed that the relation between perceived control over physical activity behavior and physical activity behavior was stronger in individuals with high income as opposed to those with low income. Similar to mediation analysis, more complex research questions regarding moderation effects can be tested by including additional variables or levels of analysis.

It is also possible to combine mediation and moderation analysis. There are several possible ways in which mediation and moderation can be combined; interested readers are referred to Hayes (2013). For example, researchers can test for moderated mediation, that is, whether the mediation of $M$ on the relation between $X$ and $Y$ is consistent across the levels of a moderator variable $Z$. It is possible that mediating effects might vary across situations or type of individuals, leading to underestimation or overestimation of such effects if observed across only some of the levels of a moderator variable. Curran, Hill, and Niemiec (2013) provided an example of moderated mediation in sport psychology research.

While it is possible to also test for mediated moderation (i.e., whether the moderating effect of $Z$ on the relation between $X$ and $Y$ is indirect via mediator $M$; e.g., see Reysen, Snider, & Branscombe, 2012), Hayes (2013) proposed that it is not particularly interesting and should not be tested. Hayes explained that this is because the product between the predictor variable $(X)$ and moderator $(Z)$, which is required to estimate a moderated regression analysis (described later) and subsequently a mediated moderation analysis, is actually meaningless. The product is included in the regression equation simply as a method to estimate the effect of $X$ on $Y$ as a function of the samples' scores on $Z$ (i.e., so that $X$'s effect on $Y$ is not constrained to be invariant across values of $Z$). However, the $XZ$ product does not quantify anything; that is, while $X$ and $Z$ represent scores on measured constructs, their product does not. Thus, because $XZ$ has no substantive meaning, the indirect effect of this product via $M$ is also meaningless (Hayes, 2013). Hayes encouraged researchers to reconceptualize questions pertaining to mediated moderation as tests of moderated mediation. In light of Hayes' arguments, we do not provide an example of mediated moderation in this chapter.

In sum, the purpose of this chapter is to illustrate some fairly rudimentary applications of mediation and moderator tests using multiple regression analysis. For more detailed treatment of mediation and moderator tests via regression analysis, we refer the readers to specialized books by Cohen, Cohen, West, and Aiken (2002), Hayes (2013), and MacKinnon (2008). Both of these tests could also be conducted via more sophisticated tests (structural equation modeling and multilevel modeling) presented in subsequent chapters of this book.

# Utility of the Methods in Sport and Exercise Science

The popularity of mediation analysis in the sport and exercise science literature is not surprising. Many theories and models describe mediating or intervening processes. For example, the theory of planned behavior (Ajzen, 1991) suggests that intention to perform a behavior (e.g., exercise) mediates the relations between attitudes toward the behavior, existing norms regarding the behavior, and perceived control over the behavior, with the behavior itself. In the sport and exercise science literature, mediation analysis has been widely used to test direct and indirect pathways by which predictor variable(s) predict outcome/criterion variable(s). Such testing, when guided by theory and sound rationale, is crucial in moving beyond a mere description of antecedents and outcomes and toward an understanding of the underlying mechanisms that connect a network of variables. In other words, mediation analysis, when underpinned by appropriate research designs, can help to fill in the "black box in the middle" and explain how some variables predict other variables in a chain of hypothesized events and networks. Hence, mediation analysis has the potential to aid the development and refinement of theoretical frameworks.

Caution, however, should be exerted in drawing causal conclusions from mediation analysis. For a causal argument regarding mediation, the $X$, $Y$, and $M$ variables should be temporally separated (i.e., should be measured sequentially at different time points), and spurious covariates should be controlled. For example, Antonakis, Bendahan, Jacquart, and Lalive (2010) outlined a procedure for dealing with spurious effects, in particular when $X$ is not experimentally manipulated and $M$ is not temporally separated from $Y$. Experimental manipulation of the $X$ and, where possible, of the $M$ makes a stronger case for causal mediation effects. In the sport and exercise science field, most mediation analyses are conducted with cross-sectional and nonexperimental data. In such cases, the ordering of the variables into $X$, $Y$, and $Z$ is based on relevant theory and theoretical models, but causal inferences should be best avoided.

Moderation analysis is also useful for sport and exercise scientists. Tests for moderation are, for example, important in terms of examining whether the relation between two variables varies across different dosages of an intervention (e.g., intense vs. minimal intervention for promoting physical activity), different demographic variables (e.g., low vs. high socioeconomic status), or different scores of a continuous variable (e.g., those with high vs. low scores on adaptive types of motivation). In this respect, moderation analysis can also assist in the development and refinement of theoretical frameworks by detecting conditions under which relations exist or not exist or are stronger as opposed to weaker. For example, Gay, Saunders, and Dowda (2011) showed that the relation between motivational factors and exercise behavior was stronger for individuals who had more favorable perceptions of their neighborhood physical environment. However, it is important that moderation analysis is conducted in a parsimonious and an ad hoc (as opposed to post hoc) manner. In other words, the choice of moderators should be done carefully and prior to the analyses. Further, only the most important moderators (on the basis of theory, or previous evidence, or other reasons that can be clearly articulated) should be tested (as opposed to all possible moderators researchers can think of). For example, subgroup analyses (i.e., splitting the original sample into subgroups and comparing findings across groups) can increase the likelihood of false negative and positive findings (Higgins & Green, 2011).

# The Substantive Example

## Mediation

The first example is an example of mediation. Drawing from self-determination theory (SDT; Deci & Ryan, 2002), we examine the extent to which perceptions of coach need support (*X*) negatively predict female athletes' concerns about their body weight (*Y*) via satisfying the athletes' need for autonomy (*M*). The sequence of testing is based on Deci and Ryan (2002) and Vallerand's (1997) conceptualizations of perceptions of the social environment as antecedent variables of individuals' psychological need satisfaction, which in turn predicts variations in individuals' cognitive, behavioral, and affective experiences. In our example, perceptions of coach need support refer to the degree to which coaches are perceived by their athletes to be empathetic and caring, respectful to their athletes' choices and decisions, and providing opportunities for them to develop skills and master important tasks. The need for autonomy refers to the degree to which athletes feel ownership and control over their behavior. Theoretical (e.g., Verstuyf, Patrick, Vansteenkiste, & Teixeira, 2012) and empirical (e.g., Thøgersen-Ntoumani, Ntoumanis, & Nikitaras, 2010) arguments suggest that weight concerns and unhealthy weight control behaviors are less likely to occur in social environments (e.g., parental, romantic) that are need supportive.

In subsequent tests of mediation, in addition to the need for autonomy, we look at two more mediators, namely, the need for relatedness (i.e., feeling accepted and valued by the coach) and the need for competence (i.e., feeling effective in producing desired outcomes). This is an example of a multiple mediator model that includes all three basic psychological needs advanced by SDT. We also present an example of mediation that has two predictor variables, coach need support and coach control. The latter variable refers to instances in which a coach undermines athletes' basic psychological needs by being coercive and distant and by devaluing athletes' contributions and opinions (Bartholomew, Ntoumanis, & Thøgersen-Ntoumani, 2009). Lastly, we briefly present an example of a moderated mediation analysis in which we examine whether age moderates the mediation sequence of need support → autonomy need satisfaction → body weight concern.

# The Synergy

## Mediation

We start our example by presenting the method that most sport and exercise scientists are familiar with, that is, the Baron and Kenny (1986) four-step approach. In Figure 3.1, we demonstrate the use of this approach by showing how athletes' perceptions of need-supportive coach behaviors negatively predict athletes' reports of body weight concerns and whether this statistical effect is mediated by autonomy need satisfaction. The data file is labeled "mediation data2.sav." Readers are advised to check the assumptions underlying regression analysis before performing mediation analyses (e.g., Cohen et al., 2002).

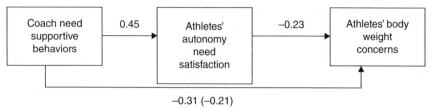

−0.31 (−0.21)
Note: All standardized path coefficients are significant at $p < 0.01$

*Figure 3.1    Testing the mediation of athletes' autonomy need satisfaction of the relation between athletes' perceptions of coach need-supportive behaviors and athletes' weight concerns, using the Baron and Kenny (1986) four-step approach.*

According to the four-step approach, mediation testing involves the following sequence:

Step 1: Test whether a need-supportive coach environment ($X$) predicts athletes' body weight concerns ($Y$). This step establishes the total predictive effect of the predictor variable on the criterion variable.

Step 2: Test whether a need-supportive coach environment predicts the mediator variable ($M$) of autonomy need satisfaction.

Step 3: Test whether autonomy need satisfaction predicts body weight concerns while statistically partialing out coach need support. In other words, both the $X$ and the $M$ are simultaneous predictors of the $Y$.

Step 4: Using the output from the analysis in Step 3, examine how much the effect of need-supportive coach behaviors on body weight concerns is reduced in Step 3, when compared to the same effect in Step 1.

Baron and Kenny (1986) suggested that when the $X$ to $Y$ statistical effect in Step 4 is nonsignificant, then evidence of complete mediation is provided. When this effect is reduced, compared to the same effect in Step 1, but is still significant, then evidence of partial mediation is shown. However, given that the significance of the regression path coefficients is affected by sample size, Kenny (e.g., see his website: http://davidakenny. net/cm/mediate.htm#BK) subsequently dropped the reference to statistical significance. Further, the terms partial and full mediation can be potentially hindering theory testing and development, as they imply additional mediators (when such variables might not exist) or no additional mediator (when such variables might exist). In fact, Hayes (2013) argues against the use of the terms full and partial mediation. Instead, it is more informative to examine the effect size of the indirect effect.

Based on Baron and Kenny's four-step approach, three regression analyses were run in SPSS (see Appendix 3.1), and the standardized path coefficients are summarized in Figure 3.1. The results indicate that autonomy need satisfaction is a mediator of the relation between need-supportive coach behaviors and athletes' body weight concerns. This is because the conditions outlined in the first three steps are met, and also, Step 4 indicates that the direct effect is reduced from $\beta = -0.31$ in Step 1 to $\beta = -0.21$ in Step 3.

The four-step approach is now considered by many methodologists as an out-dated practice. For example, Preacher and Hayes (2008) and Rucker Preacher, Tormala, and Petty (2011) have questioned whether a total effect needs to exist between the $X$ and $Y$ as a prerequisite to establish mediation (see Step 1). This is because indirect effects can be significant even if the direct or total effect from $X$ to $Y$ is not significant. Hence, the emphasis on mediation analysis has shifted from testing the four-step approach and establishing the statistical significance of the reduction in the size of the direct effect to testing the size and significance of the indirect effect. In Figure 3.1, the indirect effect of need-supportive coach behaviors on body weight concerns via autonomy need satisfaction is equal to the product of the two direct effects (i.e., from coach behaviors to autonomy and from autonomy to body weight concerns): $0.45 \times -0.23 = -0.10$. This is equivalent (in absolute terms) to the reduction in the direct effect from Step 1 to Step 3 (i.e., from $\beta = -0.31$ to $\beta = -0.21$).

The Sobel test (Sobel, 1982), based on normal theory statistics, has often been used in the past to establish the statistical significance of the indirect effect. However, it has been shown that this test is not appropriate for small sample sizes (Preacher & Hayes, 2008). Preacher and Hayes recommended the indirect effect method, namely, the use of bootstrapping procedures to construct confidence intervals (CI) around the parameter estimate of the indirect effect. Bootstrapping makes no assumptions about normal distribution and estimates the indirect effect in a number of samples randomly drawn from the original sample. Using the estimates of the indirect effect provided by bootstrapping, researchers can construct 95% CI of this effect. There are various alternatives in terms of which CI to use, but often, the bias-corrected CI are preferred, which, unlike conventional CI, can be asymmetric around the mean estimate. If the zero is outside the CI, researchers can claim evidence of an indirect effect being in operation (Preacher & Hayes, 2008). Andrew Hayes has developed custom dialog box for SPSS and SAS (labeled PROCESS and available from http://www.afhayes.com/introduction-to-mediation-moderation-and-conditional-process-analysis.html#process), which can be employed to estimate direct and indirect effects.

Using the PROCESS dialog box for SPSS (see Appendix 3.2), the lower and upper values of the bias-corrected 95% CI of the indirect effect ($\beta = -0.10$) of coach need-supportive behaviors on athlete weight concerns are calculated to be $-0.166$ and $-0.056$, respectively. Given that zero is not included in the CI, the findings provide evidence of an indirect effect from need-supportive behaviors on body weight concerns via autonomy need satisfaction. The same conclusion is reached by looking at the $z$ value of the Sobel statistic (which is presented here for illustrative purposes only): $z = -3.83, p < 0.0001$. PROCESS also presents the ratio of the indirect effect to the total effect (in our example, about a third, 33.56%, of the total effect is indirect) and the ratio of the indirect effect to the direct effect (about a half, 50.50%, in our example). Hayes (2013) warned against the use of these proportion measures unless the sample size is large (at least 500, according to MacKinnon, Warsi, and Dwyer (1995)) and the total effect is (i) larger than the indirect effect and (ii) of the same sign. Preacher and Kelley (2011) presented various effect size indices for quantifying the magnitude of indirect effects. PROCESS reports one of them, the kappa-squared effect size, which in our example is 0.0992. This statistic ranges from 0 to 1 with higher values indicating larger indirect effects. Note that PROCESS presents standardized estimates for indirect effects only. If readers want to obtain standardized estimates for other effects in the regression model, all variables need to be converted into $z$ scores before they are inputted into PROCESS.

Many theories and models applied to sport and exercise science advocate the operation of multiple intermediary or mediatory variables. Hence, the next step in this section is to present a multiple mediator model. Testing multiple mediators simultaneously is not possible using the linear regression option in SPSS; hence, the PROCESS custom dialog box is needed. Simultaneous testing of multiple mediators allows the examination of specific indirect effects via each mediator while controlling for the effects of other mediators. PROCESS can accommodate models in which none of the mediators predict each other (parallel multiple mediator model; see Figure 3.2) or when some mediators predict other mediators (serial multiple mediator model). Please note that when mediator variables are correlated with each other (as is the case more often than not), the total indirect effect in the multiple mediator model will not equal the sum of the indirect effects obtained if each mediator was tested in separate analyses. Furthermore, when mediator variables are highly intercorrelated, this might result in some indirect effects being nonsignificant due to multicollinearity. In some cases, highly intercorrelated mediators might produce models in which some indirect effects have opposite signs compared to when each mediator is tested on its own, due to statistical suppression. In such cases, one or more of these mediators could be omitted from the analysis. A more extensive treatment of this topic can be found in MacKinnon, Krull, and Lockwood (2000).

In Figure 3.2, we present a parallel multiple mediation model which includes all three psychological needs (autonomy, competence, and relatedness) proposed by Deci and Ryan's (2002) SDT. We test whether these three needs mediate the relation between

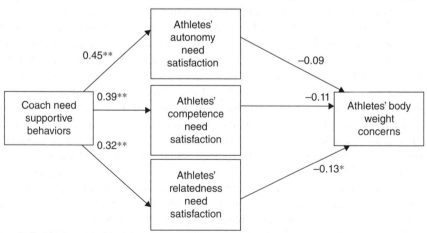

Note: Indirect effects and their bootstrapped CI are reported in the text. *$p < 0.05$, **$p < 0.01$

*Figure 3.2    Testing a multiple mediation model by including two more psychological needs in Figure 3.1.*

coach need-supportive behaviors and body weight concerns. Prior to the analysis, we converted all variables into $z$ scores (see Appendix 3.3) in order to provide standardized parameter estimates in the PROCESS outputs. It is not essential to do that; in fact, unstandardized coefficients are perfectly fine for testing mediation effects. The only reason we standardized the variables was so that we can compare the findings of the parallel multiple mediation model with those of the single mediator model.

The results indicate that the total standardized indirect effect via the three needs is $\beta = -0.13$ (0.1274 to be more precise, if readers want to replicate our analyses). Note that if we were to run separate single mediator models (not shown in this book) for each psychological need and sum up the indirect effects, the total indirect effect would be $\beta = -0.26$. This discrepancy exemplifies what we stated earlier, that is, the total indirect effect in the multiple mediator model will not equal the sum of the indirect effects obtained if each mediator was tested in separate analyses, if the mediators are correlated. In our data, the correlations among the three needs range from $r = 0.53$ to $r = 0.64$. Interestingly, the indirect effect via autonomy is $\beta = -0.04$ (whereas in the single mediator model it was $\beta = -0.10$); the indirect effects via competence and relatedness are similar in size ($\beta = -0.05$ and $\beta = -0.04$, respectively). The PROCESS output also presents the contrasts of the indirect effects via each psychological need (e.g., CI is the contrast between the indirect effect via autonomy and the indirect effect via competence). All three contrasts have values very close to zero, and their 95% bias-corrected CI includes zero. These findings indicate that the three specific indirect effects are very similar to each other and most probably not different from zero.

Note that Preacher and Hayes (2008) recommended the reporting of unstandardized indirect effects and their 95% bias-corrected CI (as opposed to $p$ values); to obtain those unstandardized indirect effects, researchers would need to run PROCESS with the original unstandardized variables. The CI of each specific indirect effect includes zero (see the second PROCESS model in Appendix 3.3). Further, if we were to use the Sobel test, all these indirect effects would be deemed as nonsignificant. In contrast, if each psychological need was tested separately in a single mediator model, their indirect effects would have been significant. The problem in our example is that the three needs are correlated quite substantially. Hence, the paradox is that the total indirect effect is significant and its 95% CI does not contain zero, whereas all three specific indirect effects are not significant. According to Hayes (2013), in such situations, researchers should focus more on the direct and specific indirect effects, not the total indirect effect. In a sense, both the single mediator and the multiple mediator models are correct, but they test different questions; the latter model tests the effect of each mediator while controlling for the other mediators. Figure 3.2 presents the direct effects only of the parallel multiple mediator model. All three psychological needs are predicted by coach need-supportive behaviors, but only relatedness need satisfaction predicts (negatively) athletes' body weight concerns.

We can extend the previous model by adding a second predictor variable, perceptions of coach controlling behaviors. SPSS PROCESS can handle only one predictor variable at the time. However, the other predictor variables can be entered in the analysis as covariates.

We then run as many models as the number of predictor variables, substituting the variables in the *independent variable* and *covariate* boxes in PROCESS. This analysis will give the effects of each $X$ on $M$, controlling for the other $X$ variables in the model. Appendix 3.4 shows the setup and the output for an expanded version of Figure 3.2 that includes coach controlling behaviors as an additional predictor variable of the three psychological needs. In the first model, coach need support is the independent variable, and coach controlling behaviors is the covariate. In the second model, the variables in the two boxes are swapped. The results indicate that need support is again a significant positive predictor of all three psychological need variables. In contrast, perceptions of coach control predict (negatively) autonomy need satisfaction ($b = -0.14$; $p = 0.015$) only. None of the three indirect effects nor the total indirect effect of coach control on body weight concerns via the three psychological needs are significant (see the second model in Appendix 3.4).

Finally, we present an example of a mediation which is moderated (see Appendix 3.5). There are various types of moderated mediation (see Hayes, 2013). In this example, we test whether both the direct and indirect effects in Figure 3.1 are moderated by age ($W$). This is model 59 in PROCESS (see http://www.afhayes. com/public/templates.pdf). Essentially, this model expands Figure 3.1 by adding the main effects of $W$ on $M$ and $Y$, the interaction $XW$ in predicting $M$ and $Y$, as well as the interaction $MW$ in predicting $Y$. In our example (see Figure 3.3), age predicts weight concerns, but it does not predict autonomy need satisfaction, and the interactions between need support and age in predicting need satisfaction and body weight concerns are not significant. The autonomy $x$ age interaction in predicting weight concerns is significant ($\beta = -0.13$; $p = 0.29$). SPSS PROCESS presents the indirect effects of need support on weight concerns at one standard deviation

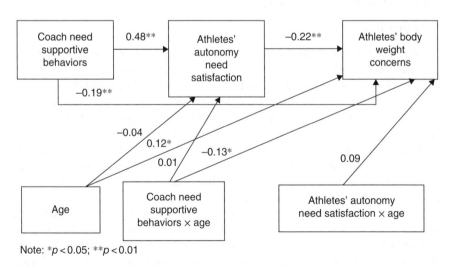

Note: *$p < 0.05$; **$p < 0.01$

*Figure 3.3    Moderated mediation; testing the moderation of age on the mediation of athletes' autonomy need satisfaction of the relation between athletes' perceptions of coach need-supportive behaviors and athletes' weight concerns.*

(SD) below the mean of the moderator, at the mean of the moderator, and at one SD above the mean of the moderator. In our example, the indirect effect is significant at the mean and at one SD above the mean for age, but is not significant at one SD below the mean. In other words, the indirect effect of need support on body weight concerns is strongest for relatively older athletes ($\beta = -17$; CI $= -0.27$ to $-0.08$).

According to Preacher and Hayes (2008), the indirect effect method, compared to the Baron and Kenny (1986) method, helps theory testing and development by examining indirect effects even when direct effects are not evident (e.g., due to measurement error or low power), by avoiding the unnecessary and often misleading distinction between partial and total mediation, and by decomposing and comparing specific indirect effects in complex models involving potentially several independent, mediator, and dependent variables. The indirect effect method can also be tested via structural equation modeling, which, unlike regression analysis, can accommodate the simultaneous testing of multiple dependent variables and can correct for measurement error by including item indicators of latent variables. The software Mplus offers the same capabilities as PROCESS (in terms of reporting specific indirect effects and the bias-corrected bootstrapped CI of these effects) and can be used to test complex mediation models with latent variables. However, structural equation modeling typically requires a much larger sample than regression analysis. Mediation analysis can also be conducted with multilevel models to examine mediation at different levels of the hierarchy (e.g., see Preacher, Zhang, & Zyphur, 2011). Selig and Preacher (2009) gave examples of advanced statistical techniques that can be used to examine mediation with longitudinal data.

# The Substantive Example

## Moderation

The first moderation example considers a continuous moderator. Grounded in SDT, this example considers whether the relation between controlling coaching ($X$) and athletes' positive affect ($Y$) is moderated by coach autonomy support ($M$). Controlling coaching behavior has been characterized by controlling use of rewards, negative conditional regard, intimidation, and excessive personal control (Bartholomew, Ntoumanis, & Thøgersen-Ntoumani, 2010) and has been shown to undermine athletes' well-being (Bartholomew, Ntoumanis, Ryan, Bosch, & Thøgersen-Ntoumani, 2011). However, because a coach can employ controlling and autonomy supportive strategies concurrently, it is possible that the detrimental effects of the former type of coaching strategies will be buffered when the coach also employs the latter type of strategies.

The second moderation example considers a dichotomous moderator. Specifically, we consider the moderating role of athletes' gender ($M$) in the relation between mothers' other-oriented perfectionism (OOP) ($X$) and athletes' perfectionistic cognitions ($Y$). OOP is characterized by the belief that significant others should attain perfection and a critical response when others fail to achieve desired standards (Hewitt & Flett, 1991). The perfectionism literature (Frost, Lahart, & Rosenblate, 1991) has proposed a "same-sex" hypothesis of perfectionism development, which assumes that athletes' perfectionistic tendencies develop as a result of same-sex parental perfectionistic demands. In our example, we predict a positive relation between mothers' OOP and female athletes' but a nonsignificant or negative correlation between mothers' OOP and male athletes' perfectionistic cognitions. Continuing with the same-sex perfectionism hypothesis, the final example in this section is a moderated moderation analysis (also known as three-way interaction). Here, the moderation of $X$'s effect by $M$ is itself moderated (by $W$; Hayes, 2013). Specifically, we consider whether the hypothesized difference between males and females in the mothers' OOP–athlete perfectionistic cognitions relation is moderated by athletes' age. The SPSS data file for the three moderation examples is "moderation data.sav."

# The Synergy

## Moderation

Prior to outlining the steps involved with conducting a moderation analysis, a word about sample size. There are a number of resources that provide guidance on the appropriate sample size for conducting a moderation analysis. For example, in their classic text on moderated regression, Aiken and West (1991) provide a table that identifies the sample size required when statistical power is 0.80 and $\alpha = 0.05$. More recently, Shieh (2009) developed syntax to determine appropriate sample sizes for specific levels of power and effect size when conducting moderated regression with continuous variables. The reader is encouraged to consult these texts prior to collecting data associated with tests of moderation. As with mediation, the assumptions underlying regression analysis should also be checked before performing tests of moderation.

The first and second moderation examples consider two-way interactions, in which the relation between an independent variable ($X$) and a dependent variable ($Y$) changes according to the value of a moderator ($M$). The regression equation for a two-way moderation is

$$Y = b_0 + b_1 X + b_2 M + b_3 XM + \varepsilon \qquad (3.1)$$

where $b_0$ is the intercept, $b_1$ is the coefficient of $X$, $b_2$ is the coefficient of the moderator, $b_3$ is the coefficient of the interaction variable (i.e., the outcome of multiplying $X$ and $M$), and $\varepsilon$ is the residual. When $b_3$ is statistically significant (i.e., $p < 0.05$), we say $M$ moderates the $X$–$Y$ relation.

The PROCESS dialog box in SPSS for our first example is presented in Appendix 3.6. In order to conduct a moderation analysis, the researcher *must* include $X$, $M$ and the interaction between $XM$ in the regression equation. When using PROCESS, the $XM$ interaction variable is created automatically for the researcher (labeled as "int_1" in the output). In addition, the researcher has the option of including covariates should he/she desire. In the current example, the "Mean center for products" has been selected in the "Options" tab. It is not essential to mean center $X$ and $M$ (i.e., subtracting the mean from the value of the original variable so that it has a mean of 0), despite popular belief in the sport and exercise science literature that doing so is necessary to prevent multicollinearity between $X$ and $M$ with $XM$. The reason we choose the "mean center for products" option in PROCESS is to ensure that the coefficients $b_1$ and $b_2$ are meaningful. For example, in the regression equation for the moderation outlined earlier, $b_1$ concerns the difference between participants' scores on $Y$ who also differ by one unit on $X$ when $M=0$. Equally, $b_2$ concerns the difference between participants' scores on $Y$ who also differ by one unit on $M$ when $X=0$. The $b_1$ and $b_2$ can only be interpreted, however, if 0 is a meaningful value in the response system for $M$ or $X$, respectively (which is not the case for autonomy support and controlling coaching in our example; Hayes, 2013). In contrast, a mean-centered version of $X$ ($M$) results in $b_1$ ($b_2$) estimating the difference between two participants' scores on $Y$ who also differ in one unit on $X$ ($M$) among cases *average* on $M$ ($X$), which is more meaningful and can be interpreted (Hayes, 2013). In sum, the decision to mean center $X$ and $M$ variables will depend on whether 0 is a meaningful value in a data set, but not as a strategy to reduce multicollinearity (Hayes, 2013).

Hierarchical moderated regression analysis (HRMA) has been the dominant approach to testing moderation in sport and exercise science, which involves researcher entering the $X$ and $M$ in model (also called "step") one, followed by the interaction variable $XM$ in model (step) two. Model two is generally favored in the HRMA approach when the $XM$ variable is significant and the $R^2$ value in model two is greater than the $R^2$ value associated with model one (i.e., the change in $R^2$ from model one to two was significant). PROCESS does not rely on the hierarchical approach, but rather automatically calculates the unique variability accounted for by $XM$ in $Y$ (Hayes, 2013).

The PROCESS output (see Appendix 3.6) indicates the regression coefficient (unstandardized) for the $XM$ variable is $b_3=0.4319$; $p<0.01$. This coefficient quantifies how the effect of controlling coaching on athletes' positive affect changes as coach autonomy support changes by one unit. We can conclude that the effect of controlling coaching for athletes' positive affect depends on the extent to which the coach is autonomy supportive. If the interaction variable is nonsignificant, it is best to remove the interaction and estimate a model with $X$ and $M$. In contrast, $X$ and $M$ should always be retained even if not statistically significant; excluding $X$ or $M$ will bias the estimate of moderation effect. The PROCESS output also shows us that 3.31% (i.e., "R2-chng") of the variance in positive affect is accounted for by the $XM$ variable. However, Dawson (2014) suggested that $R^2$ is not an ideal metric for measuring the size of an interaction effect due to the shared variance between $X$, $M$, and $XM$. Instead, Dawson suggested the $f^2$, which can be calculated using the following equation:

$$f^2 = \frac{R_2^1 - R_2^2}{1 - R_2^2} \tag{3.2}$$

where $R_2^1$ and $R_2^2$ represent the variance explained by the models including and excluding the interaction term, respectively (Aiken & West, 1991). In our example, $f^2=0.05$. Dawson suggested that many significant interaction effects only have small effect sizes; hence, he recommended that researchers emphasize the practical relevance of significant interactions.

The PROCESS output also indicates that the coefficients associated with controlling coaching ($b_1 = -0.2594$) and autonomy support ($b_2 = 0.3585$) are statistically significant. In other words, among athletes average in their perceptions of controlling coaching (because $M$ was mean centered), two athletes who differ by one unit in their perceptions of autonomy support are estimated to differ by 0.36 units in their positive affect. Likewise, among athletes average in their perceptions of autonomy support (because $X$ was also mean centered), two athletes who differ by one unit in their perceptions of controlling coaching are estimated to differ by −0.26 units in their positive affect.

Having established that $b_3$ is significant, the next step is to graphically plot the interaction. When plotting an interaction, a common method is to use the sample mean value plus one SD above and below the mean. PROCESS assists by producing a table of estimates of $Y$ for combinations of $X$ and $M$ (under the heading "Data for visualizing conditional effect of X on Y"; see Appendix 3.6). The values in this table can be copied into an SPSS syntax command (see also Appendix 3.6) to graphically plot the significant interaction. Alternatively, various online resources can be used, such as www.jeremydawson.com/slopes.htm or http://quantpsy.org/interact/mlr2.htm. As recommended by Hayes (2013), in the current example, $X$ and $M$ have been transformed from their centered versions back into the original scores in the syntax (see the "compute" commands) to ensure the plotted interaction can be interpreted without having to mentally convert the metrics. Figure 3.4 shows that when controlling coaching increases, athletes report lower positive affect when autonomy support is at the sample mean and 1 SD below the mean. Figure 3.4 also shows that positive affect remains stable, despite increases in controlling coaching, when autonomy support is 1 SD above the sample mean.

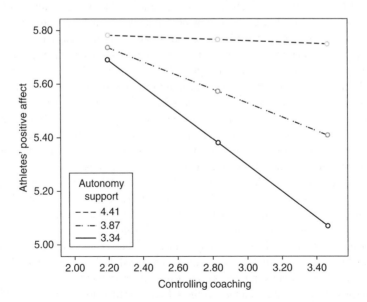

*Figure 3.4   A visual representation of the moderation of the effect of coaches' controlling behavior (X) on athletes' positive affect (Y) by coach autonomy support (M).*

It has been common to follow up this graphical representation by "probing" the interaction to establish where in the distribution of the moderator $X$ has an effect on $Y$ that is different from zero (and where it does not). A popular approach to "probing" an interaction is the pick-a-point strategy (also labeled "simple slopes analysis"). When conducting an analysis of simple slopes, a researcher conducts an inferential test (which can include CI) of the conditional effect of $X$ on $Y$ at certain values of $M$. In PROCESS, the results from the pick-a-point approach are automatically produced whenever a moderation analysis is conducted. Consistent with the graphic representative of the interaction in Figure 3.4, PROCESS produces values of the moderator equal to the sample mean as well as one SD below and above this mean. However, should the researcher wish, it is possible to override this pick-a-point strategy by selecting "Percentiles" in the "Conditioning" box. By selecting "Percentiles," PROCESS estimates the conditional effect of $X$ at values of $M$ corresponding to the 10th, 25th, 50th, 75th, and 90th percentiles in the sample distribution of $M$.

Using the default pick-a-appoint method in PROCESS, the output (see Appendix 3.6, under the heading "Conditional effect of X on Y at values of the moderator(s)") reveals that controlling coaching has an effect on athletes' positive affect at one SD below the mean ($b = -0.49$; $p < 0.01$) for autonomy support and the sample mean autonomy support ($b = -0.26$; $p < 0.01$). In contrast, the relation between controlling coaching and athletes' positive affect was nonsignificant when autonomy support was 1 SD above the sample mean ($b = -0.03$; $p > 0.05$).

An analysis of simple slopes is a popular approach to probing a significant interaction in the sport and exercise science literature. However, Dawson (2014) and Hayes (2013) cautioned against employing this pick-a-point probing analysis. Both authors proposed that in the past, researchers have selected somewhat arbitrary values of $M$, such as one SD above and below the sample mean. Often, there is nothing particularly meaningful about values that are one SD above and below the mean. That is, these values are sample specific, and thus, what is low autonomy support in our current example may be different in another sample. Dawson argued that rather than selecting arbitrary values, researchers should (if possible) choose meaningful values of the moderator at which to examine the slopes. This may be possible when the moderator is categorical where specific values (e.g., 0, 1) are assigned to conditions or groups of individuals or when specific values of a continuous moderator have been universally accepted as "high" and "low." However, if there are no meaningful values to choose, Dawson argued that it is probably unwise to conduct a pick-a-point probe of simple slopes.

Two approaches that address some of the limitations of the pick-a-point strategy, but which have been underemployed in the sport and exercise literature, are the Johnson–Neyman (J–N) technique (Bauer & Curran, 2005) and an evaluation of regions of significance (Aiken & West, 1991; Curran, Bauer, & Willoughby, 2006). The J–N technique, which can only be used when $M$ is a continuous variable, centers on different methods for describing the variability about the estimate produced by the regression analysis. For example, the J–N technique produces confidence bands around the simple slope which are interpreted in a similar manner to the CI associated with regression coefficients (Dawson, 2014). It is possible to implement the J–N technique in PROCESS which, according to Hayes, will produce one of possible three outputs (see section heading

"Johnson–Neyman Technique" in Appendix 3.6). The first possible outcome is a single J–N value within the range of $M$. In this instance, the conditional effect of $X$ on $Y$ is statistically significant when $M$ is $\leq$ or $\geq$ the J–N value, but not both. In other words, the region of significance of $X$'s effect on $Y$ is defined as either $M \leq$ or $\geq$ the J–N value. The second possible outcome is two values (J–N value[1] and J–N value[2]). In this instance, the region of significance of $X$'s effect on $Y$ is either J–N value[1]$\leq M \leq$J–N value[2] or $M \leq$J–N value[1] and $M \geq$J–N value[2]. The former means that the conditional effect of $X$ on $Y$ is statistically significant when $M$ is between, but not beyond, the two J–N values. The latter means that the conditional effect of $X$ on $Y$ is statistically significant when $M$ is less than or equal to J–N value[1] and when $M$ is greater than or equal to J–N value[2], but not between these two values. A third possible outcome is for no J–N value to be reported. No J–N value either means the effect of $X$ on $Y$ is statistically significant across the entire range of the moderator or the effect is not statistically significant anywhere in the observed distribution of the moderator (Hayes, 2013). In our example, one J–N value is produced (0.1981). The table below the J–N value (labeled "Conditional effect of X on Y at values of the moderator (M)") confirms that only when autonomy support is $\leq$0.1981 (or 4.062 when noncentered) is the conditional effect of coaches' controlling behavior on athletes' positive affect statistically significant ($p=0.05$).

It is also possible to plot the region of significance identified by the J–N technique along with confidence bands (see Bauer & Curran, 2005; Rogosa, 1980) using the syntax provided by Hayes (see page 267 for an example) and presented in Appendix 3.6. Figure 3.5 displays the region of significance in this example. As can be seen, when $M>4.0619$, the lower confidence band crosses zero.

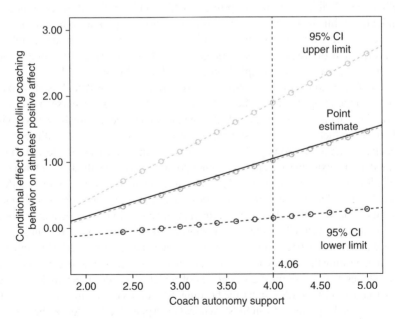

*Figure 3.5    The conditional effect of controlling coach behavior on athletes' positive affect as a function of coach autonomy support.*

The second alternative approach to the pick-a-point strategy is an evaluation of regions of significance (Aiken & West 1991), which seeks to identify the values of $M$ for which the $X$–$Y$ relation is statistically significant. Evaluating the regions of significance is valuable because it identifies values of $M$ at which $X$ is more or less likely to be important (Dawson, 2014). In order to identify the regions of significance, the PROCESS output can be inputted into the online utility at http://quantpsy.org/interact/mlr2.htm (Preacher, Curran, & Bauer, 2006). Specifically, the user is required to input the coefficients and asymptotic variances (i.e., the squared standard errors) for the intercept, $X$, $M$, and $XM$; the asymptotic covariances of $M$ with intercept of $XM$ with $X$; and the degrees of freedom, which are determined by the formula $df = N - k - 1$ where $N$ is the sample size and $k$ is the number of predictors (including interactions and any covariates). The default value is $\alpha = 0.05$, but this can be adjusted. A screenshot of the online utility with the required information entered to test for regions of significance for the current example is provided in Appendix 3.6.

If no errors are found, the results will be presented in the first output window (labeled "Two-way interaction simple slopes output"; see Appendix 3.6). Scrolling down this first output window reveals information pertaining to the "region of significance" which confirms the relation between controlling coaching and athletes' positive affect would be significant for any values of autonomy support lower than 4.0854 or higher than 5.6364. The final output window in the utility includes $R$ syntax for graphically representing the regions of significance. Clicking "Submit above to Rweb" will produce the graph presented in Figure 3.6. As Dawson (2014) pointed out, there is nothing special about these values. Rather, these are the values at which the relation between controlling coaching and positive affect are found to be significant within this particular data set. As with the pick-a-point approach, the values produced from the regions of significance test are dependent on sample size. However, when the regions of significance are interpreted with this point in mind, they are of greater use than simple slopes tests alone (Dawson, 2014).

In the first example of moderation, $M$ was a continuous variable. It is also possible to test the moderating effects of a dichotomous variable, and thus, in this second example, we examine the moderating role of athletes' gender ($M$) in the relation between mothers' OOP ($X$) and athletes' perfectionistic cognitions ($Y$). The steps involved with conducting the analysis with a dichotomous $M$ in PROCESS are the same as those described in the first moderating example, except that it is not possible to employ the J–N technique. The PROCESS output (see Appendix 3.7) shows an unstandardized regression coefficient for the $XM$ variable of $b_3 = -1.914$ ($p < 0.001$). Thus, we can conclude that the relation between mothers' OOP and athletes' perfectionistic cognitions is moderated by the athletes' gender. The PROCESS output also shows us that 18.75% (i.e., "R2-chng") of the variance in athletes' perfectionistic cognitions is accounted for by the $XM$ variable.

When plotting the significant $XM$ interaction in this second example, we are limited to two slopes that represent the categories of athletes' gender (0 = female, 1 = male). The output from PROCESS under the heading "Data for visualizing conditional effect of X on Y" can be pasted into an SPSS syntax (see Appendix 3.7). As can be seen from Figure 3.7, the relation between mothers' OOP and athletes' perfectionistic cognitions is positive for female athletes, but negative for male athletes.

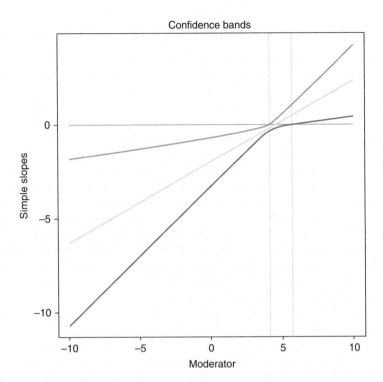

*Figure 3.6   Regions of significance for the conditional effect of controlling coach behavior on athletes' positive affect as a function of coach autonomy support.*

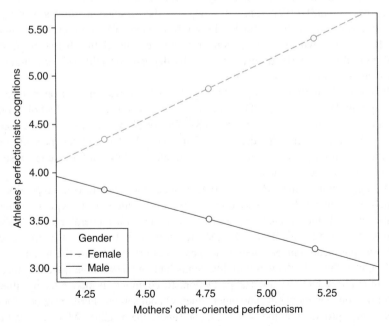

*Figure 3.7   A visual representation of conditional effects of mothers' other-oriented perfectionism (X) on athletes' perfectionistic cognitions (Y) among female and male athletes.*

We can also probe this interaction, albeit we are limited to the pick-a-point approach that estimates the conditional effect of $X$ on $Y$ for the two values of the dichotomous moderator (Hayes, 2013). PROCESS automatically recognizes that $M$ is a dichotomous variable and calculates the effect of $X$ for the two values of $M$. As outlined in the section of the output (see Appendix 3.7) labeled "Conditional effect of X on Y at values of the moderator(s)" the relation between $X$ and $Y$ is statistically different from zero at both values of the moderator.

So far, the analyses have been limited to one moderator variable. The final exercise in this section is a moderated moderation analysis (also known as three-way interaction), in which the moderation of $X$'s effect by $M$ is itself moderated (by $W$). Interpreting a moderated moderation analysis is complicated, compared to when the analysis contains one $M$ variable (for a detailed overview, see Aiken & West, 1991, and Jaccard & Turrisi, 2003). Fortunately, PROCESS is able to conduct a moderated moderation interaction and provide the output required to graphically plot and probe significant three-way interactions. The PROCESS dialog box in SPSS for conducting a moderated moderation is shown in Appendix 3.8.

For our moderated moderation example, we will extend the analysis conducted earlier concerning the moderating role of athletes' gender in the relation between mothers' OOP and athletes' perfectionistic cognitions by including athletes' age as $W$. Variables were again mean centered in this example using the option in PROCESS. The PROCESS output in Appendix 3.8 reveals that the regression coefficient for the $XMW$ interaction term is statistically significant (see "int_4"), $b=-0.0681$, $t(191)=-2.5817$, $p=0.011$. This suggests the interaction between mothers' OOP and athletes' gender and age is statistically different from zero. The PROCESS output also shows us that 0.0089% (i.e., "R2-chng") of the variance in athletes' perfectionistic cognitions is accounted for by the $XMW$ variable. We can therefore conclude that the extent to which athletes' gender moderates the relation between mothers' OOP and athletes' perfectionistic cognitions depends on athletes' age, albeit the three-way moderation is very weak.

It is possible to graphically plot the significant three-way interaction by inserting the output under the heading "Data for visualizing the conditional effect of X on Y" into an SPSS syntax (see Appendix 3.8). The resulting graphs are presented in Figure 3.8, which reveals that the effect of mothers' OOP on athletes' perfectionistic cognitions is different for female and male athletes, and this difference is consistent in younger and older athletes.

An inspection of the PROCESS output under the heading (see Appendix 3.8) "Conditional effect of X*M interaction at values of W" allows us to begin to probe the significant $XMW$ interaction. Given we have a continuous $W$ moderator, PROCESS has estimated the conditional effect of the $XM$ interaction on $Y$ at values of $W$ corresponding to the sample mean, one SD above the mean, and one SD below the mean (Hayes, 2013). Given that all effects are highly significant ($p<0.001$), we conclude that the effect of mothers' OOP on athletes' perfectionistic cognitions is moderated by athletes' gender for younger, moderate, and older athletes in our sample. Further support for this conclusion is provided by the J–N technique (under the heading "Moderator value(s) defining Johnson–Neyman significance region(s)"). The J–N technique reveals that the interaction between mothers' OOP and athletes' gender becomes nonsignificant at age

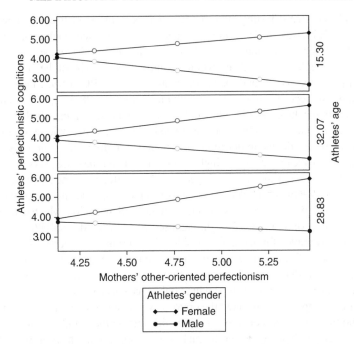

*Figure 3.8    The conditional effect of mothers' other-oriented perfectionism on athletes' perfectionistic cognitions as a function of gender and age. (The three panels for age correspond to values of age equal to one standard deviation below the mean, the sample mean, and one standard deviation above the mean).*

below −13.2532 (mean centered from 8.71 years). However, this finding should be interpreted with caution given there were only two athletes aged 8 and 9 years in the sample. Thus, contrary to the hypothesis, we conclude the athletes' age does not moderate the interaction between mothers' OOP and athletes' gender.

# Summary

Applications of mediation and moderation, and to a lesser extent their combination via moderated mediation, using regression analysis can be found within many influential journals in sport and exercise science. The specific strategies employed, however, often differ from study to study with many researchers still relying on outdated techniques. The purpose of this chapter was to demonstrate mediation and moderated analyses using current recommendations with relevant examples.

In the section on mediation, we began with an example of a single mediator using Baron and Kenny's now outdated four-step approach and the associated Sobel test. The four-step approach encourages the researcher to make conclusions regarding full and partial mediation, although it is now recognized that this terminology may hinder theory testing and development. In light of these limitations, we suggest sport and exercise scientists abandon the four-step approach in favor of more recent developments centered on testing indirect effects. Testing indirect effects has been made relatively straightforward since PROCESS was made readily available to the research community. We used PROCESS to calculate the indirect effects (plus the associated CI) for the single mediator in our first example and considered how to quantify the effect size of the indirect effects. We then presented our second mediation example using PROCESS, which examined the specific indirect effects of (three) multiple mediators. PROCESS also enabled a comparison of the three specific indirect effects using CI to determine which (if any) was the strongest mediator in our hypothesized model. This second example also presented an opportunity to consider the implications of conducting multiple mediator analyses using PROCESS when the mediators are (highly) correlated. In this instance, it is recommended the researcher interprets the direct and specific indirect effects, not the total indirect effect (Hayes, 2013). We then extended the second example to include an additional predictor variable. Finally, we presented an example of moderated mediation, which demonstrated the indirect effect of $X$ on $Y$ via $M$ at different scores on the moderator ($W$).

The first example of moderation considered a continuous moderator in the relation between $X$ and $Y$. The rationale behind whether centering $X$ and $M$ in creating the product term was considered, dispelling the myth that doing so is a required step in conducting moderated regression analysis. Having established the product term was significantly different from zero, we considered the options available to the researcher when graphically plotting, and subsequently probing, the interaction. Traditionally, sport and exercise scientists have relied on the pick-a-point approach, which graphically plots and probes significant interactions at somewhat arbitrary values of $M$ (e.g., sample mean, one SD above this mean, and one SD below this mean). However, given the values selected in the pick-a-point approach are sample specific, its value in probing a significant interaction is somewhat limited. We illustrated two alternative options, the J–N technique and the regions of significance. The benefits of, and the steps involved in, conducting both techniques were discussed in the first example of moderation.

The second example of moderation considered a single dichotomous moderator (i.e., gender) in the relation between $X$ and $Y$. Many of the steps involved with conducting a regression analysis with a dichotomous moderator are identical to those discussed in example one, except the probing of a significant interaction via a graphical representation is limited to the pick-a-point approach (given there are only two values of the dichotomous moderator). The third example we presented was that of moderated moderation, a strategy that is useful when the moderation of $X$'s effect by $M$ is itself moderated (by $W$). Although mathematically less straightforward than the first and second moderation examples, moderated moderation is relatively easy to implement in PROCESS. As with example one of moderation, it is also possible to graphically plot and subsequently probe a three-way interaction using a variety of strategies.

Although it is possible to extend the analyses covered in this chapter to include additional variables (e.g., moderated mediation could include multiple mediators and moderators), we envisage that the techniques and strategies outlined within the synergy sections of this chapter should provide a clear framework for sport and exercise scientists to conduct mediation and moderation analyses (in simple and more complex forms) in SPSS using PROCESS. We hope the advancements in these techniques will help the development and testing of theory in sport and exercise sciences.

# References

Aiken, L. S., & West, S. G. (1991). *Multiple regression: Testing and interpreting interactions.* Newbury Park, UK: Sage.

Ajzen, I. (1991). The theory of planned behavior. *Organizational Behavior and Human Decision Processes, 50,* 179–211.

Amireault, S., Godin, G., Vohl, M. C., & Pérusse, L. (2008). Moderators of the intention-behaviour and perceived behavioural control-behaviour relationships for leisure-time physical activity. *International Journal of Behavioral Nutrition and Physical Activity, 5*(1), 7.

Antonakis, J., Bendahan, S., Jacquart, P., & Lalive, R. (2010). On making causal claims: A review and recommendations. *The Leadership Quarterly, 21,* 1086–1120.

Baron, R. M., & Kenny, D. A. (1986). The moderator–mediator variable distinction in social psychological research: Conceptual, strategic, and statistical considerations. *Journal of Personality and Social Psychology, 51,* 1173.

Bartholomew, K., Ntoumanis, N., Ryan, R., Bosch, J., & Thøgersen-Ntoumani, C. (2011). Self-determination theory and diminished functioning: The role of interpersonal control and psychological need thwarting. *Personality and Social Psychology Bulletin, 37,* 1459–1473.

Bartholomew, K. J., Ntoumanis, N., & Thøgersen-Ntoumani, C. (2009). A review of controlling motivational strategies from a self-determination theory perspective: Implications for sports coaches. *International Review of Sport and Exercise Psychology, 2,* 215–233.

Bartholomew, K., Ntoumanis, N., & Thøgersen-Ntoumani, C. (2010). The controlling interpersonal style in a coaching context: Development and initial validation of psychometric scale. *Journal of Sport & Exercise Psychology, 32,* 193–216.

Bauer, D. J., & Curran, P. J. (2005). Probing interaction in fixed and multilevel regression: Inferential and graphical techniques. *Multivariate Behavioral Research, 40,* 373–400.

Cohen, J., Cohen, P., West, S. G., & Aiken, L. S. (2002). *Applied multiple regression-correlation analysis for the behavioral sciences* (3rd ed). Mahwah, NJ: Lawrence Erlbaum Associates.

Curran, P. J., Bauer, D. J., & Willoughby, M. T. (2006). Testing and probing interaction in hierarchical linear growth models. In C. S. Bergeman & S. M. Boker (Eds.), *The Notre Dame series on quantitative methodology:* Vol. *1.* Methodological issues in Aging research (pp. 99–129). Mahwah, NJ: Erlbaum.

Curran, T., Hill, A. P., & Niemiec, C. P. (2013). A conditional process model of children's behavioural engagement and behavioural disaffection in sport based on self-determination theory. *Journal of Sport and Exercise Psychology, 35,* 30–43.

Dawson, J. F. (2014). Moderation in management research: What, why, when and how. *Journal of Business and Psychology, 29,* 1–19.

Deci, E. L., & Ryan, R. M. (2002). *Handbook of self-determination research.* Rochester, NY: University of Rochester Press.

Frost, R. O., Lahart, C., & Rosenblate, R. (1991). The development of perfectionism: A study of daughters and their parents. *Cognitive Therapy and Research, 15,* 469–489.

Gay, J. L., Saunders, R. P., & Dowda, M. (2011). The relationship of physical activity and the built environment within the context of self-determination theory. *Annals of Behavioral Medicine, 42,* 188–196.

Hayes, A. F. (2013). *Introduction to mediation, moderation, and conditional process analysis.* New York: The Guilford Press.

Hewitt, P. L., & Flett, G. L. (1991). Perfectionism in the self and social contexts: Conceptualization, assessment, and association with psychopathology. *Journal of Personality and Social Psychology, 60*, 456–470.

Higgins, J. P. T., & Green, S. (Eds). *Cochrane handbook for systematic reviews of interventions* Version 5.1.0 [updated 2011]. The Cochrane Collaboration, 2011. Available from www. cochrane-handbook.org.

Jaccard, J., & Turrisi, R. (2003). *Interaction effects in multiple regression* (2nd ed.). Thousand Oaks, CA: Sage Publications.

MacKinnon, D. P. (2008). *Introduction to statistical mediation analysis*. Mahwah, NJ: Erlbaum.

MacKinnon, D. P., Krull, J. L., & Lockwood, C. M. (2000). Equivalence of the mediation, confounding and suppression effect. *Prevention Science, 1*, 173–181.

MacKinnon, D. P., Warsi, G., & Dwyer, J. H. (1995). A simulation study of mediated effect measures. *Multivariate Behavioral Research, 30*, 41–62.

Preacher, K. J., Curran, P. J., & Bauer, D. J. (2006). Computational tools for probing interaction in multiple linear regression, multilevel modelling, and latent curve analysis. *Journal of Educational and Behavioral Statistics, 31*, 437–448.

Preacher, K. J., & Hayes, A. F. (2008). Contemporary approaches to assessing mediation in communication research. In A. F. Hayes, M. D. Slater, and L. B. Snyder (Eds.), *The Sage sourcebook of advanced data analysis methods for communication research* (pp. 13–54). Thousand Oaks, CA: Sage Publications.

Preacher, K. J., & Kelley, K. (2011). Effect size measures for Mediation models: Quantitative strategies for communicating indirect effects. *Psychological Methods, 16*, 93–115.

Preacher, K. J., Zhang, Z., & Zyphur, M. J. (2011). Alternative methods for assessing mediation in multilevel data: The advantages of multilevel SEM. *Structural Equation Modeling, 18*, 161–182.

Reysen, S., Snider, J. S., & Branscombe, N. R. (2012). Corporate renaming of stadiums, team identification, and threat to distinctiveness. *Journal of Sport Management, 26*, 350–357.

Rogosa, D. (1980). Comparing nonparallel regression lines. *Psychological Bulletin, 88*, 307–321.

Rucker, D. D., Preacher, K. J., Tormala, Z. L., & Petty, R. E. (2011). Mediation analysis in social psychology: Current practices and new recommendations. *Social and Personality Psychology Compass, 5*, 359–371.

Selig, J. P., & Preacher, K. J. (2009). Mediation models for longitudinal data in developmental research. *Research in Human Development, 6*, 144–164.

Shieh, G. (2009). Sample size determination for confidence intervals on interaction effects in moderated multiple regression with continuous predictor and moderator variables. *Behavior Research Methods, 42*, 824–835.

Sobel, M. E. (1982). Asymptotic confidence intervals for indirect effects in structural equation models. *Sociological Methodology, 13*, 290–312.

Thøgersen-Ntoumani, C., Fox, K. R., & Ntoumanis, N. (2002). Testing the mediating role of physical acceptance in the relationship between physical activity and self-esteem: An empirical study with Danish public servants. *European Journal of Sports Sciences, 2*, 1–10.

Vallerand, R. J. (1997). Toward a hierarchical model of intrinsic and extrinsic motivation. In M. P. Zanna (Ed.), *Advances in experimental social psychology* (pp. 271–360). New York, NY: Academic Press.

Verstuyf, J., Patrick, H., Vansteenkiste, M., & Teixeira, P. J. (2012). Motivational dynamics of eating regulation: A self-determination theory perspective. *International Journal of Behavioral Nutrition and Physical Activity, 9* (1), 21.

# 4

# Item response theory and its applications in Kinesiology

## Weimo Zhu and Yan Yang

*Department of Kinesiology & Community Health, University of Illinois at Urbana-Champaign, Urbana, IL, USA*

## General Introduction

To be able to measure anything we are interested in (e.g., fitness, motor skill, knowledge, etc.), a "yardstick" that can measure the construct of interest must be available. In measurement practice, we often call this "yardstick" a "test," "scale," "instrument," etc. Through the interaction between a test and testees, scores can be generated, which in turn are used to estimate the construct we are interested in. To make a test score meaningful, a measurement system has to have been defined for the test so that a score of "30" or "300" has quantitative meaning. The process of defining a measurement system for a test is called test calibration, which sets a frame of reference for interpreting test results. A specific test calibration approach is usually associated with a testing theory, which refers to the procedures for estimating the key characteristics of the test or test scores, such as validity and reliability, dictated by the measurement model, which has a unique set of assumptions and is based on a statistical or mathematical model (Suen, 1990). Many test theories, such as the true-score theory, strong true-score theory, criterion-referenced measurement, and item response theory (IRT) (Berk, 1980; Crocker & Algina, 1986; Gulliksen, 1950; Lord, 1952, 1980; Lord & Novick, 1968; McDonald, 1999, Rasch, 1960/1980; Wright & Stone, 1979) have been developed since the beginning of the twentieth century.

*An Introduction to Intermediate and Advanced Statistical Analyses for Sport and Exercise Scientists*, First Edition.
Edited by Nikos Ntoumanis and Nicholas D. Myers.
© 2016 John Wiley & Sons, Ltd. Published 2016 by John Wiley & Sons, Ltd.
Companion website: www.wiley.com/go/ntoumanis/sport

Among them, the true-score theory, also known as the classical test theory (CTT), has been used most often in measurement, and it is still the most commonly used testing theory in the field of Kinesiology today.

Calibration approaches in test development can generally be classified into three categories: subject centered, item centered, and response centered (Torgerson, 1958). The primary purpose of the subject-centered approach is to locate testees at different positions on a continuum, for example, on a norm. The major advantages of this approach are its simplicity and wide range of applications. The major disadvantages are that calibrations are often sample and test dependent, and testing items and testees are calibrated on different reference frameworks. In addition, this approach assumes that the measurement scales employed are already at interval-scale levels and that scores are additive, which, unfortunately, is often not the case. The primary purpose of the item-centered approach, in contrast to the subject-centered approach, is to locate items on a continuum. This approach was originally developed by psychophysicists who were interested in developing quantitative relationships between responses and physical stimuli (e.g., lights, weights, and pressure). Therefore, it is also known as the "stimulus-centered" approach. Because it focuses only on the calibration of items, its applications are limited. Finally, the primary purpose of the response-centered approach is to locate both testees and testing items on a common continuum according to the strength or amount of the trait possessed by both. The major advantage of this approach is that, because testing items and testee are set on the same scale, testing results can be interpreted in a single-reference framework, and the major disadvantage is that it is typically more complex than the subject-centered and item-centered approaches.

Most tests in Kinesiology are constructed using the conventional subject-centered approach. More specifically, to calibrate these tests, total scores, which are the sums of response scores, are usually computed first. Based upon the total scores, the tests are calibrated using norm-referenced measurements in which percentiles by sex and chronological age are determined. Unfortunately, several serious flaws exist in this conventional practice. First, calibrations based on norm-referenced measurements are often sample and test dependent. For example, the commonly used CDC's overweight/obese standard used 1960s/1970s samples/data as their reference population. As the population became heavier over the next several decades, it is now not uncommon to see strange statements such as "17% at or above the 95th percentile" (Zhu, 2012a). Second, all facets (e.g., testees and testing items) involved in the testing cannot be taken into account in the calibration simultaneously, and the facets are calibrated on different metrics, which makes it difficult to interpret testing results. Finally, many motor development and skill instruments use ordinal scales in which response categories are ordered. Therefore, total raw scores from ordinal scales may be misleading, because ordinal scales are not additive (Zhu, 1996). Furthermore, testees' scores derived from a norm-referenced measurement, for example, percentile ranks, are also ordinal scores. Thus, an ideal calibration should meet the following conditions: (i) parameter estimations are independent from both testees and tests employed; (ii) all facets involved in the calibration are taken into account and the calibrated facets share the same metric; and (iii) calibrated measurement scales are additive. The IRT-based calibration, a response-centered approach, meets all these conditions.

# What Is IRT?

IRT is a set of statistical models that represents the relationship between facets involved in testing, or simply, the models predict the probability of a specific item response as a function of the latent ability variable and item characteristics. An explanation of the most basic IRT model, the Rasch (1960/1980) or one-parameter model, will help clarify what IRT is. Let's start with a testee and testing item, the two most important facets in a testing interaction. If the testee's ability $(\theta_1)$ is lower than the level of difficulty $(b)$ (see Figure 4.1), the possibility, or chance, that the testee will successfully complete the item should become lower; when the testee's ability $(\theta_2)$ is at the same level as the difficulty, the chance should be half-and-half; finally, if a testee's ability $(\theta_3)$ is higher than the level of difficulty of a testing item, the likelihood that the testee will successfully complete the item should be higher. This two-faceted relationship is represented mathematically. The equation requires that we first determine the difference between the testee's ability $(\theta_j)$ and the level of difficulty of a test item $(b_i)$, which can, theoretically, range from minus infinity to plus infinity. By taking this difference $(\theta_j - b_i)$ as an exponent of the natural constant $e = 2.71828$, then $e^{(\theta_j - b_i)}$ falls in a range between zero and plus infinity. We can then bring $e^{(\theta_j - b_i)}$ into an interval between zero and one by using the following ratio:

$$P_i(\theta) = \frac{e^{(\theta_j - b_i)}}{1 + e^{(\theta_j - b_i)}} \tag{4.1}$$

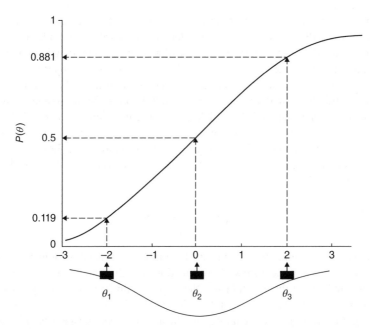

*Figure 4.1    Relationship between testees' abilities and probability of success.*

This equation (4.1) expressed literally:

$$\text{Chance of a person to get an item right} = \frac{e\left(\text{Ability of person } j - \text{Difficulty of item } i\right)}{1 + e\left(\text{Ability of person } j - \text{Difficulty of item } i\right)}$$

Equation 4.1 is the Rasch or one-parameter model, which denotes the probability, $P_i(\theta)$, of a testee $j$ with ability $\theta$ to successfully complete an item $i$ with a level of difficulty of $b$. For example, an item has a level of difficulty equal to 0, where the level of difficulty for the Rasch model is defined as the point on the ability scale where the probability of a correct response to the item is 0.5. If a testee's ability is 2, his/her probability to complete this item successfully is 0.881. If a testee's ability is $-2$, his/her probability to complete this item successfully decreases to 0.119 (see Figure 4.1). Through this equation, the relationship between testees and an item can be summarized into an $S$-shaped curve (see Figure 4.1). The curve is called the item characteristic curve (ICC), also known as the trace line. The ICC is a regression function that relates the probability of success on an item to the testee's ability measured by the test. Note that, although ICC is a monotonically increasing function, the relationship described is not linear since change in ability at both the lower and upper ability range is not linear with the change of probability in successfully completing an item correctly.

# Other Commonly Used IRT Models

With an understanding of the Rasch model, it should not be difficult to learn other commonly used IRT models. Besides the location or level of difficulty of an item described in the Rasch model, the ICC shape of an item also could have an impact on the probability of a testee answering the item correctly. The steeper the ICC, the greater the sensitivity of an item is to the change in the testees' abilities. Figure 4.2 summarizes two ICCs with the same difficulty, but with different steepness. ICC-A has a steeper shape than ICC-B, which means that in a certain range of ability, a slight change in ability will lead to a larger possibility in scoring Item A correctly than Item B. This steepness feature is called "discrimination" in IRT literature. A new discrimination parameter can be added to the Rasch model to describe this feature mathematically:

$$P_i(\theta) = \frac{e^{a_i(\theta_j - b_i)}}{1 + e^{a_i(\theta_j - b_i)}}, \tag{4.2}$$

where $a_i$ is the discrimination parameter of the model. To make the logistic function as close as possible to the normal ogive function, a scaling factor ($D = 1.7$) is sometime added in front of the $a_i$ parameter. Nevertheless, this practice is only associated with certain IRT software (e.g., LOGIST, Wingersky, Barton, & Lord, 1982).

In cognitive testing, a testee may guess the answer when he/she is not sure of the correct answer for a multiple-choice or true–false question. In ICC, the guess

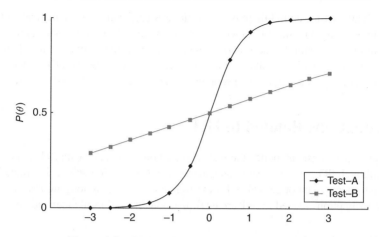

*Figure 4.2    ICC and discrimination parameters.*

behavior is usually on the lower asymptote of the ICC tail. The higher the tail, the more guessing. This guessing behavior can be modeled by adding another parameter $C$ to Equation 4.2:

$$P_i(\theta) = c_i + (1 - c_i) \frac{e^{a_i(\theta_j - b_i)}}{1 + e^{a_i(\theta_j - b_i)}}. \tag{4.3}$$

As a result, the model becomes a three-parameter model (4.3). It should be noted that because other factors are involved in guessing (e.g., attractive alternatives in a multiple-choice item), some researchers have proposed not wholly accurate to label the $C$-parameter the guessing parameter. The aforementioned three logistic models are the most common ones in cognitive testing dealing with dichotomous scores.

In practice, especially in effective survey research, the data are often not only scored dichotomously. In fact, most of the data in the field of Kinesiology are scored into more than three or more categories or scored continuously. Fortunately, multiple-category models, known as polytomous, have been developed to meet these practice needs. For example, a number of polytomous models have been developed from the Rasch model, such as the rating scale (Andrich, 1978) and the partial credit model (Wright & Masters, 1982). A more detailed treatment of the polytomous models can be found in IRT books edited by van der Linden and Hambleton (1997) and Nering and Ostini (2010). When more than two facets (e.g., raters or other subgroup characteristics) get involved in testing, many-facets models are needed (Linacre, 1989). Finally, if more than one dimension has been included in the measurement, there are a few multidimensional models, which will be discussed later, available for this modeling purpose.

Selection and preference of a particular model for IRT application are often dependent on users' training, experience, their beliefs of the model, and the data available. The difference in preference sometimes even leads to heated debates concerning which model should be employed. A rational view is that no model will fit every situation all the time and, if there is no additional significant measurement advantages that can be brought in, the model whose cost is low (e.g., requiring small sample size) and can provide a simple and practical interpretation of the testing results should be chosen. In the most high-stake testing practices, for example, TOFEL, GRE, SAT, ACT, etc., one- or three-parameter models are usually used for the test construction.

# Assumptions Related to IRT

Like any other statistical model, there are assumptions associated with IRT. This means that, although IRT has a number of advantages over CTT, which will be described later, these advantages cannot be realized if the IRT models' assumptions are not met. Two major assumptions related to IRT are unidimensionality and local independence.

## Unidimensionality

Except for a few new multidimensional models, most of IRT models assume that all testing items in the instrument measure a single latent trait or ability (e.g., gross motor function). In reality, this assumption may not be met perfectly because more than one trait, such as motivation and familiarity with the motor task, may be involved in the performance of a motor task. The common practice, therefore, is that the assumption can be considered adequately met as long as there is a dominant factor or component that determines the performance of the task (Hambleton, Swaminathan, & Rogers, 1991). However, when there are clearly more than one factor or components influencing the performance, the assumption may be violated and multidimensional IRT models are needed.

## Local Independence

Local independence means that a testee's responses to the testing items are statistically independent, that is, the probability of a testee response to an item will only depend on this testee's ability, not the connection among the items. In reality, a testee's responses to several test items are likely related to each other when the items share some common traits, for example, measure the same knowledge. This seems contradictory to the local independence assumption. However, after these common traits are removed or held constant, the items should become uncorrelated. Thus, local independence more accurately should be called "conditional independence" (Hambleton et al., 1991). Whether or not the data meet the assumptions should be examined first before interpreting the results of an IRT analysis, which is described later.

# Addressing Model-Data Fit

Obtained item and ability estimates, however, may not be able to be used to evaluate items and testees employed if lacking close matches between the model selected and the test data. Generally, the question of whether a model fits the data or not should be addressed in three general ways. First, the assumptions of the model should be examined to determine if the data satisfy them; secondly, the features of the model should be examined; and lastly, a goodness of fit should be conducted to determine the closeness of fit between prediction and observable outcomes. Hambleton and Swaminathan (1985) have provided an extensive review about this topic and only a brief summary will be included below.

## Inspecting Model Assumptions

Although the IRT is characterized by its strong assumptions, these assumptions often will not be completely met by any set of test data (Lord, 1980; Lord & Novick, 1968). Evidence has shown that the models are robust to moderate concerning departures from their assumptions (Hambleton & Cook, 1983; Wainer & Wright, 1980). The extent of this kind of robustness, however, has not been well understood because the assumptions could be violated in different ways, and the seriousness of the violations depends on the nature of the testee sample and the related application. Commonly inspected assumptions are unidimensional, local independence, equal discrimination indices, minimal guessing, and nonspeeded test administration. Only the first two will be discussed here because of their importance. For dimensionality, a comprehensive review is provided by Hattie (1984) in which 88 different indexes for assessing dimensionality are examined. For local independence, often four common statistical approaches—the odds ratio test, the proportion of correct under independence, the Mantel–Haenszel chi-square test, and the Goodman–Kruskal gamma test—were used (Rosenbaum, 1984). Both the odds ratio and the proportion of correct under independence were developed on the same algebraic base, and both are used only when an item or a subset of items are scored dichotomously. The Mantel–Haenszel procedure is similar to a chi-square test for independence as an overall significance test (Mantel & Henszel, 1959). Finally, the Goodman–Kruskal Gamma test is an index of relationships for discrete ordinal data arranged in a bivariate frequency table (Roscoe, 1975).

## Inspecting Expected Model Features

Invariance, or estimation that is sample or item free, is one of the most important features of IRT. When item parameters in the IRT are not dependent upon the ability level of the testees responding to the item, the group is invariant in item estimation (Baker, 1985; Hambleton, 1989). To test the feature of group invariance, the item parameter estimates that are from different subgroups of the population must be compared. If the estimates are invariant, the plot should be linear with an amount of scatter that only reflects sample size error (Hambleton, 1989). The common way to test group invariance is to compare ICC from different estimations. First, the item parameters need to be estimated from different subgroups; then the ICC can be developed from these parameters. Since ability scales are often arbitrary in an IRT analysis, the ICCs must be matched on the same scale, for example, using a linear transformation, before comparing.

## Inspecting Overall Model-Data Fit

Perhaps the majority of statistical procedures or other procedures developed for model-data fit are used to determine the overall fit of model, item, and testee. These tests can be generally classified into two categories: chi-square related and residuals based. Although chi-square-related procedures have been extensively studied and widely applied to test data, the effect of sample size on the statistical model fit has a serious flaw. It has been noted that these statistical fit tests should not be overlaid (Hambleton, 1989) since "when sample sizes are large, nearly all departures between a model and a data set (even those where the practical significance of the differences is minimal) will lead to rejection of the null hypothesis of model-data fit" (Hambleton & Murray, 1983, p. 72).

Residual analysis, combined with graphical analysis, is considered a good alternative for chi-square-based tests (Ludlow, 1986; Murray & Hambleton, 1983). Two indexes, raw residual (RR) and standardized residuals (SR), are often used in the residual analysis. The indexes reflect the degree of misfit between the test data and the expected item performance based on the chosen model. The major difference between raw and SR is that RR are simpler to calculate and easier to interpret while SR take into account the associated sampling error. The experimental comparison of these two indexes (Murray & Hambleton, 1983) has shown that both provide very useful fit information, but the SR presents a more accurate model-data fit picture (see also Baker & Kim, 2008 on model-data fit-related issues).

## Computer Simulation for Model-Data Fit Testing

Finally, the development of computer and software has provided measurement specialists with useful new tools to study model-data fit and help determine the effect on the model-data fit of different factors, such as sample size, length of test, and item difficulty. The value of employing a computer simulation analysis, which is often called a Monte Carlo study, is that the true or underlying parameters are already known and can be compared with those estimated by an IRT model. Two indexes, the correlation coefficients and the root-mean-squared error (RMSE), are most often used in this procedure. The correlation coefficient measures the intercorrelations between the known item or ability parameters and the estimated parameters, but it is not sensitive to systematic error if there is one. RMSE, in contrast, is used to detect the absolute deviation between known and estimated parameters, which is computed by averaging the squared difference between known and estimated parameters and then taking the square root. The accuracy of parameters estimation is sometimes described as recovery of item parameters, in the sense of recovery of true parameters by estimation. Research applying a computer simulation analysis including the accuracy of parameter estimations (Lord, 1975; Swaminathan & Gifford, 1979), effect of sample size (Hambleton & Cook, 1983), selection of IRT model (Yen, 1981), and so on. However, caution should be taken when applying the finding of the computer simulation since the simulated data may not accurately resemble real data (Harwell, Stone, Hsu, & Kirisci, 1996).

# Unique Features and Advantages of IRT

Comparing CTT, there are several features that make IRT unique and useful, namely, estimation invariance, common metric scale, item and testing information, and not "global" reliability.

## Estimation Invariance

First, parameter estimations in the calibration are independent from testees and testing items employed. In the IRT literature, this feature is referred to as the *invariance* of parameters (Lord, 1980). The idea of invariance is very much like the invariant estimation of any regression function, that is, a regression function is unchanged even if the distribution of the predictor variable is changed. In the context of the Rasch calibration, for example, an item response function can be viewed as the regression of an item score on a latent ability.

## Common Metric Scale

In contrast to the different scales for items (e.g., *p*-value for level of difficulty) and testees (e.g., raw or standardized scores) in a CTT-based test construction, IRT employs a common scale, called the ability scale (Hambleton et al., 1991), for both items and testee. Because the ability is a latent trait and cannot be measured directly, an arbitrary metric scale must be set up so that the relationship between items and testees can be placed along the scale accordingly. This setup is completed through the estimation procedures described previously. In theory, because of the nature of invariance, this process should not be impacted by item difficulty level and/or testees' ability. In practice, since the scale has to be set up on either the mean of the items or testees, there will be a scale difference when different items or groups of testee are employed. This difference, however, can be easily adjusted for using statistical methods.

The ability scale can also be considered as a log-odds scale. The unit of a log-odds scale is called *logits*, the contraction of *log-odds unit*. The log-odds scale is a scale with ratio scale properties, simply logits can be thought of as probabilities, the probability that a testee with a given ability will successfully complete an item. For example, a difference of 0.7 (more accurately, 0.693) logits between two testees corresponds to a doubling of the odds ($e^{(0.693)} = 2.0$) for the higher ability testee's success compared to the other testee, while a difference of 1.4 corresponds to a quadrupling of the odds. The log-odds scale, therefore, has the following two important features: (i) it is a "linear" model because all facets (e.g., testee's ability and item difficulty level, in this case) can be represented as fixed positions along one straight line, and (ii) logits are of equal intervals, thus additive. In measurement, additive measures are also called *linear measures*. For more information about the log-odds scale and logits, as well as the scaling issue under more complex IRT models, see Wright (1977) and Hambleton and Swaminathan (1985, pp. 57–61).

## Item and Test Information

Another very special feature of IRT is the item and test information function. Information in general is defined as to "know something about a particular object or topic" (Baker, 1985). Testing thus can be considered a process to get information about testees. In statistics, defined by Sir R.A. Fisher, the information ($I$) is the reciprocal of the precision with which a parameter could be estimated: $I = 1/\sigma^2$, where $\sigma^2$ is the variance of the parameter estimators, a precision measure of the variability of around the parameter.

In IRT, information related to an item is called "item information function"; it is defined specifically for each IRT model. For example, item information function of the two-parameter model is defined as

$$I_i(\theta) = a_i^2 P_i(\theta) Q_i(\theta).$$ (4.4)

Because $a = 1$ all the time in the Rasch model, the item information function in the model becomes

$$I_i(\theta) = P_i(\theta) Q_i(\theta).$$ (4.5)

Test information function, $I_T(\theta)$, can be computed very easily—simply add all item information functions in a test at a particular ability level together:

$$I_T(\theta) = \sum_{i=1}^{N} I_i(\theta),$$ (4.6)

where $N$ is the number of items in the test. According to Equation 4.4, the test information function of the two-parameter logistic model can then be expressed as follows:

$$I_T(\theta)_{\text{for two-parameter model}} = \sum_{i=1}^{N} a_i^2 P(\hat{\theta}) Q(\hat{\theta})$$ (4.7)

The test information thus is exactly the same as within the square root of the standard error (SE) equation in IRT:

$$SE(\hat{\theta}) = \frac{1}{\sqrt{\sum_{i=1}^{N} a_i^2 P(\hat{\theta}) Q(\hat{\theta})}}$$ (4.8)

Similar to using reliability and SE measurement ($SD\sqrt{t(1-r)}$, where SD = Standard Deviation and $r$ = reliability) to determine the quality of a measure or score in CTT, we can also compute a precision index called the SE in IRT to determine the accuracy of the ability estimation using Equation 4.8. Like SEmeas in CTT, $SE(\hat{\theta})$ is a measure of the variability of the values of $\hat{\theta}$ around the testee's latent parameter value $\theta$, that is, if we use the same test to measure the testee many times, most of a testee ability estimates will be close to the testee's true ability value with a few very low and high variations. Unlike SEmeas, however, $SE(\hat{\theta})$ is a local precision index, which is associated with a specific ability value ($\theta$). The idea that the measurement precision is determined locally is a very useful feature of IRT, which will be described more thoroughly later. Based on Equations 4.7 and 4.8, the relationship between the $SE\left(\hat{\theta}\right)$ and test information function can be expressed as

$$SE\left(\hat{\theta}\right) = \frac{1}{\sqrt{I_T\left(\theta\right)}} \tag{4.9}$$

To illustrate this, assume that there two tests with five items each. The difficulty levels of the items ($b$s) are as follows:

|         | Item 1 | Item 2 | Item 3 | Item 4 | Item 5 |
|---------|--------|--------|--------|--------|--------|
| Test A  | −1     | −0.05  | 0      | 0.05   | 1      |
| Test B  | 2      | 2.2    | 2.4    | 2.6    | 2.8    |

Using Equations 4.5 and 4.6, item and test information functions were computed, summarized in Table 4.1. As we expect, because of the distributions of items (i.e., more variability in item difficulties in Test A and more difficult items in Test B), Test A has a large range test information function with a focus at the center, and Test B, a more difficult test, could provide more information at the high end of the ability scale (see the top of Figure 4.3).

Table 4.1   An example of item information "$I_i(\theta)$" and test information "$I_T(\theta)$" function.

| Ability | Item 1 | Item 2 | Item 3 | Item 4 | Item 5 | $I_T(\theta)$ |
|---------|--------|--------|--------|--------|--------|--------------|
| | | | $I_i(\theta)$ | | | |
| *Test A* | | | | | | |
| −3 | 0.104994 | 0.070104 | 0.045177 | 0.028453 | 0.017663 | 0.266390 |
| −2 | 0.196612 | 0.149146 | 0.104994 | 0.070104 | 0.045177 | 0.566032 |
| −1 | 0.250000 | 0.235004 | 0.196612 | 0.149146 | 0.104994 | 0.935756 |
| 0 | 0.196612 | 0.235004 | 0.250000 | 0.235004 | 0.196612 | 1.113231 |
| 1 | 0.104994 | 0.149146 | 0.196612 | 0.238651 | 0.250000 | 0.939403 |
| 2 | 0.045177 | 0.070104 | 0.104994 | 0.173343 | 0.196612 | 0.590229 |
| 3 | 0.017663 | 0.028453 | 0.045170 | 0.075347 | 0.104994 | 0.271633 |
| *Test B* | | | | | | |
| −3 | 0.006648 | 0.005456 | 0.004476 | 0.003671 | 0.003009 | 0.023260 |
| −2 | 0.017663 | 0.014556 | 0.011981 | 0.009853 | 0.008096 | 0.062149 |
| −1 | 0.045177 | 0.037632 | 0.031252 | 0.025890 | 0.021402 | 0.161353 |
| 0 | 0.104994 | 0.089800 | 0.076255 | 0.064358 | 0.054038 | 0.389445 |
| 1 | 0.196612 | 0.177894 | 0.158685 | 0.139764 | 0.121729 | 0.794684 |
| 2 | 0.250000 | 0.247517 | 0.240261 | 0.228784 | 0.213910 | 1.180471 |
| 3 | 0.196612 | 0.213910 | 0.228784 | 0.240261 | 0.247517 | 1.127083 |

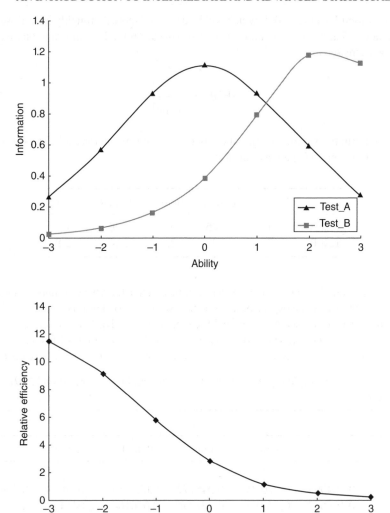

*Figure 4.3    Item and test information function (top); relative efficiency of Tests A and B (bottom).*

## Test Relative Efficiency

One of the useful applications of test information function is to compare efficiency of tests or subtests for either evaluation or selection purpose (Lord, 1977, 1980). Relative efficiency (RE) can be computed simply by comparing information function of one test with another at a particular ability level:

$$RE(\theta) = \frac{I_A(\theta)}{I_B(\theta)} \tag{4.10}$$

Using the previous example again, RE(−3, −2, −1, 0, 1, 2, 3) = 11.45271, 9.107661, 5.799434, 2.858506, 1.182109, 0.4999945, and 0.2410053, respectively (see the bottom of Figure 4.3). With RE and the information targeting to the testee population, a more appropriate test can be easily selected.

## Global "Reliability" Is no Longer a Concern

Because IRT is able to provide precision information of a measure at a specific ability level, test reliability used in traditional CTT test construction is no longer a concern. As introduced earlier, the SE in IRT is associated with an ability level, and there is no guarantee that a test can be reliable within the whole range of the scale. In fact, because of the development in local precision measurement in IRT, there is a call for the change in treatment of "reliability": (i) reliability has to be interpreted under the framework of the measurement theory employed, and (ii) test developers should try to provide local precision measure even if a test is constructed under CTT, for example, using conditional SE coefficient (American Educational Research Association, American Psychological Association, & National Council on Measurement in Education [AERA, APA, & NCME], 1999).

Finally, IRT and its unique features have made many other measurement practices possible and convenient, such as examining item bias and differential item functioning (Gao & Zhu, 2011a, 2011b) and conducting test equating (Zhu, 2001).

## Item Bank and IRT-Based Test Construction

With IRT features and advantages, test construction has become more convenient and efficient. Test construction based on a calibrated item bank is a major successful IRT application in modern test construction. An item bank is a collection of items or questions organized and catalogued to take into account the content of each item, as well as other measurement characteristics (e.g., validity, reliability, and level of difficulty; Umar, 1997). More importantly, all of the items in the bank share a common scale after IRT calibration. With an item bank, several measurement advantages can exist.

First, since all of the items are set on the same scale, the problem of score unequivalence among different tests is automatically eliminated, and scores can be directly compared with each other. Second, a stable scale can be developed even if new versions or items are added to the bank later on, that is, the mean and standard deviation of the scale are consistent across different times even if new items are used. Again, a stable scale is essential to measure a test across occasions and to communicate the results in a readily understandable manner. Third, since the characteristics of the items are already known, constructing new tests for different purposes of testing becomes much easier. For example, if a researcher is interested in constructing a test to screen a group's ability, items that cover a broad range of the ability can be selected (see the top of Figure 4.4). If, on the other hand, the interest is to construct a test to determine if a testee is qualified for professional certification (e.g., mastery vs. nonmastery), only items around a theoretical cutoff point will be selected. As a result, a shorter test, but one with peaked information at the cutoff point, can be constructed (see the middle of Figure 4.4). Having a stable scale allows for more accurate classification.

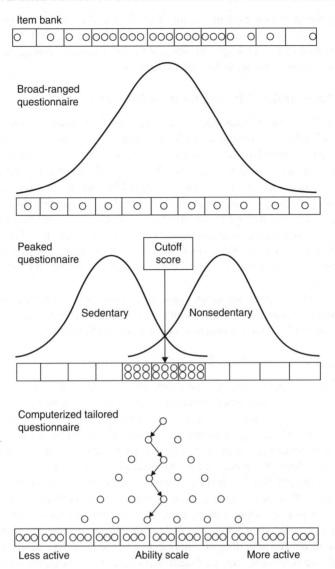

*Figure 4.4    IRT item bank-based test construction.*

Finally, with a well-developed item bank, a new and tailored way to administer a survey using computers, known as "computerized adaptive testing" (CAT, Wainer, 1990), becomes possible. CAT, which was originally developed in educational measurement practice, is very similar to a high-jump competition, in which competitors choose their jumping heights depending on their perceived abilities. In CAT, a question is first asked in the middle of an ability range that an item bank has defined. If it is answered correctly, the next question asked is more difficult; if it is incorrectly answered, the next question is easier. This continues until the testee's proficiency is established to within a predetermined level of accuracy. Because of IRT invariance, testees' abilities can be estimated even if they respond to different items within CAT. In fact, a more accurate estimation is expected since items selected are closer to a testee's ability. Because responses have been entered into a computer during the test administration, the final estimation of a testee's ability can be reported as soon as the test is finished (see the bottom of Figure 4.4).

## Parameter Estimation and Software

One of the major tasks in applying IRT is to estimate item and ability parameters. Depending on the IRT models employed, parameters such as level of difficulty, discrimination, and guessing really represent characteristics of an item. To be able to develop a good test, the item characteristics have to fit the needs of the test to be constructed. Because the purpose of developing tests is to determine the latent abilities of the testees and the differences among them, ability parameters of the testees also have to be estimated. In practice, the estimation procedures for these parameters have often already been embedded in the IRT software employed and, as a result, the software user/researchers often have limited choices in terms of which estimation procedure to use. For a general understanding, Baker's (1985) classical introduction (pp. 35–44, 65–77) is still the best. For a more comprehensive description, please refer to Baker and Kim (2008).

Like most other advanced measurement techniques, software is necessary for IRT applications. The software varies depending on the chosen models, estimation procedure, and fit statistic employed. Operation systems and prices also vary. Many websites provide an overview on these software now and interested readers are suggested to conduct some searches for the latest development and detailed information.

# Utility of the Methodology in Kinesiology

Spray (1987) called for research to determine whether the application of IRT can offer some improvement over the measurement techniques then used in Kinesiology when she introduced IRT to the field of Kinesiology. Based on the relatively limited IRT research efforts in the field of Kinesiology, two conclusions can be drawn addressing Spray's call. First, when data are dichotomous or polytomous, all existing IRT models can be applied (e.g., Safrit, Zhu, Costa, & Zhang, 1992; Zhu, 1996; Zhu & Kurz, 1994) and associate measurement advantages can be taken (e.g., Zhu & Cole, 1996; Zhu, Timm, & Ainsworth, 2001). In fact, Kinesiology researchers have been actively exploring IRT's advantages in solving critical measurement problems, for example, in determining optimal categorization (Zhu, 2002; Zhu, Updyke, & Lewandowski, 1997) and detecting judge bias in competitive sports such as figure skating (Loony, 1997). Because of its relative small sample size requirement and ease of interpreting results, almost all IRT applications in Kinesiology are of the Rasch model or its extensions. Considering most of the data in Kinesiology are continuous, there is still a significant gap in exploring the continuous IRT model. Except for a few attempts (see e.g., Spray,

1990; Zhu & Safrit, 1993), there has been little progress in developing and applying the continuous IRT models (Ferrando, 2002; Wang & Zeng, 1998).

The second conclusion drawn is the field of Kinesiology has not availed itself of the measurement advantages of IRT. In fact, the IRT method has been basically ignored in the regular measurement practice in Kinesiology except for a few applications ("FitSmart" fitness knowledge test (Zhu, Safrit, & Cohen, 1999) and "PEMetrics" for the assessment of physical education standard (Zhu, Fox, et al., 2011; Zhu, Rink, et al., 2011)). Although it was originally hoped (Wood, 1987) that subareas such as Sport Psychology, which typically has polytomous data, would take up the method first, it never happened even though there are many "needs improvement" areas in Sport Psychology's measurement practice (Zhu, 2012b). IRT could provide significant measurement advantages to measurement practice in Psychology (Embretson & Reise, 2000) and there even was a call for the IRT application made within Sport Psychology (Tenenbaum & Fogatry, 1998). The lack of a progress may still be due to three major reasons recognized by Wood (1987) many years ago: lack of training in the field, the complex nature of IRT, and the nature of psychomotor measurement. The lack of demand for stake tests in physical education is perhaps another reason. Beside fitness tests, few schools, if any, require a stake test for physical education and link the testing results in physical education with students' graduation or teachers' accountability. To take full advantages of IRT, the field of Kinesiology must start addressing these issues.

Finally, to help illustrate IRT and its application, the raw data and software command employed in a study by Zhu and Cole (1996) are in Appendices 4.1 and 4.2, respectively. Interested readers may run the data and learn the interpretation of the results from the paper by Zhu and Cole.

# IRT Limitations and Future Direction

Although many advantages have been demonstrated in IRT-based test construction, IRT is not without limitations. Strong assumption requirements, need for large sample size, and lack of continuous model applications are perhaps the major limitations associated with IRT. As mentioned earlier, there are several critical assumptions required by IRT models. Although the violation of an assumption may not cause critical threats to the credibility of the results, we have to be very careful in interpreting the finding whenever a violation occurs. Understanding the data and taking steps to prevent violation early is perhaps the best approach in dealing with this limitation. Large sample sizes needed for IRT is another limitation. In general, $n = 200$ and 20 items are needed for the Rasch model. When two- and three-parameter models are employed, the sizes become $n = 500$ for 30 items and $n = 1000$ for 60 items, respectively (Suen, 1990). For large-scale testing, this requirement is not a problem. However, it may be a major threat when applying IRT in Kinesiology laboratory research, in which a sample of 30 or above could be problematic due to cost and time concerns. Finally, as mentioned earlier, most of IRT models are developed for dichotomous and polytomous data, while the majority of the motor performance data in Kinesiology are continuous. Although

Spray (1990) introduced a set of models that can analyze "multiple-attempt, single-item" data and a few continuous IRT models (see e.g., Ferrando, 2002; Samejima, 1973) and software (Zopluoglu, 2012) exist, there is still a significant shortage in the availability of IRT continuous models, related software, and applications. Measurement specialists in Kinesiology must make an effort to explore and develop new models and related application software to better address our continuous data.

Although IRT has been around for 60+ years, IRT research efforts and development are ongoing and can be summarized into three areas: new models, new components, and new applications. Because test performance and score is often determined by more than one single trait, the unidimensionality assumption of IRT is often a limitation in practice; efforts have been made in developing new multidimensional IRT (MIRT) models. In fact, a set of MIRT models (e.g., McDonald, 2000; Reckase, 2009; van der Linden & Hambleton, 1997) and related software (e.g., Chalmers, 2012; Han & Paek, 2014; Wu, Adams, & Wilson, 1998) have been developed. It is expected that more new models and software will become available soon. To loosen the restriction of IRT assumptions, efforts have also been made to develop a set of nonparametric IRT models (Sijtsma & Molenaar, 2002). Although no major applications have been reported, it is worthwhile to pay attention to its development.

Another area of new IRT developments is to integrate cognitive, trait, or data characteristics into the modeling. For a long time, the development of psychometric modeling has been criticized for paying too much attention on the "metric" aspect of a model (i.e., quantitative, statistical, or mathematical aspect of a model) and too little on its "psycho" features or characteristics (see Suen, 1990). Fortunately, some significant efforts (e.g., Nichols, Chipman, & Brenna, 1995; van der Linden & Hambleton, 1997) have been made to integrate cognitive components into newly developed IRT models. Furthermore, some more recently developed IRT models have taken data characteristics into considerations. For example, to take the clustered nature of school research data, a set of new multilevel IRT models was developed (see Pastor, 2003). It is expected that these developments will lead to new areas of IRT application, for example, mixture IRT modeling (Bolt, Cohen, & Wollack, 2001). Finally, IRT applications have been moved out of the traditional box of educational measurement, or knowledge testing, in which measuring testees' cognitive abilities are the only interest. Today, IRT has been applied to measurement practices in various areas, such as Medicine, Biology, Sociology, etc. Applications of IRT have extended also to address many untraditional measurement issues, for example, optimal categorization (Zhu, 2002), artistic judgment (Bezruczko, 2002), and genomic measurement (Markward, 2004). Expectation is that the extension of IRT will continue as IRT further develops in its applicability.

# Conclusion

In conclusion, because of its measurement advantages, IRT has become a major measurement theory used in measurement practice in many fields. New development in both theory and practice makes it a very useful measurement theory for measurement in Kinesiology. Unfortunately, although IRT's introduction to the field happened back in 1987 (Spray, 1987), it still has not been regularly employed in Kinesiology measurement practice. Kinesiology urgently needs to make more efforts in developing IRT applications and in training all Kinesiology graduate students IRT, not only the field's measurement specialists.

# References

American Educational Research Association, American Psychological Association, & National Council on Measurement in Education. (1999). *Standards for educational and psychological testing*. Washington, DC: Author.

Andrich, D. (1978). A rating formulation for ordered response categories. *Psychometrika, 47*(1), 561–573.

Baker, F. B. (1985). *The basics of item response theory*. Portsmouth, NH: Heinemann.

Baker, F. B., & Kim, S.-H. (2008). *Item response theory: Parameter estimation techniques* (2nd ed.). New York, NY: CRC Press.

Berk, A. R. (Ed.). (1980). *Criterion-referenced measurement: The state of the art*. Baltimore, MD: Johns Hopkins University Press.

Bezruczko, N. (2002). A multi-factor Rasch scale for artistic judgment. *Journal of Applied Measurement, 3*, 360–399.

Bolt, D. M., Cohen, A. S., & Wollack, J. A. (2001). A mixture item response for multiple-choice data. *Journal of Educational and Behavioral Statistics, 26*, 381–409.

Chalmers, R. P. (2012). MIRT: A multidimensional item response theory package for the R environment. *Journal of Statistical Software, 48*(6), 1–29. Retrieved from http://www.jstatsoft.org/v48/i06/paper

Crocker, L., & Algina, J. (1986). *Introduction to classical and modern test theory*. New York, NY: Harcourt Brace Jovanovich College.

Embretson, S. E., & Reise, S. P. (2000). *Item response theory for psychologists*. Mahwah, NJ: Lawrence Erlbaum Associates.

Ferrando, P. J. (2002). Theoretical and empirical comparisons between two models for continuous item response. *Multivariate Behavioral Research, 37*(4), 521–542. doi:10.1207/S15327906MBR3704_05

Gao, Y., & Zhu, W. (2011a). Differential item functioning analysis of 2003–2004 NHANES physical activity questionnaire. *Research Quarterly for Exercise and Sport, 82*, 381–390.

Gao, Y., & Zhu, W. (2011b). Identifying group sensitive physical activities: A DIF analysis of NHANES data. *Medicine & Science in Sports & Exercise, 43*(5), 922–929.

Gulliksen, H. (1950). *Theory of mental tests*. New York, NY: John Wiley & Sons.

Hambleton, R. K. (1989). Principles and selected applications of item response theory. In R. L. Linn (Ed.), *Educational measurement* (pp. 147–200). New York, NY: Macmillan.

Hambleton, R. K., & Cook, L. L. (1983). The robustness of item response models and effects of length and sample size on the precision of ability estimation. In D. Weiss (Ed.), *New horizons in testing* (pp. 31–49). New York, NY: Academic Press.

Hambleton, R. K. & Murray, L. (1983). Some goodness of fit investigations for item response models. In R. K. Hambleton (Ed.), *Application of item response theory* (pp. 71–94). Vancouver, BC: Educational Research Institute.

Hambleton, R. K., & Swaminathan, H. (1985). *Item response theory: Principles and applications.* Boston, MA: Kluwer-Nijhoff.

Hambleton, R. K., Swaminathan, H., & Rogers, J. H. (1991). *Fundamentals of item response theory.* Newbury Park, CA: Sage.

Han, K. T., & Paek, I. (2014). A review of commercial software packages for multidimensional IRT modeling. *Applied Psychological Measurement, 38*(6), 486–498. doi:10.1177/0146621614536770

Harwell, M., Stone, C. A., Hsu, T.-C., & Kirisci, L. (1996). Monte Carlo studies in item response theory. *Applied Psychological Measurement, 20*(2), 101–125.

Hattie, J. A. (1984). An empirical study of various indices for determining unidimensionality. *Multivariate Behavioral Research, 19*, 49–78.

Linacre, J. M. (1989). *Many-faceted Rasch measurement.* Chicago, IL: MESA Press.

Loony, M. A. (1997). Objective measurement of figure skating performance. *Journal of Outcome Measurement, 1*, 143–163.

Lord, F. M. (1952). *A theory of test scores* (Psychometric Monograph No. 7). Iowa City, IA: Psychometric Society.

Lord, F. M. (1975). *Evaluation with artificial data of a procedure for estimating ability and item characteristic curve parameters* (ETS RB 75-33). Princeton, NJ: Educational Testing Service.

Lord, F. M. (1977). Practical applications of item characteristic curve theory. *Journal of Educational Measurement, 14*, 117–138.

Lord, F. M. (1980). *Applications of item response theory to practical testing problems.* Hillsdale, NJ: Lawrence Erlbaum Associates.

Lord, F. M., & Novick, M. R. (1968). *Statistical theories of mental test scores.* Reading, MA: Addison-Wesley.

Ludlow, L. H. (1986). Graphical analysis of item response theory residuals. *Applied Psychological Measurement, 10*, 217–229.

Mantel, N., & Henszel, W. (1959). Statistical aspects of the analysis of data from retrospective studies of disease. *Journal of the National Cancer Institute, 22*, 719–748.

Markward, N. J. (2004). Establishing mathematical laws of genomic variation. *Journal of Applied Measurement, 5*, 1–14.

McDonald, R. P. (1999). *Test theory: A unified treatment.* Mahwah, NJ: Lawrence Erlbaum Associates.

McDonald, R. P. (2000). A basis for multidimensional item response theory. *Applied Psychological Measurement, 24*, 99–114.

Murray, L. N., & Hambleton, R. K. (1983). *Using residual analyses to assess item response model-test data fit* (Laboratory of Psychometric and Evaluative Research Report No. 140). Amherst, MA: University of Massachusetts.

Nering, M. L., & Ostini, R. (Eds.). (2010). *Handbook of polytomous item response theory models.* New York, NY: Routledge.

Nichols, P. D., Chipman, S. F., & Brennan, R. L. (Eds.). (1995). *Cognitively diagnostic assessment.* Hillsdale, NJ: Lawrence Erlbaum Associates.

Pastor, D. A. (2003). The use of multilevel item response theory modeling in applied research: An illustration. *Applied Measurement in Education, 16*, 223–243.

Rasch, G. (1980). *Probabilistic models for some intelligence and attainment tests.* Chicago, IL: University of Chicago Press. (Original work published 1960).

Reckase, M. D. (2009). *Multidimensional item response theory* (Statistics for Social and Behavioral Sciences). New York, NY: Springer.

Roscoe, J. T. (1975). *Fundamental research statistics for the behavioral sciences* (2nd ed.). Chicago, IL: Holt, Rinehart & Winston.

Rosenbaum, P. R. (1984). Testing the conditional independence and monotonicity assumptions of item response theory. *Psychometrika, 49*(3), 425–435.

Safrit, M. J., Zhu, W., Costa, M. G., & Zhang, L. (1992). The difficulty of sit-up tests: An empirical investigation. *Research Quarterly for Exercise and Sport, 63*, 277–283.

Samejima, F. (1973). Homogeneous case of the continuous response model. *Psychometrika, 38*, 203–219.

Sijtsma, L., & Molenaar, I. W. (2002). *Introduction to nonparametric item response theory.* Thousand Oaks, CA: Sage.

Spray, J. A. (1987). Recent developments in measurement and possible applications to the measurement of psychomotor behavior. *Research Quarterly for Exercise and Sport, 58*, 203–209.

Spray, J. A. (1990). One-parameter item response theory models for psychomotor tests involving repeated, independent attempts. *Research Quarterly for Exercise and Sport, 61*, 162–168.

Suen, H. K. (1990). *Principles of test theories.* Hillsdale, NJ: Lawrence Erlbaum.

Swaminathan, H., & Gifford, J. A. (1979). *Estimation of parameters in the three-parameter latent-trait model* (Laboratory of Psychometric and Evaluation Research, Report No. *90*). Amherst, MA: University of Massachusetts.

Tenenbaum, G., & Fogarty, G. (1998). Application of the Rasch analysis to sport and exercise psychology measurement. In J. L. Duda (Ed.), *Advances in sport and exercise psychology measurement* (pp. 409–421). Morgantown, WV: Fitness Information Technology.

Torgerson, W. S. (1958). *Theory and methods of scaling.* New York, NY: John Wiley & Sons.

Umar, J. (1997). Item banking. In J. P. Keeves (Ed.), *Educational research, methodology, and measurement: An international handbook* (2nd ed., pp. 923–930). New York, NY: Elsevier Science.

van der Linden, W. J., & Hambleton, R. K. (Eds.). (1997). *Handbook of modern item response theory.* New York, NY: Springer.

Wainer, H. (1990). *Computerized adaptive testing: A primer.* Hillsdale, NJ: Lawrence Erlbaum.

Wainer, H. & Wright, B. D. (1980). Robust estimation of ability in the Rasch model. *Psychometrika, 45*(3), 373–391.

Wang, T., & Zeng, L. (1998). Item parameter estimation for a continuous response model using an EM algorithm. *Applied Psychological Measurement, 22*(4), 333–344.

Wingersky, M. S., Barton, M. A., & Lord, F. M. (1982). *LOGIST user's guide.* Princeton, NJ: Educational Testing Service.

Wood, T. M. (1987). Putting item response theory into perspective. *Research Quarterly for Exercise and Sport, 58*, 216–220.

Wright, B. D. (1977). Solving measurement problems with the Rasch model. *Journal of Educational Measurement, 14*, 97–116.

Wright, B. D., & Masters, G. N. (1982). *Rating scale analysis: Rasch measurement.* Chicago, IL: MESA Press.

Wright, B. D., & Stone, M. H. (1979). *Best test design.* Chicago, IL: MESA Press.

Wu, M. L., Adams, R. J., & Wilson, M. R. (1998). *ACER ConQuest: Generalised item response modeling software manual.* Melbourne, Australia: Australian Council for Educational Research.

Yen, W. M. (1981). Using simulation results to choose a latent trait model. *Applied Psychological Measurement, 5*, 245–262.

Zhu, W. (1996). Should total scores from a rating scale be used directly? *Research Quarterly for Exercise and Sport, 67*, 363–372.

Zhu, W. (2001). An empirical investigation of Rasch equating of motor function tasks. *Adapted Physical Activity Quarterly, 18*(1), 72–89.

Zhu, W. (2002). A confirmatory study of Rasch-based optimal categorization of a rating scale. *Journal of Applied Measurement, 3*(1), 1–15.

Zhu, W. (2012a). "17% at or above the 95th percentile"—What is wrong with this statement? *Journal of Sport and Health Science, 1*(2), 67–69.

Zhu, W. (2012b). Measurement practice in sport and exercise psychology: A historical, comparative and psychometric view. In G. Tenenbaum, R. Eklund, & A. Kamata (Eds.), *Measurement in sport and exercise psychology* (pp. 9–21). Champaign, IL: Human Kinetics.

Zhu, W., & Cole, E. L. (1996). Many-faceted Rasch calibration of a gross-motor instrument. *Research Quarterly for Exercise and Sport, 67*(1), 24–34.

Zhu, W., Fox, C., Park, Y., Fisette, J. L., Dyson, B., Graber, K. C., ... Raynes, D. (2011a). Development and calibration of an item bank for PE metrics assessments: Standard 1. *Measurement in Physical Education and Exercise Science, 15*, 119–137.

Zhu, W., & Kurz, K. A. (1994). Rasch partial credit analysis of gross motor competence. *Perceptual and Motor Skills, 79*, 947–961.

Zhu, W., Rink, J., Placek, J. H., Graber, K. C., Fox, C., Fisette, J. L., ... Raynes, D. (2011b). Physical education metrics: Background, testing theory, and methods. *Measurement in Physical Education and Exercise Science, 15*, 87–99.

Zhu, W., & Safrit, M. J. (1993). The calibration of a sit-ups task using the Rasch Poisson Counts model. *Canadian Journal of Applied Physiology, 18*, 207–219.

Zhu, W., Safrit, M. J., & Cohen, A. S. (1999). *FitSmart test user manual: High school edition.* Champaign, IL: Human Kinetics.

Zhu, W., Timm, G., & Ainsworth, B. A. (2001). Rasch calibration and optimal categorization of an instrument measuring women's exercise perseverance and barriers. *Research Quarterly for Exercise and Sport, 72*(2), 104–116.

Zhu, W., Updyke, W., & Lewandowski, C. (1997). Post-hoc Rasch analysis of optimal categorization of an ordered-response scale. *Journal of Outcome Measurement, 1*(4), 286–304.

Zopluoglu, C. (2012). EstCRM: An R package for Samejima's continuous IRT model. *Applied Psychological Measurement, 36*(2), 149–150. doi:10.1177/0146621612436599

# 5

# Introduction to factor analysis and structural equation modeling

## Katie E. Gunnell[1], Alexandre Gareau[2], and Patrick Gaudreau[2]

[1] Healthy Active Living and Obesity (HALO) Research Group, the Children's Hospital of Eastern Ontario Research Institute, Ottawa, ON, Canada
[2] École de Psychologie/School of Psychology, Université d'Ottawa/University of Ottawa, Ottawa, ON, Canada

## General Introduction

How can we measure something we cannot see, hear, or touch? In sport and exercise psychology, researchers are often faced with the daunting task of measuring variables that are not readily observable. For example, motivation is not something a researcher can tangibly observe or directly quantify. Instead, researchers must develop theories about motivation and make inferences about how it can be measured. Arguably, questionnaires are one of the most common forms of assessment for variables that are not directly observable in sport and exercise psychology. Items (or indicators) in a questionnaire are typically developed based on a theory, and researchers often ask participants to evaluate the extent to which each of the items is true, applies, or corresponds to them. Typically, these items are then aggregated, and the resulting score is thought to reflect the construct that the items were developed to measure. Aggregating

*An Introduction to Intermediate and Advanced Statistical Analyses for Sport and Exercise Scientists*, First Edition.
Edited by Nikos Ntoumanis and Nicholas D. Myers.
© 2016 John Wiley & Sons, Ltd. Published 2016 by John Wiley & Sons, Ltd.
Companion website: www.wiley.com/go/ntoumanis/sport

items, by summing or averaging, creates what is called a *composite score* (or an observed variable). Composite scores are typically used in the traditional analysis of variance (ANOVA), regression analyses, multilevel modeling, and path analyses. However, the problem associated with using composite scores is that they produce attenuated (i.e., smaller) correlations between study variables. Moreover, using composite scores in path analysis has been shown to cause valid models to appear invalid, change substantive conclusions, and reduce power needed to reject invalid models (see Cole & Preacher, 2014). Measurement error can be corrected and a true correlation between two variables can be estimated by modeling latent variables.

The first step for resolving the issue of measurement error is to acknowledge that there could be one overarching factor or *latent variable* that is responsible for why items in a questionnaire are closely related (i.e., items that measure one construct typically *covary*). A *latent variable* is an undefined variable that is inferred and assumed to be the cause of the covariance between a set of clustered (or similar) items. Therefore, a latent variable cannot be directly assessed nor tangibly touched—it is inferred through the covariation between items that were, most of the time, designed to measure a theoretical concept (e.g., psychological and social). The latent factor is hypothesized (when we create a pool of items) and inferred (when we interpret the covariance among the items). The factor is said to be indeterminate because several alternative factor solutions could account for the same covariance between clusters of items. As such, a latent concept should be interpreted as an abstraction or an inference rather than a tangible object that readily exists in the real world. Latent factors are analyzed through a family of statistical procedures known as factor analysis.

# Utility of the Method in Sport and Exercise Science

In sport and exercise psychology, researchers are often interested in predicting variance in latent theoretical constructs such as motivation or anxiety. The two primary advantages of factor analysis and structural equation modeling (SEM) are that they allow researchers to examine (i) the validity of the scores to their questionnaires (as is done through exploratory factor analysis (EFA) and confirmatory factor analysis (CFA)) and (ii) the associations between latent variables without the undue influence of measurement error (as is done through SEM). Factor analysis is a broad term used to describe techniques such as EFA, CFA, SEM, and exploratory SEM (ESEM; see Chapter 8). Each of these analyses can play a unique role in different parts of the research process as you will see in this chapter.

In its inception, measurement theory was rooted in *classical test theory*. Within classical test theory, observations are the result of the sum of a true score and its associated error:

$$\text{Observed score} = \text{true score} + \text{error} \qquad (5.1)$$

The errors are said to be nonsystematic with a theoretical normal distribution with a mean of zero and a normal standard deviation. Also, it is assumed that true scores are uncorrelated with the errors. In factor analysis, two types of variance are estimated: (i) the common variance associated with the latent factor itself—this variance is estimated with the indicators shared variance—and (ii) the unique variance, the part of an indicator that is not explained by the factor or not common with other items defining the factor. More simply stated, the error for each item and each latent factor is estimated in a factor analysis.

The main goals of EFA and CFA are to reproduce the relationships between indicators with the smallest number of factors and to determine the weight of each item to obtain a latent variable score. EFA is often used in the early stages of instrument development or instrument modification. EFA enables researchers to examine the communality between items and how they can be grouped together to create the smallest number of latent factors present in the data. EFA can also be helpful for determining the structure of the responses because it provides researchers with a tool to determine how many latent factors are being estimated by the items and to identify items that might be measuring more than one latent factor. That is, EFA allows for *item cross-loadings* (i.e., items that were designed to measure one latent variable may also load onto another latent factor), and therefore, the researcher can determine if an item is a "simple" measure of one latent factor or if the item is assessing more than one latent variable because it cross-loads onto multiple latent factors. As such, the main difference between EFA and CFA lies in the a priori hypothesis about the structure underlying the items. EFA allows researchers to infer the simplest factor structure by reducing the number of latent factors based on the shared variance of indicators without the stringent hypothesis of zero cross-loadings that is characteristic of CFA (see panel A in Figure 5.1). Hence, a common myth of EFA is that it is typically viewed as data driven because it allows for cross-loadings— yet it is important to recognize that ultimately, researchers determine the number of latent factors that best explain the common thread (i.e., covariance) among indicators. Furthermore, hypothesis testing can be carried out in an EFA framework. A complete description of EFA is beyond the scope of this chapter, but interested readers are encouraged to see Brown (2006) for more information on EFA principles.

The idea behind CFA is to test a stringent hypothesis that certain items are tapping a latent factor without any cross-loadings onto other latent factors. To test a CFA, each indicator will usually be hypothesized to load onto only one factor; all other factor loadings (i.e., all cross-loadings) are fixed to zero (see panel B in Figure 5.1). Therefore, this model is different from the EFA model because researchers using CFA apply a set of constraints based on stringent a priori hypotheses about the number of latent factors and the pattern of items (i.e., primary loadings and cross-loadings) that describe them (compare panels A and B in Figure 5.1). Stated differently, in EFA, researchers assume that most items will have a certain amount of cross-loading, and therefore, small cross-loadings are tolerated. In CFA, researchers assume that most items will measure only one thing and cross-loadings are not tolerated because they are fixed to zero. For this reason, CFA is usually estimated when researchers have a clear hypothesis about the number of latent factors and specific pattern of fixed and free factor loadings.

CFA can also be used to simultaneously examine multiple instruments in one model. A model that contains many latent factors from more than one instrument is commonly

Panel A: Exploratory factor analysis (EFA) with oblique rotation

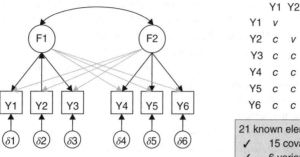

|    | Y1 | Y2 | Y3 | Y4 | Y5 | Y6 |
|----|----|----|----|----|----|----|
| Y1 | $v$ |   |   |   |   |   |
| Y2 | $c$ | $v$ |   |   |   |   |
| Y3 | $c$ | $c$ | $v$ |   |   |   |
| Y4 | $c$ | $c$ | $c$ | $v$ |   |   |
| Y5 | $c$ | $c$ | $c$ | $c$ | $v$ |   |
| Y6 | $c$ | $c$ | $c$ | $c$ | $c$ | $v$ |

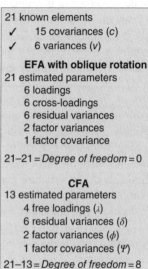

21 known elements
✓    15 covariances ($c$)
✓    6 variances ($v$)

**EFA with oblique rotation**
21 estimated parameters
  6 loadings
  6 cross-loadings
  6 residual variances
  2 factor variances
  1 factor covariance
21–21 = *Degree of freedom* = 0

**CFA**
13 estimated parameters
  4 free loadings ($\lambda$)
  6 residual variances ($\delta$)
  2 factor variances ($\phi$)
  1 factor covariances ($\Psi$)
21–13 = *Degree of freedom* = 8

Panel B: Confirmatory factor analysis (CFA)

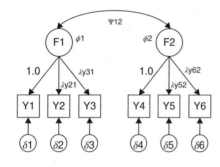

Panel C: Structural equation model (SEM)

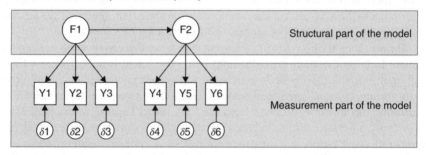

*Figure 5.1    Graphical representation of the differences between EFA, CFA, and SEM.*

referred to as a *measurement model* and is typically examined for the following two reasons: on the one hand, the results of the measurement model provide researchers with the bivariate correlations between all latent variables. These correlations have the advantage of not being attenuated by measurement error compared to correlations based on composite scores. On the other hand, examining a measurement model provides researchers with an indication of how well their data are fitting the hypothesized factor structure (i.e., pattern of loadings and latent variables). For example, the measurement model provides researchers with evidence that indicators used to measure a predictor or an antecedent variable are not loading on the latent variable created to measure a criterion or a dependent variable, and/or vice versa. It is sometimes easier to test a measurement model before examining models that contain regression pathways as would be done in testing a SEM to ensure that any sources of misfit are not the result of measurement problems (rather than structural problems).

Once researchers have established a good measurement model to ensure that the measures conform to the hypothesized factor structure, they can then examine the direction of the relationships between latent variables using SEM (see panel C in Figure 5.1). SEMs contain a measurement portion and a structural portion where regression paths are specified between latent factors. SEM allows researchers to specify the paths from the *exogenous variable(s)* (i.e., the independent variable in regression language) to the *endogenous variable(s)* (i.e., the dependent variable in regression language) while accounting for measurement error. Furthermore, SEM is flexible because it allows researchers to examine complex models using both composite scores and latent factors. For example, scores from an accelerometer measuring physical activity are typically modeled as composite scores, whereas scores on motivation are typically modeled as latent variables. In this example, a researcher can use SEM to examine if the latent variable of motivation predicts the composite score of exercise. Another advantage of SEM is that researchers can examine multiple exogenous variables, multiple mediators and/or moderators, and multiple endogenous variables simultaneously within one model. Overall, SEM is a flexible analytic tool that can be used to study complex models while accounting for measurement error.

# Terminology and Methodology

Before delving into the substantive example, it is important to briefly describe additional key terminologies (see Table 5.1), assumptions, and principles used in factor analyses (including EFA, CFA, SEM, and other methods described in this book such as ESEM). The first term you will see throughout this textbook is a *variance/covariance matrix* (a correlation matrix is a standardized variance/covariance matrix). A variance/covariance matrix is the foundation of EFA, CFA, and SEM. Other important terms are outlined in Table 5.1. According to Kline (2010), the general approach for testing a factor analysis model and a SEM includes six steps: (1) specification, (2) identification, (3) collect data, (4) estimation, (5) respecification, and (6) report of results. The first five steps will now be outlined, and details about step 6 will be provided in the synergy section through an example of writing up the results of EFA, CFA, and SEM:

(1) *Specification.* Model specification begins before the data are obtained and involves creating a priori hypotheses based on theory about the relationships between observed and latent variables. Moreover, researchers should devote considerable attention to the theoretical and conceptual definition of key constructs that will be examined in the model prior to collecting data (see Mackenzie, Podsakoff, & Podsakoff, 2011). Specification also includes consideration of instruments that will be used, if the

Table 5.1  Terms and definitions commonly used in factor analysis.

| Term usually used | Alternative terms | Greek symbol | Definition | Model symbol |
|---|---|---|---|---|
| Covariance matrix | Sample matrix | $\Sigma$ | Unstandardized association between all variables in the analysis | |
| Factor variance | | $\phi$ | Reflects the sample variability | Double arrow around the factor |
| Residual variance | Uniqueness, errors | $\delta$ or $\varepsilon$ | Unique variance from the item that is not predicted by the latent factor. Typically thought to reflect measurement error | $\theta$ |
| Explained variance | | | Amount of variance in a dependent variable that is explained by an independent variable(s) | $R^2$ |
| Factor loadings | Coefficient | $\lambda$ | Regression paths from the latent factor to the item. Expected change in the observed score per unit of latent variable | $\rightarrow$ |
| Intercept | | $\tau$ | Value of an indicator when its corresponding factor ($y$) is 0. | |
| Factor mean | | $\kappa$ | Corresponds to the mean of an indicator or any endogenous variable A factor is by definition exogenous with its indicators, the mean of the factor reflects the unstandardized path with the constant | |
| Latent factor | Latent variable | $\zeta$ | Variable that accounts for the covariation among observed variables | $\bigcirc$ |
| Indicators | Items, questions | | An observed variable used to represent a latent construct | $\square$ |
| Observed variable | Manifest variable, composite score | | An item, or a set of items (summed or averaged), that assumes no measurement error | $\square$ |
| Endogenous | Dependent variable | | Variable caused by one or more variables in the model | |
| Exogenous | Independent variable | | Variable that has no cause modeled | |

model is identified (discussed in the following), and the structure of the relationships between variables. Common parameters that are altered (i.e., freed or constrained) during model specification include *factor loadings*, *residual variances*, and *factor variance* (see Table 5.1). Specification is the most important step because once researchers have established their model through specification, subsequent steps carry the assumption that the retained parameters are needed and/or correct. For this reason, it is suggested that researchers make a list of possible changes to the initial model that are aligned with theory or empirical results to ensure that changes to the model made after initial specification are well justified (Kline, 2010). This list can also be achieved through specifying alternative models that can be compared against the original model.

(2) *Identification*. The second step is to identify the model based on the chosen specification. Identification asks the question: is there enough information for the computer to estimate unknown parameters (e.g., a latent factor variance)? A model is identified if the known information (e.g., the variances and covariances in the data) is sufficient to derive a unique set of parameter estimates for unknown parameters (e.g., factor loadings, factor covariances; see Figure 5.1 panel on the left). A model must have at least the following two requirements for identification. Firstly, the degrees of freedom (*df*; the number of known elements minus the number of free parameters) must be zero or higher. Researchers should strive to find the most parsimonious (i.e., simple) model possible in order to maximize df. Specifically, researchers should aim to have an overidentified model (i.e., $df > 0$). When the model is just identified ($df = 0$), the goodness-of-fit statistics cannot be interpreted because they will be perfect. As well, an underidentified model (usually $df < 0$) cannot be estimated (see Brown (2006) and Kline (2010) for more information on identification). Secondly, setting the metric of the latent variable is important because latent factors are not *real* (i.e., they are created and inferred based on items). Because they are not real, they have no inherent scale of measurement and must be given one by the researcher. There are two methods for identifying the metric of a latent variable: (i) the factor loading of one of the items (usually the first) can be constrained to 1.0 or (ii) the factor variance can be constrained to 1.0. Both approaches to setting the metric of a latent factor generally result in similar overall fit with slightly different parameter estimates. However, in some circumstances, setting a factor loading to 1.0 could cause misfit if that item is a poor indicator of the latent factor. Similarly, setting the variance of the latent factor to 1.0 could cause misspecification if the variance is much larger or smaller than 1.0. Finally, an additional concern for identification is that it is important to consider the number of items per latent factor when considering identification. For example, when the latent factors are correlated, each latent factor requires at least two items to achieve identification. When latent factors are not correlated, at least three items per latent factor are needed to achieve identification. These conditions are necessary but not always sufficient to achieve model identification. For more information on df and establishing identification, readers are encouraged to consult Kline (2010) or Brown (2006).

(3) *Collect data*. Once the model has been specified, the researcher must collect data to test the model. Factor analysis and SEM with maximum likelihood estimation (detailed in the following) require large sample sizes for proper model estimation and

convergence. Rules of thumb (e.g., 10 participants per free parameter) and minimal sample size requirements ($N \geq 200$) have been proposed to help researchers in estimating their needed sample size. However, the appropriate sample size needed is influenced by many factors such as the size of correlations in the data, model complexity, and estimation procedures. Further discussion about sample size is beyond the scope of this chapter, but readers are encouraged to read Chapter 13 of this book on power estimation.

(4) *Estimation.* There are many estimation procedures that can be used to run factor analytic models (EFA, CFA, and SEM). Different estimation procedures may generate slightly different results; therefore, the method of estimation should be selected with care depending on the circumstances of the sample data. For CFA and SEM, the most commonly used estimation method is maximum likelihood estimation (ML). When data are nonnormally distributed, it is recommended that the researcher employ robust estimators such as robust maximum likelihood estimation (MLR), which corrects the standard errors of each parameter. Because ML and MLR assume the data are continuous, researchers who are using scales with five points or fewer should consider alternative estimation methods such as weighted least square means and variances adjusted (WLSMV; see Finney & DiStefano, 2006) or Bayesian estimation (see Chapter 8).

## Evaluating Model Fit

The null hypothesis when using ML or MLR estimation in factor analysis or SEM is that the hypothesized covariance matrix (i.e., with constraint; $\Sigma$) is equal to the observed covariance matrix in the population (i.e., observed from the sample $\Sigma(\Theta)$). Put differently, the null hypothesis is $\Sigma - \Sigma(\Theta) = 0$. Hence, in SEM, we are not attempting to reject the null hypothesis, but rather we are attempting to *minimize the discrepancy* between the two matrices (the observed matrix based on the data and the estimated/hypothesized matrix with constraints that is specified by the researcher). When estimating a factor analysis or a SEM, we can evaluate the results by examining (i) if the proposed model reproduced the covariances among items (e.g., null hypothesis testing and goodness-of-fit indices); (ii) the size, statistical significance, and confidence intervals of the parameter coefficients (e.g., examining the size of factor loadings); and (iii) how much variance in an item is accounted for by the latent variable (e.g., $R^2$).

Traditionally, the most commonly used index to examine if the proposed model reproduced the covariances among items is the chi-square test. Recall that the null hypothesis is an exact fit of the hypothesized model. Therefore, if the observed model of a chi-square test is not statistically significant ($p > 0.05$), the results indicate that the null hypothesis is *not* rejected—meaning that the model is a good fit to the data. The chi-square test is often regarded as the only true statistical test for model fit. If the chi-square test is significant (e.g., indicating misfit), it should prompt researchers to examine their model to understand the source of misfit. Despite its prominence in the factor analysis literature, some researchers have argued that the chi-square test has important limitations. First, a model with an exact fit is rare, and therefore, the null hypothesis is rarely realistic. Second, large sample sizes increase the statistical power of the chi-square test, and small variations from the exact fit will increase with larger sample sizes—a problem given that larger sample sizes are needed for factor analysis and SEM. Nevertheless, it is important to acknowledge that a significant chi-square test signifies lack of fit and should prompt researchers to identify the cause of the misfit. In doing so, researchers can interpret parameter estimates and other fit indices to help identify the misspecification (see Brown, 2006). Other goodness-of-fit indices are useful because they offer complementary information about model fit. It is important to note however that goodness-of-fit indices are not testable through null hypothesis testing (i.e., there is no statistical significance test) and they do not solve the problem associated with large sample sizes and power.

There are three types of goodness-of-fit statistics: (i) absolute fit indices, (ii) incremental fit indices, and (iii) parsimony correction indices. The standardized root mean square residual (SRMR) is an absolute fit index and represents the average discrepancy between the correlations in the observed matrix and the correlations in the predicted matrix. The SRMR value is informative; however, examining the pattern of residuals *as well as* the SRMR value is important because there may be many high residuals—which is not good—and many low residuals, resulting in an adequate value indicating a well-fitting model even though there are many high residuals. SRMR values range from 0.0 to 1.0 with smaller values representing better fit. The comparative fit index (CFI) is an example of an incremental fit index that performs reasonably well with small sample sizes. The CFI model compares the hypothesized model with a more restricted model that typically consists of a model where all the covariances are constrained to zero. CFI values typically range between 0.0 and 1.0, with values closer to 1.0 indicating a well-fitting model. Similarly, the Tucker–Lewis index (TLI) also typically ranges from 0.0 to 1.0 and can be negative; however, the TLI incorporates a penalty for overly complex models and is therefore considered a parsimony correction index. Another parsimony correction index is the root mean square error of approximation (RMSEA).[1] A perfect RMSEA is denoted by a value of 0.0, and a confidence interval can be calculated offering more precision for larger samples. Ideally, the lower bound should be close to 0.0 and the upper bound should not exceed 0.10. Finally, it should be noted that RMSEA tends to favor models with a higher number of df. For example, models with three items per subscale and 2–3 latent factors often yield RMSEA confidence intervals outside the recommended range.

There are no gold standards for evaluating model fit based on goodness-of-fit indices (see Marsh, Hau, & Wen, 2004), and therefore, their evaluation is interpretative and should always be substantiated by theoretical justifications. Nonetheless, general guidelines have been offered such as values *close* to or above 0.95 for CFI and TLI (Hu & Bentler, 1999) and values *close* to or below 0.06 and 0.08 for the RMSEA and SRMR, respectively. Other investigators have offered more refined guidelines, for example, values of RMSEA < 0.08 represent adequate fit, of RMSEA < 0.05 represent good fit, and of RMSEA > 0.10 should lead the researcher to reject the model (Browne & Cudek, 1993). As you can see, there is no precise recipe for

---

[1] Many alternative fit indices exist. Please see Hu and Bentler (1999) or Brown (2006) for a list of alternative goodness-of-fit statistics.

evaluating goodness of fit, and there are considerable debates in the SEM literature. Researchers should determine guidelines for how they will evaluate fit *before* they analyze their data. Values that fall outside of guidelines should signify misfit and prompt researchers to examine its source.

## Interpreting Parameter Estimates

All parameters in the model should be carefully inspected to identify possible "Heywood cases" (i.e., out-of-range values) as these are indications of specification errors or small sample sizes. For example, a completely standardized factor correlation above 1.0 or negative residual variances could signify an out-of-range value (see Jöreskog, 1999 for an exception to standardized values over 1.0).The direction of the parameter estimate should also be considered with regard to substantive theory. In addition to examining the direction of the parameter estimates, researchers should examine the statistical significance associated with the unstandardized point estimates to determine if the estimate is significantly different from zero. Factor loadings should be examined to determine if items are reasonable indicators of the latent factors (e.g., standardized values should be above 0.30 or 0.40 and statistically significant; Brown, 2006). Researchers should also identify localized areas of ill fit and standardized residuals that are too high (i.e., what is not accounted for in the hypothesized model but exists in the observed covariance matrix). The standardized residual matrix provides researchers with information about how well the variances and covariances were reproduced. If the value is above 1.96, the residual is considered statistically significant. Moreover, a positive residual indicates that the model's parameters underestimated the zero-order relationship and vice versa. Areas of ill fit could also be identified using modification indices (M.I.'s). M.I.'s are calculated for all fixed parameters (e.g., in a CFA, item cross-loadings are likely fixed to zero) and represent the expected change in chi-square if the parameter was freely estimated.

(5) *Respecifying and comparing models.* Often, researchers will need to respecify or make post hoc modifications to their models based on the observations and inferences made through evaluating chi-square, goodness-of-fit indices, and parameter estimates. Post hoc modifications (or specification searches) to models without strong theoretical justification should be avoided because data-driven model modifications could capitalize on sample-specific idiosyncrasies in the data and therefore be difficult to replicate or generalize (see Kline, 2010). In respecifying a model, Byrne (2012) suggested that researchers must consider (i) if the respecification has theoretical and substantive meaning, (ii) if the M.I.'s are substantially large enough to signify a serious problem, and (iii) if making the change would lead to an overfitted model and therefore artificially improve model fit. If there is justification for respecifying a model such as by adding a residual covariance (e.g., if the item wording is nearly identical, if the items appear adjacent to each other on the instrument), sometimes, it is essential that the respecification be allowed to avoid biasing the estimation of other key parameters in the model (see Cole, Ciesla, & Steiger, 2007 for a discussion about correlated residual variances). A classical case is in longitudinal data using identical questionnaires over time which often requires an added residual between time 1 and

time 2 items. Omitting the correlated residual would artificially increase the test–retest correlation between time 1 and time 2 latent variables. Another example with cross-sectional research would be if the same item was rated twice by participants, which sometimes occurs when researchers wish to examine contextual versus general variables by varying instructional stems (i.e., vitality in general and vitality while exercising).

If a researcher has sufficient justification to respecify a model, their respecified model will often involve a comparison to the first. Most often, researchers will have to compare models that are either nested or nonnested. A nested model is a model that contains fixed or free parameters from a more complex model. For example, if a specified model requires an additional constraint on a parameter such as estimating a cross-loading or adding a correlation between two residuals, the revised model with the constraint is considered nested within the first model. The typical case of a nonnested model is when a researcher deletes one variable from the covariance matrix. In this case, although the two models are no longer nested because a variable has been deleted from the covariance matrix, many researchers may falsely assume that the models remain nested.

Comparing two nested models can be accomplished through the chi-square difference and Akaike information criterion (AIC) test, whereas comparing two nonnested models can be accomplished through AIC. The chi-square difference test generally involves calculating the differences in chi-square between two nested models along with the difference in df. The obtained chi-square difference values and df have the same distribution of the chi-square and can therefore be used to examine statistical significance. If a chi-square difference value is statistically significant, it indicates that the nested model is statistically significantly better than the constrained model. There are situations when the regular chi-square difference test cannot be calculated such as when robust estimation procedures are used (e.g., MLR). In this case, the Satorra–Bentler scaled chi-square difference test can be used (see Colwell, 2014 for an online calculator). The AIC is used for comparing two alternative models and is a parsimony-adjusted index that favors a simpler model. A model with a smaller AIC value is chosen as the model that is most likely to replicate in future studies because that model will have fewer free parameters and a better fit compared to the more complex model.

# The Substantive Example

In sport and exercise psychology, researchers often try to determine factors that predict behavior, emotions, and cognitions. For example, there is a large body of research that has focused on examining why exercise makes people experience greater psychological well-being. To showcase the utility of factor analysis and SEM techniques, we will examine the following research questions: (1) how many theoretically driven motivation factors can we obtain by examining the reasons people do physical activity? and (2) which motivational factors for physical activity predict subjective vitality? Before proceeding, it is necessary to briefly outline the theory underpinning motivation and the source of the data and instruments used to assess motivation and vitality.

Self-determination theory (Deci & Ryan, 2000) was developed to explain why and how motivation predicts outcomes such as vitality (among other outcomes). In this theory, motivation can be categorized based on quality rather than simply examining quantity of motivation. In factor analysis terms, motivation can be regrouped into six related yet distinct factors. The Behavioural Regulation in Exercise Questionnaire (BREQ; Mullan, Markland, & Ingledew, 1997) was developed to assess 4 of these 6 factors of motivation proposed within self-determination theory (external, introjected, identified, and intrinsic motivation). *External motivation* occurs when an individual is engaging in the behavior because of external pressures such as pressure from a doctor or teammate. *Introjected motivation occurs* when an individual engages in the behavior because of internal pressures or contingencies. For example, an individual motivated by introjected regulation could engage in the behavior because he or she feels guilty if they do not. *Identified motivation* occurs when an individual identifies with or values the behavior. For example, an individual motivated by identified motivation could engage in the behavior because he or she truly values the behavior. Finally, *intrinsic motivation* occurs when an individual is engaging in the behavior because it is enjoyable and fun. Each quality of motivation is theorized to differentially relate to positive or negative outcomes. For instance, intrinsic and identified motivations are hypothesized to be positively associated with outcomes such as behavioral persistence, performance, and psychological well-being. In contrast, extrinsic and introjected forms of motivation are theorized to lead to outcomes such as behavioral disengagement, poor performance, and greater ill-being. Self-determination theory has been studied extensively, and researchers have found support for the factor structure of instruments designed to measure the theoretically driven factors of motivation and the relationships between motivation and vitality (Deci & Ryan, 2000; Mullan et al., 1997).

Research question 1 will be answered through EFA and CFA. Research question 2 will be answered through SEM. We will use the data that were partially presented in Gunnell, Crocker, Mack, Wilson, and Zumbo (2014). Briefly, people ($N=203$) aged 17–65 ($M_{age}=32.57$ years, SD$=15.73$ years) were asked to participate in two online questionnaires. The handling of missing data and assumptions is presented in Gunnell et al. (2014). For this illustration, only time one data were used, and the supplemented integrated motivation items were omitted. Motivation was measured with the BREQ (Mullan et al., 1997). This instrument was used to assess external (4 items), introjected (3 items), identified (4 items), and intrinsic motivation (4 items) on a scale of 1 (*not true for me*) to 5 (*very true for me*). The word "exercise" was replaced with "physical activity" for the purposes of the original study. Subjective vitality was assessed with the Subjective Vitality Scale (SVS; Ryan & Frederick, 1997). The SVS is a 7-item scale that was used to assess the amount of vitality experienced in exercise contexts. Participants were asked to rate each item on a scale of 1 (*not at all true*) to 7 (*very true*).

The data used in this example can be accessed through the online supplemental material. All of our analyses were conducted in Mplus 7.3. All syntax in the appendices contains comments (i.e., green text after an exclamation point) to guide readers on how to specify models using Mplus. Readers are encouraged to consult the Mplus User's Guide and Byrne (2012) for more details on Mplus language. Input files used to run the analyses have been placed in the online appendices (see Appendices 5.1–5.11). In the data file and input files, you will notice the following variable labels: (i) motivation, BR1–BR15 (which stands for BREQ1–BREQ15), and (ii) vitality, SV1–SV7 (which stands for SVS1–SVS7).

# The Synergy

## EFA: Establishing the Factor Structure

An EFA can be performed on the BREQ items to examine (i) if the proposed number of latent variables emerges and (ii) if any of the items have any substantial cross-loadings on nonintended latent variables. In this example, EFA is being used in a more "confirmatory" way because of our a priori expectations (see Morin, Marsh, & Nagengast, 2013). Because we know that the BREQ was developed to assess four motivations (external, introjected, identified, and intrinsic), we conducted our EFA by specifying a 4-factor solution (see Appendix 5.1). If we were using a newly created instrument and did not know how many latent factors would emerge, we could have conducted the analysis and specified a range of possible latent factors (1–6 for examples; see comments in Appendix 5.1) and examined the fit of each solution. For ease of interpretation, geomin rotation (the default in Mplus) was used. Geomin rotation is a type of oblique rotation, meaning that we anticipated the latent factors to be correlated based on previous research (see Brown, 2006 for more information on rotations). We used MLR to account for the possibility of nonnormality of the data.

To interpret our output, we examined the eigenvalues and scree plot (see Appendices 5.2 and 5.3). When examining the scree plot, we looked at the number of factors that have an eigenvalue over one and a large bend in the scree plot, respectively. Next, we examined the goodness-of-fit indices and the rotated factor loadings. Because we employed EFA, each item was allowed to cross-load onto each factor, yet we expected that items would only load significantly on their intended latent factor. Often, researchers use the values of 0.30 or 0.40 to signify salient loadings onto a factor and values below or close to zero to signify nonsalient loadings (see Brown, 2006). We followed recommendations by Preacher and MacCallum (2003) in that we present each primary and secondary loading for readers to interpret. Furthermore, our inferences about primary and secondary loadings were not strictly guided by commonly used cutoff criteria (see Preacher & MacCallum, 2003) but rather an evaluative judgment consistent with theory. For example, we considered a latent factor as "simple" if all secondary loadings were substantially lower (e.g., <0.40) than all the primary loadings (e.g., >0.70). These values could vary depending on the context of research, and therefore, researchers are encouraged to use their judgment when making decisions about primary and secondary loadings.

### Example Write-Up of EFA Results

The results of the EFA indicated that there were three latent factors with eigenvalues over 1 and a fourth latent factor with an eigenvalue very close to 1. Visual inspection of the scree plot corroborated the possibility of four latent factors. Interpretation of the goodness-of-fit statistics indicated that the model was a good fit to the data, despite the significant MLR chi-square value: $\text{MLR}\chi^2_{(51)} = 75.176$, $p = 0.015$, $\text{CFI} = 0.982$, $\text{TLI} = 0.963$, $\text{RMSEA} = 0.048$, 90% CI [0.022, 0.070]. The rotated loadings (Table 5.2) indicated that each item loaded on its intended latent factor $\geq .584$ ($p < 0.050$) except for the identified motivation item "I get restless if I don't exercise" (BR8). This item did not significantly load onto the identified latent factor (estimate $= 0.279$, $p > 0.050$) and statistically significantly loaded onto intrinsic motivation (estimate $= 0.326$, $p < 0.050$) and introjected motivation (estimate $= 0.324$, $p < 0.050$). Therefore, this item was identified as problematic. Based on previous research that has identified this item as particularly problematic, and also based on the conceptual meaning of this item in comparison to the definition of identified motivation from self-determination theory, item 8 was removed from

Table 5.2    EFA results for BREQ scores.

| Item | Factor loadings | | | | | | | |
|------|------|------|------|------|------|------|------|------|
| | 1 | | 2 | | 3 | | 4 | |
| | External | SE | Introjected | SE | Identified | SE | Intrinsic | SE |
| BR1 | **0.832***  | 0.057 | 0.109 | 0.075 | −0.043 | 0.055 | 0.028 | 0.038 |
| BR2 | **0.934***  | 0.046 | −0.092 | 0.069 | 0.014 | 0.041 | 0.005 | 0.031 |
| BR3 | **0.833***  | 0.067 | 0.010 | 0.040 | 0.102 | 0.067 | −0.122 | 0.104 |
| BR4 | **0.777***  | 0.057 | 0.039 | 0.060 | −0.042 | 0.056 | −0.021 | 0.045 |
| BR5 | 0.253*  | 0.118 | **0.670***  | 0.116 | −0.092 | 0.075 | 0.086 | 0.058 |
| BR6 | 0.038 | 0.061 | **0.734***  | 0.113 | 0.086 | 0.110 | −0.078 | 0.077 |
| BR7 | −0.007 | 0.050 | **0.584***  | 0.097 | 0.070 | 0.089 | −0.157 | 0.101 |
| BR8 | −0.152 | 0.082 | 0.324*  | 0.105 | **0.279** | 0.150 | 0.326*  | 0.132 |
| BR9 | 0.022 | 0.062 | 0.047 | 0.089 | **0.770***  | 0.151 | 0.149 | 0.116 |
| BR10 | −0.051 | 0.077 | −0.006 | 0.075 | **0.743***  | 0.099 | −0.033 | 0.059 |
| BR11 | 0.029 | 0.060 | −0.021 | 0.072 | **0.718***  | 0.126 | 0.048 | 0.064 |
| BR12 | 0.015 | 0.057 | −0.048 | 0.068 | 0.043 | 0.088 | **0.868***  | 0.055 |
| BR13 | −0.004 | 0.051 | 0.001 | 0.059 | 0.238 | 0.126 | **0.697***  | 0.099 |
| BR14 | −0.031 | 0.070 | 0.045 | 0.086 | −0.027 | 0.058 | **0.831***  | 0.041 |
| BR15 | 0.011 | 0.041 | −0.004 | 0.048 | 0.014 | 0.051 | **0.927***  | 0.042 |

| Factor correlations | 1 | 2 | 3 | 4 |
|------|------|------|------|------|
| 1. External | − | | | |
| 2. Introjected | 0.339* | − | | |
| 3. Identified | −0.256* | 0.353* | − | |
| 4. Intrinsic | −0.311* | 0.180* | 0.530* | − |

*Note*: Bolded values represent items that should load onto their respective latent factors.
BR, BREQ item number; SE, standard error.
*$p < 0.05$.

further analysis, and the EFA was reestimated because deletion of an item changes the covariance matrix (see Appendix 5.4). In other words, it is necessary to ensure that removing BR8 did not cause other items to become problematic. The results indicated a good fit to the data despite the slight increase in RMSEA and decrease in TLI: MLR$\chi^2_{(41)}$ = 63.353, $p$ = 0.014, CFI = 0.982, TLI = 0.960, RMSEA = 0.052, 90% CI [0.024, 0.076]. The pattern of rotated loadings indicated that each item loaded significantly onto its intended latent factor without any significant cross-loadings (see Appendix 5.5 for the rotated loadings). However, a cross-validation sample was not obtained to confirm the modified BREQ model, so caution is warranted when interpreting the results.

## CFA: Testing the Measurement Models

Ideally, a second sample would be collected to cross-validate the results of the EFA before moving onto a CFA framework. For the purposes of this example, we will continue with the same sample using the BREQ without item BR8. The next important step in the research process would be to examine the responses obtained from each instrument to determine if they fit the hypothesized model without any cross-loadings and removing any identified problematic items. We ran separate CFAs for BREQ (see Appendix 5.6) and SVS[2] (see Appendices 5.7 and 5.8) scores, setting the metric of the latent variable with the first indicator approach (for an example of CFA syntax in which the metric of the latent variable was set by specifying the latent variable to have a variance of 1, please see Appendix 5.9). Each item was specified to load onto its target latent factor only, and cross-loadings were not permitted (i.e., constrained to 0). Residual variances and factor variances were freely estimated, and no residual covariances were added between indicators. In the BREQ CFA, all latent factors were free to correlate with each other. MLR estimation was used. Finally, using each separate CFA, we examined score reliability for each latent factor. Below, we present the composite reliability formula from Diamantopoulos and Siguaw (2000):

$$\rho_c = \frac{\left(\Sigma\lambda\right)^2}{\left[\left(\Sigma\lambda\right)^2 + \left(\Sigma\delta\right)\right]} \tag{5.2}$$

where $\lambda$ represents the standardized factor loadings and $\delta$ represents the standardized residual variance. All models were interpreted using the guidelines presented previously for interpreting model fit. In addition, 95% confidence intervals for parameter estimates were interpreted and reported.

---

[2] We did not use EFA because the SVS was hypothesized to have only one latent factor. If the SVS was a new instrument and the researcher was unsure about the items and the pattern of loading onto latent variables, EFA could be performed as an exploratory option.

**Example Write-Up of CFA Results for the BREQ**

The data provided a good fit to the model MLR$\chi^2_{(71)}$ = 109.860, $p$ = 0.002, CFI = 0.968, TLI = 0.960, RMSEA = 0.052, 90% CI [0.032, 0.070]. The model was identified (i.e., $df > 0$), and there were no convergence problems or Heywood cases. Examination of the parameter estimates and confidence intervals (see Table 5.3) indicated that each standardized factor loading was above the recommended 0.300 ($\lambda = 0.557$–0.919) value and all factor loadings were statistically significant ($p < 0.050$ and confidence intervals did not cross zero). Each latent factor was correlated ($r$'s range from |0.250| to |0.506|, $p < 0.050$) except for the correlation between intrinsic motivation and introjected motivation ($r = 0.102$, $p = 0.313$). Item residual variances ranged from

Table 5.3    CFA results for BREQ and SVS responses.

| | Factor loading $\lambda$ | 95% CI | SE | Residual $\delta$ |
|---|---|---|---|---|
| Extrinsic motivation | | | | |
| BR1 | 0.871* | [0.808, 0.934] | 0.032 | 0.241 |
| BR2 | 0.888* | [0.837, 0.938] | 0.026 | 0.212 |
| BR3 | 0.850* | [0.783, 0.918] | 0.035 | 0.277 |
| BR4 | 0.813* | [0.739, 0.888] | 0.038 | 0.339 |
| Introjected motivation | | | | |
| BR5 | 0.780* | [0.671, 0.889] | 0.056 | 0.392 |
| BR6 | 0.742* | [0.623, 0.861] | 0.061 | 0.449 |
| BR7 | 0.557* | [0.414, 0.700] | 0.073 | 0.690 |
| Identified motivation | | | | |
| BR9 | 0.891* | [0.807, 0.976] | 0.043 | 0.206 |
| BR10 | 0.716* | [0.603, 0.829] | 0.058 | 0.488 |
| BR11 | 0.706* | [0.484, 0.927] | 0.113 | 0.502 |
| Intrinsic motivation | | | | |
| BR12 | 0.886* | [0.830, 0.942] | 0.029 | 0.215 |
| BR13 | 0.843* | [0.766, 0.919] | 0.039 | 0.290 |
| BR14 | 0.828* | [0.765, 0.891] | 0.032 | 0.315 |
| BR15 | 0.919* | [0.878, 0.960] | 0.021 | 0.155 |
| Vitality | | | | |
| SV1 | 0.838* | [0.774, 0.903] | 0.033 | 0.297 |
| SV2¥ | 0.593* | [0.449, 0.736] | 0.073 | 0.649 |
| SV3 | 0.615* | [0.519, 0.711] | 0.049 | 0.622 |
| SV4 | 0.862* | [0.801, 0.923] | 0.031 | 0.257 |
| SV5 | 0.663* | [0.569, 0.758] | 0.048 | 0.560 |
| SV6 | 0.651* | [0.551, 0.752] | 0.051 | 0.576 |
| SV7 | 0.816* | [0.748, 0.884] | 0.035 | 0.335 |

95% CI, 95% confidence interval; ¥, item is reverse scored; BR, BREQ item number; SV, subjective vitality item number.
*$p < 0.05$.

$\delta = 0.155$ to 0.690. Standardized residuals were examined next, and results indicated that there were 11 out of 91 (12%) values over 1.96 ($p < 0.050$). Finally, M.I.'s suggested the presence of two-item cross-loadings (external motivation onto BR5 and identified motivation onto BR13; M.I.'s = 10.715 and 14.629, respectively) and two error covariances (BR14 with BR13 and BR15 with BR14; M.I.'s = 15.482 and 12.584, respectively). Neither previous research nor the wording of these items provided substantial justification for estimating the cross-loadings. We also provided evidence of score reliability for external ($\rho_c = 0.916$), introjected ($\rho_c = 0.738$), identified ($\rho_c = 0.817$), and intrinsic ($\rho_c = 0.925$) motivation using CFA. Overall, the responses provided to the BREQ appear to conform to a 4-factor latent solution based on the interpretation of (i) goodness-of-fit statistics, (ii) high factor loadings, (iii) low residual variances, and relatively (iv) few standardized residuals.

## Example Write-Up of CFA Results for the SVS

Based on the chi-square, TLI, and RMSEA, results indicated that the data provided an unacceptable fit: $MLR\chi^2_{(14)} = 43.552, p = 0.001, CFI = 0.945, TLI = 0.918, RMSEA = 0.102,$ 90% CI [0.069, 0.137]. Examination of the parameters and associated confidence intervals indicated no Heywood cases, plus the standardized factor loadings were all above the recommended 0.300 ($\lambda = 0.593$–0.856) and were statistically significant ($p < 0.050$ and the confidence intervals did not contain zero). Item residual variances ranged from $\delta = 0.267$–0.648. There were three standardized residuals out of 21 (14%) that were above 1.96 ($p < 0.05$). Examination of the modification indices suggested that correlating the errors of the item SV7 ("I feel energized") and SV6 ("I nearly always feel alert and awake") would result in a significantly better fitting model (M.I. = 28.084). Conceptually, the item wording of item 6 and 7 is very similar in that they are both asking about a sense of energy and may be causing this correlated error to be estimated. Furthermore, the items appeared on the questionnaire in adjacent positions, which could also lead to correlated errors. As such, we reran the analysis and included the error covariance between items SV7 and SV6 based on conceptual and methodological justification. Considering that the two models were nested within each other, we conducted a chi-square difference test using an online calculator, since the MLR estimator was used (Colwell, 2014). Results indicated that the second model resulted in a significantly better fitting model: $\Delta MLR\chi^2_{(1)} = 19.981, p < 0.001, MLR\chi^2_{(13)} = 17.713,$ $p = 0.169$, CFI = 0.991, TLI = 0.986, RMSEA = 0.042, 90% CI [0.000, 0.087]. The model was identified (i.e., $df > 0$), and there were no convergence problems or Heywood cases. Standardized factor loadings were all $\geq 0.593$, $p < 0.001$, and confidence intervals did not cross zero (see Table 5.3), the error correlation between SV6 and SV7 was significant ($r = 0.437$, $p < 0.001$), the item residual variances were all $\leq 0.649$, and there were only two standardized residuals over 1.96. Overall, the original hypothesized model for SVS scores did not fit the data well. Adding an error covariance between two items that appeared to be assessing very similar components and were positioned adjacent on the questionnaire of SVS provided a superior fit to the data. Therefore, based on the (i) goodness-of-fit statistics, (ii) high factor loadings, (iii) low residual variances, and relatively (iv) few standardized residuals, the second SVS model with the correlated error between SV6 and SV7 fits the hypothesized model well. However, a cross-validation sample was not obtained to confirm the modified SVS model, so caution is warranted when interpreting the results.

## Structural Equation Modeling: Adding the Regression Paths

Having established validity evidence for the factor structure of the data from both instruments, we have more confidence that the responses provided to the questionnaires reflect the latent factors that we intended to measure, and we can proceed to test our main research question using SEM. Before proceeding to test a SEM, we first test a full measurement model which is similar to the individual CFAs we ran previously; however, in this CFA, we simultaneously included BREQ and SVS scores. This model should have a good fit to the data (based on goodness-of-fit statistics, factor loadings, residual variances, standardized residuals, and modification indices). If it does not have a good fit to the data, then the structural portion of the SEM could be biased. More fundamentally, it would also suggest that the two constructs are conceptually undistinguishable (lack of discriminant validity). As such, a better explanation for their correlation could be that they belong to the same underlying latent factor. Therefore, their correlation should not be interpreted as evidence for the fact that one influences the other. They potentially covary only because they are explained by a common cause or belong to the same latent variable.

First, a full measurement model (see Appendix 5.10) was tested specifying each item to load only onto their respective target latent factors, and the only residual covariance estimated was between SV6 and SV7 as it was identified in the previous CFA. The first indicator approach was used to set the metric of each latent variable. After having demonstrated a good model fit of the measurement model, we proceeded to test the structural part of the SEM (see Appendix 5.11) by adding regression paths from each motivation latent factor to the latent factor of subjective vitality and removing the covariances between latent variables (Mplus does this automatically when regression paths are added). Goodness-of-fit statistics, parameter estimates, 95% confidence intervals, modification indices, and effect sizes ($R^2$) were interpreted.

### Example Write-Up for SEM

Results indicated that the measurement model was a good fit to the data: $MLR\chi^2_{(178)} = 235.014$, $p = 0.0027$, CFI = 0.972, TLI = 0.966, RMSEA = 0.040, 90% CI [0.024, 0.053]. The model was identified (i.e., $df > 0$), and there were no convergence problems or Heywood cases. Standardized factor loadings were all ≥0.556 ($p < 0.050$ and confidence intervals did not cross zero), residual variances were all ≤0.691, and there were 23 out of 210 (11%) standardized residuals over 1.96. Latent variable correlations between all latent variables are presented in Table 5.4. Vitality was statistically significantly related to external, identified, and intrinsic motivations, and confidence intervals did not include zero. Next, we ran the model with regression paths in a SEM (see Figure 5.2). Examination of the fit statistics indicated that this new model fit the data well: $MLR\chi^2_{(178)} = 235.014$, $p = 0.0027$, CFI = 0.972, TLI = 0.966, RMSEA = 0.040, 90% CI [0.024, 0.053]. Only intrinsic motivation was

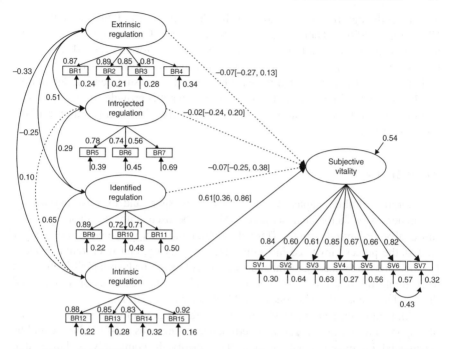

*Figure 5.2    SEM. Solid lines p < 0.05. Dashed lines p > 0.05. Ninety-five confidence intervals are shown in brackets. For diagram clarity, 95% confidence intervals are not shown for factor loadings, exogenous covariances, or residual covariance.*

Table 5.4    Latent variable correlations.

| Variable | 1 | 2 | 3 | 4 |
|---|---|---|---|---|
| | r (95% CI) | r (95% CI) | r (95% CI) | r (95% CI) |
| 1. Vitality | – | | | |
| 2. External motivation | −0.301* [−0.451, −0.150] | – | | |
| 3. Introjected motivation | 0.026 [−0.173, 0.224] | 0.507* [0.351, 0.663] | – | |
| 4. Identified motivation | 0.470* [0.319, 0.621] | −0.251* [−0.427, −0.075] | 0.293* [0.114, 0.471] | – |
| 5. Intrinsic motivation | 0.671* [0.555, 0.788] | −0.334* [−0.508, −0.160] | 0.103 [−0.096, 0.301] | 0.645* [0.481, 0.809] |

95% CI, 95% confidence interval.
*$p < 0.05$.

a statistically significant predictor of subjective vitality ($\beta = 0.607$, $p < 0.01$, 95% CI [0.358, 0.856]). Therefore, at the bivariate level of analysis (i.e., in the measurement model results), each motivation except for introjected motivation was associated with vitality, whereas in the multivariate SEM, only intrinsic motivation predicted vitality. The difference between the measurement model and the SEM is that in the SEM, the addition of regression paths provides researchers with an indication of how motivation accounts for vitality while controlling for all the other motivations.

# Summary

The purpose of this chapter was to showcase to sport and exercise psychology researchers how factor analysis and SEM can be used with real data to answer substantive research questions. Through providing a synergy, we were able to show readers the process involved in estimating, respecifying, and interpreting models. Now that the reader has a general understanding of factor analysis and SEM, we wish to highlight the importance of theory and validation processes as operationalized through factor analytic techniques (see MacKenzie et al., 2011).

Although factor analytic techniques are useful for examining the factor structure of responses to questionnaires, an overreliance on goodness-of-fit indices could be detrimental. For example, within classical test theory, the commonly used method of assessing score reliability through internal consistency (i.e., alpha) assumes that *increasing* the number of items is a good way to improve reliability of a test. In contrast, CFA favors parsimony and *fewer* items which results in the creation and selection of models with a small number of indicators per subscale. The contradiction lies within the misfit between CFA models and estimates of internal consistency whereby an instrument with very few indicators (favored by a CFA) would need to have indicators that have highly similar items (i.e., synonyms, slight variations of an idea, and partially redundant items) in order to be favored by internal consistency. Creating items with highly similar wording only serves to narrow the scope of the latent variable under investigation at the cost of sacrificing the coherence between method and theory. Despite the popularity of CFA models (and their fit indices), it is important to strike a balance between validity evidence based on content (having all the needed elements of a construct within a subscale) and validity evidence of factor structure (empirical demonstration that the model is a good fit to the data). Newly created questionnaires with 10 items per subscale are becoming sparse in recent exercise and sport psychology literatures because subscales with several items are almost systematically failing to reach traditional "acceptable level of model fit." Yet, these questionnaires would potentially offer a more comprehensive coverage of the construct they are trying to measure while providing higher and (nonartificially boosted) levels of internal consistency (a needed condition to minimize the problems associated with measurement error).

Given our strict usage of CFA, subscales with a larger number of items per subscale tend to be washed out of the literature because they typically divide into minuscule subfactors that might be semantically distinct (similar words or ideas loading together) but empirically related to a large extent. To this end, it is not rare to see factors correlating between 0.70 and 0.90. These high correlations call into question the distinction between such latent factors while creating many challenges in the creation of multivariate theory and empirical models trying to examine their unique effect to predict consequential outcome variables. In some cases, incorporating method factors (e.g., all the items starting with the words "I" or all items incorporating a similar stem "My goal is") to account for semantic similarity might enable the proper estimation of "good fitting" subscales with several indicators. In other cases, other factor analytic techniques such as ESEM (see Chapter 8) might be needed to reduce latent factor correlations caused by small item cross-loadings.

# References

Brown, A. (2006). *Confirmatory factor analysis for applied research.* New York, NY: Guilford Press.

Browne, M. W., & Cudek, R. (1993). Alternative ways of assessing model fit. In K. A. Bollen & J. S. Long (Eds.), *Testing structural equation models* (pp. 136–162). Newbury Park, CA: Sage.

Byrne, B. M. (2012). *Structural equation modeling with Mplus: Basic concepts, applications, and programming.* New York, NY: Routledge.

Cole, D. A., Ciesla, J. A., & Steiger, J. H. (2007). The insidious effects of failing to include design-driven correlated residuals in latent-variable covariance structure analysis. *Psychological Methods, 12,* 381–398. doi:10.1037/1082-989X.12.4.381

Cole, D. A., & Preacher, K. J. (2014). Manifest variable path analysis: Potentially serious and misleading consequences due to uncorrected measurement error. *Psychological Methods, 19,* 300–315. doi:10.1037/a0033805

Colwell, S. R. (2014). Chi-Square difference testing using the Satorra–Bentler Scaled Chi-Square. Retrieved from http://www.uoguelph.ca/~scolwell/difftest.html

Deci, E. L., & Ryan, R. M. (2000). The "what" and "why" of goal pursuits: Human needs and the self-determination of behavior. *Psychological Inquiry, 11,* 227–268. doi:10.1207/S15327965PLI1104_01

Diamantopoulos, A., & Siguaw, J. (2000). *Introducing LISREL.* Thousand Oaks, CA: Sage.

Finney, S. J., & DiStefano, C. (2006). Nonnormal and categorical data in structural equation modeling. In G. R. Hancock & R. O. Mueller (Eds.), *Structural equation modeling: A second course. A volume in quantitative methods in education and the behavioral sciences: Issues, research and teaching.* (pp. 269–314). Greenwich, CT: Information Age Publishing.

Gunnell, K. E., Crocker, P. R., Mack, D. E., Wilson, P. M., & Zumbo, B. D. (2014). Goal contents, motivation, psychological need satisfaction, well-being and physical activity: A test of self-determination theory over 6 months. *Psychology of Sport & Exercise, 15,* 19–29. doi:10.1016/j.psychsport.2013.08.005

Hu, L., & Bentler, P. M. (1999). Cutoff criteria for fit indexes in covariance structure analysis: Conventional criteria versus new alternatives. *Structural Equation Modeling, 6,* 1–55.

Jöreskog, K. G. (1999). How large can a standardized coefficient be? Retrieved from http://www.ssicentral.com/lisrel/techdocs/HowLargeCanaStandardizedCoefficientbe.pdf

Kline, R. B. (2010). *Principles and practice of structural equation modeling* (3rd ed.). New York, NY: The Guilford Press.

MacKenzie, S. B., Podsakoff, P. M., & Podsakoff, N. P. (2011). Construct measurement and validation procedures in MIS and behavioural research: Integrating new and existing techniques. *MIS Quarterly, 35*(2), 293–334.

Marsh, H. W., Hau, K., & Wen, Z. (2004). In search of golden rules: Comment on hypothesis-testing approaches to setting cutoff values for fit indexes and dangers in overgeneralizing Hu and Bentler's (1999) Findings. *Structural Equation Modeling: A Multidisciplinary Journal, 11*, 320–341. doi:10.1207/s15328007sem1103_2

Morin, A. J. S., Marsh, H. W., & Nagengast, B. (2013). Exploratory structural equation modeling. In G. R. Hancock, & R. O. Mueller (Eds.), *Structural equation modeling: A second course* (2nd ed., pp. 395–436). Charlotte, NC: Information Age Publishing.

Mullan, E., Markland, D., & Ingledew, D. (1997). A graded conceptualization of self-determination in the regulation of exercise behavior: Development of a measure using confirmatory factor analytic procedures. *Personality and Individual Differences, 23*, 745–752. doi:10.1016/S0191-8869(97)00107-4

Preacher, K. J., & MacCallum, R. C. (2003). Repairing Tom Swift's electric factor analysis machine. *Understanding Statistics, 2*, 13–43. doi:10.1207/S15328031US0201_02

Ryan, R. M., & Frederick, C. (1997). On energy, personality, and health: Subjective vitality as a dynamic reflection of well-being. *Journal of Personality, 65*, 529–565. doi:10.1111/j.1467-6494.1997.tb00326.x

Weston, R., & Gore, P. A. (2006). A brief guide to structural equation modeling. *The Counseling Psychologist, 34*, 719–751. doi:10.1177/0011000006286345

# 6

# Invariance testing across samples and time: Cohort-sequence analysis of perceived body composition

**Herbert W. Marsh, Philip D. Parker, and Alexandre J. S. Morin**

*Institute for Positive Psychology and Education, Australian Catholic University, Strathfield, NSW, Australia*

Some 20 years ago, Schutz and Gessaroli (1993) argued that while for many applications, confirmatory factor analysis (CFA) and structural equation modeling (SEM) should be the methodology of choice, they had seen almost no application in sport/exercise psychology. Even a casual perusal of the major sport/exercise journals shows that the popularity of CFA/SEM has increased substantially. However, in the 2007 *Handbook of Sport Psychology*, Marsh (2007) argued that despite this growing popularity, there appears to be an ever-widening gap between "state-of-the-art" methodological and statistical techniques that should be part of the repertoire of quantitative researchers and the actual skill levels of many applied researchers in sport/exercise sciences. Among other issues described by Marsh were tests of factorial invariance of parameter estimates across independent groups (e.g., men and women, different age groups, or elite vs. nonelite athletes) or over time, which can be

*An Introduction to Intermediate and Advanced Statistical Analyses for Sport and Exercise Scientists*, First Edition.
Edited by Nikos Ntoumanis and Nicholas D. Myers.
© 2016 John Wiley & Sons, Ltd. Published 2016 by John Wiley & Sons, Ltd.
Companion website: www.wiley.com/go/ntoumanis/sport

formulated as a set of fully (or partially) nested set of models in which the endpoints are models with no invariance constraints and models with all parameter estimates invariant (i.e., constrained to be equivalent) across all groups or occasions. In this chapter, we expand upon the presentation of invariance across groups and time, introducing new and evolving design issues and strategies for evaluating these data.

We briefly introduce the importance of invariance testing generally and its relevance in sports and exercise science. In particular, we focus on the use of the cohort-sequence design (also called accelerated longitudinal design; Bell, 1953; Mehta & West, 2000; Nesselroade & Baltes, 1979) to evaluate longitudinal invariance over time and multigroup invariance over samples. Then we briefly review substantive issues that underpin the demonstrations in this chapter. Finally, we demonstrate evolving statistical approaches to the evaluation of cohort-sequence designs.

# General Introduction to the Importance of Measurement Invariance

Tests of measurement invariance evaluate the extent to which measurement properties generalize over multiple groups, situations, or occasions. Of particular substantive importance for sport/exercise research are the evaluations of differences across multiple groups (e.g., athlete vs. nonathlete, male vs. female, age groups, exercise treatment groups vs. control groups) or over time (i.e., observing the same group of participants on multiple occasions, perhaps before and after an intervention). The need for rigorous tests of whether the underlying factor structure is the same for different groups or occasions has often been ignored in sport/exercise research. However, such comparisons assume the invariance of at least factor loadings and, in some cases, item intercepts. Indeed, unless the underlying factors are measuring the same construct in the same way and the measurements themselves are operating in the same manner across groups or time, the comparison of parameter estimates is potentially invalid. For example, if gender or longitudinal differences vary substantially for different items used to infer a construct, in a manner unrelated to respondents' true levels on the latent construct, then the observed differences might be idiosyncratic to the particular items used. From this perspective, it is important to be able to evaluate the full measurement invariance of participants' responses.

Marsh et al. (2009, 2010) operationalized a taxonomy of 13 models (see Appendix 6.1) designed to test measurement invariance that integrates traditional CFA approaches to factor invariance (e.g., Jöreskog & Sörbom, 1988, 1993; Marsh, 1994, 2007; Marsh & Grayson, 1994) with item-response-theory approaches to measurement invariance (e.g., Meredith, 1964, 1993; also see Millsap, 2011; Vandenberg & Lance, 2000). Key models test the goodness of fit of models with no invariance constraints (configural invariance, Model 1), invariance of factor loadings (metric or weak invariance, Model 2), factor loadings and item intercepts (scalar or strong invariance, Model 5), or factor loadings, item intercepts, and item uniquenesses (strict invariance, Model 7). The final four models (Models 10–13) all constrain mean differences between groups to be zero—in combination with the invariance of other parameters.

Essentially the same logic and taxonomy of models can be used to test the invariance of parameters across multiple occasions for a single group. One distinctive feature of longitudinal analyses is that they should normally include correlated uniquenesses between responses to the same item on different occasions (see Jöreskog, 1979; Marsh, 2007; Marsh & Hau, 1996). Although occasions are the most typical test of invariance over a within-person construct like time (i.e., multiple occasions), this is easily extended to include other within-subject variables (e.g., coach or teammates' ratings of the same athlete; e.g., Marsh, Liem, Martin, Morin, & Nagengast, 2011; Marsh, Morin, Parker, & Kaur, 2014; Marsh, Nagengast et al., 2011). Indeed, it is possible to extend these models to test the invariance over multiple grouping variables or combinations of multigroup (between-person) and within-person variables (e.g., Marsh, Abduljabbar, Morin et al., 2015; Marsh, Abduljabbar, Parker et al., 2014; Marsh, Abduljabbar, Parker et al., 2015; Marsh, Morin et al., 2014; Marsh, Nagengast, & Morin, 2013; Morin, Marsh, & Nagengast, 2013).

Although application of the full taxonomy of models is useful, in the present investigation, we focus primarily on three models that are central for latent variable models and the evaluation of latent means:

- Configural invariance (whether the a priori factor structure fits when no invariance constraints are imposed over time or groups; see Model Con-1a and 1b in Table 6.1 and Mplus syntax in Appendix 6.2)

- Metric or weak factorial invariance (tests of the invariance of factor loadings over time and/or groups; Model Met-2a, 2b, and 2c in Table 6.1 and Mplus syntax in Appendix 6.3)

- Scalar or strong (tests of the invariance of factor loadings and item intercepts over time and/or groups; see Models Scl-3a to Scl-3d in Table 6.1 and Mplus syntax in Appendices 6.4 and 6.5)

*Differential item functioning* (DIF) is a critical issue in tests of invariance: whether item-level parameter estimates are the same over groups, time, or combinations of groups and time. The metric invariance model tests for DIF in relation to factor loadings, whereas the scalar invariance model tests for DIF in relation to item intercepts. If the purpose of a research study is merely to evaluate how relations among constructs vary over multiple groups or occasions, then factor loading (metric) invariance may be sufficient. However, if the purpose of the study is to compare latent means over groups or occasions, then scalar (factor loading and intercept) invariance is required. For example, if differences over groups or time are not consistent across the items associated with a particular latent factor, then the results are likely to depend on the mix of items considered. A subset of the items actually used, or a new sample of items designed to measure the same factor, could give different results.

We note that it is also possible to test the invariance of the uniqueness terms (including random measurement error) associated with individual items (see Model Unq-4a in Table 6.1 and Mplus syntax in Appendix 6.6). However, if the focus is on the evaluation of latent relations or latent means based on latent variable models, then

Table 6.1 Goodness of fit for alternative cohort-sequence models.

| Model | ChiSq | df | RMSEA | CFI | TLI | Description |
|---|---|---|---|---|---|---|
| Comparison of models with no invariance (configural) | | | | | | |
| Con-1a | 291 | 192 | 0.040 | 0.979 | 0.971 | No invariance, no correlated uniquenesses |
| Con-1b[a] | 120 | 120 | 0.008 | 0.999 | 1.000 | Con-1a with correlated uniquenesses |
| Comparison of models with cohort invariance of factor loadings (metric) | | | | | | |
| Met-2a | 138 | 136 | 0.010 | 0.999 | 0.999 | Con-1b with FIs invar over cohorts |
| Met-2b | 147 | 144 | 0.012 | 0.998 | 0.999 | Con-1b with Fl invar over waves |
| Met-2c[b] | 155 | 150 | 0.013 | 0.998 | 0.998 | Con-1b with Fl invar over waves and cohorts |
| Comparison of models with cohort invariance factor loadings and intercepts (scalar) | | | | | | |
| Scl-3a | 177 | 174 | 0.011 | 0.998 | 0.999 | Met-2c with intercepts (In) invar over cohorts |
| Scl-3b[c] | 180 | 174 | 0.012 | 0.998 | 0.998 | Met-2c with Int invar over waves |
| Scl-3c | 188 | 180 | 0.013 | 0.997 | 0.997 | Met-2c with Int invar over waves and cohorts |
| Scl-3d[d] | 197 | 186 | 0.014 | 0.997 | 0.997 | Met-3c with Int invar over matching latent means |
| Comparison of models with cohort invariance factor loadings, intercepts uniquenesses | | | | | | |
| Unq-4a[e] | 225 | 342 | 0.040 | 0.975 | 0.971 | Met-3c with Uniq invar over waves and cohorts |
| Comparison of models with cohort invariance factor loadings, intercepts no growth | | | | | | |
| Ngr-5a | 210 | 195 | 0.015 | 0.996 | 0.995 | Met-3c with means=0 |
| Comparison of mimic models of differences associated with gender, athlete group and their interaction | | | | | | |
| Mim-6a | 343 | 282 | 0.026 | 0.989 | 0.984 | Met-3c with Mimic=Free |
| Mim-6b[f] | 368 | 300 | 0.026 | 0.988 | 0.983 | Met-3c with Mimic Inv over matching cells |
| Mim-6c | 548 | 330 | 0.046 | 0.960 | 0.951 | Met-3c with Mimic=0 |
| Mim-6d | 199 | 186 | 0.015 | 0.997 | 0.994 | Met-3c Mimic Mns = 0 Mimic Intercepts = Free |
| Latent growth models with MIMIC variables | | | | | | |
| LGC-7a | 503 | 353 | 0.036 | 0.973 | 0.969 | Met-3c + Mns = 0, latent growth |

| | | | | | | |
|---|---|---|---|---|---|---|
| LGC-7b1[g] | 346 | 0.031 | 0.981 | 0.978 | | LGC-7a+quadratic growth, intercept=M1 |
| | 448 | | | | | |
| LGC-7b2 | 448 | 346 | 0.031 | 0.981 | 0.981 0.978 | LGC-7b1 + with intercept = zero centered |

CFI, comparative fit index; ChiSq, chi-square; df, degrees of freedom ratio; CUs, a priori correlated uniquenesses based on the negatively worded items; FL, factor loadings; IN=intercepts; RMSEA, root mean square error of approximation; TLI, Tucker–Lewis index.

[a] See syntax in Appendix 6.2: Mplus Syntax for Configural Model Con-1b and how to specify correlated uniqueness.

[b] See syntax in Appendix 6.3: Mplus Syntax for Metric Invariance Model Met-2c and how to specify factor loading invariance over within-group constructs (waves) and between-group constructs (cohort group).

[c] See syntax Appendix 6.4: Mplus Syntax for Scalar Invariance Model Scl-3b; specification of intercept invariance over waves (a within-person construct).

[d] See syntax Appendix 6.5: Mplus Syntax for Scalar Invariance Model Scl-3d.

[e] See syntax Appendix 6.6: Mplus Syntax for Scalar Invariance Model Unq-4a.

[f] See syntax Appendix 6.7: Mplus Syntax for MIMIC Model with Orthogonal Polynomial Growth Components Model Mim-6b.

[g] See syntax Appendix 6.8: Mplus Syntax for Model LGC-7b1 (see Tables 6.1 and 6.4 in main text). Latent growth curve model with MIMIC variables.

uniqueness invariance is not a necessary condition. This follows in that measurement error is controlled in latent variable models in which each of the constructs is based on multiple indicators (typically items). Nevertheless, although the valid comparison of latent means does not depend on the invariance of item uniquenesses, there are limitations associated with the noninvariance of item uniquenesses (e.g., manifest means, item variances, and scale variances, as well as relations across manifest constructs, are not comparable across groups). Thus, if the comparison over groups or occasions is based on manifest variables (or scale scores), then the necessary assumptions are the invariance of item uniquenesses, together with the invariance of the factor loadings and item intercepts. Hence, the comparison of manifest variables is considerably more demanding than comparisons based on latent variable models controlling for measurement error.

It is also possible to test the invariance over groups or occasions of latent factor variances and covariances, particularly when there are multiple factors. Although the invariance of factor variances and covariances is not a necessary assumption underlying the comparison of latent means, relations among factors (or the latent factors and other variables) are likely to be of fundamental interest in many applied research studies.

## Cohort-Sequential Designs: Longitudinal Invariance across Samples and Time

As argued by Marsh (1998; Marsh, Craven, & Debus, 1998, 1999; Parker, Marsh, Seaton, & Van Zanden, 2015), a multiwave-multicohort design often provides a stronger basis for evaluating developmental differences than cross-sectional comparisons based on many age cohorts, or longitudinal comparisons based on a single age cohort. While educational and particularly developmental psychologists often extol the virtues of true longitudinal designs over cross-sectional designs, ultimately, support for the generality of developmental effects requires convergence of results across multiple approaches. Hence, juxtaposition of longitudinal and cross-sectional approaches to developmental change provides an important basis for cross-validating the results based on each approach. For example, multicohort-sequential designs, as in the present investigation, have the advantage of providing tests for history and cohort effects (i.e., based on overlapping data collection waves collected from multiple cohorts of participants) that would not be possible with pure longitudinal designs based on a single cohort or in pure cross-sectional designs based on multiple cohorts.

Increasingly, developmental research with school-aged children relies on large-scale longitudinal data sets. However, many of these databases extend over no more than 2 or 3 years, making it difficult to fully explore the growth of key educational constructs over the course of major developmental periods such as high school/adolescence. Here, we address this issue through the use of cohort-sequential designs in which multiple waves of data are collected simultaneously from multiple age cohorts. This strategy provides sport and exercise researchers with a feasible, cost-effective alternative to exploring growth over the course of an entire developmental period (see Brodbeck, Bachmann, Croudace, & Brown, 2012; Enders, 2010; Graham, 2012; Marsh, 1998; Marsh et al., 1999). Furthermore, simulation studies have shown that cohort-sequential designs have greater power than standard longitudinal designs when the same number of time waves is collected in each cohort (Graham, 2012). The increasing prevalence of such designs and the development of statistical procedures for analyzing such data is a substantive-methodological synergy (Marsh & Hau, 2007) in which complex substantive issues stimulate the development of stronger methodological tools.

In our demonstration, four waves of data were collected, 6 months apart, for each of four age cohorts. The cohort-sequential design thus provided a total of 10 waves of data covering 5 years of high school, in which the multiple waves of data overlap for each successive cohort (see Figure 6.1a for structure and Figure 6.1b for measurement model for this design). One of the most critical aspects of such a design, however, is how to deal with the inevitable large amount of data that is missing by design (white cells in Figure 6.1), even in the absence of sample attrition and data holes. The advantage of cohort-sequential designs, however, is that the missing time points in all cohorts are missing due to the design of the study, not as a function of participants' characteristics. Thus, these missing data fully correspond to missing-completely-at-random assumptions of modern missing data techniques (Enders, 2010). This suggests that modern missing data techniques can provide unbiased parameter estimates even in the presence of missing data (Enders, 2010). There are essentially two approaches to estimating growth models with cohort-sequential data that aim to overcome this missing by design component. A common approach is to use full information maximum likelihood estimation on data that is stacked and merged across cohorts. In other words, this approach involves reorganizing the data set so that each participant (each line) is specified as having 10 measurement points, with 6 of those being missing (see Figure 6.1). In this approach, however, some cells of the variance–covariance matrix have zero coverage (i.e., all cases are missing for the entire cohort), and thus, full information maximum likelihood estimation of these covariances becomes problematic (see Enders, 2010).

A second approach, and that used here, is to make use of a multigroup approach to model estimation. Modern SEM packages are becoming increasingly powerful and flexible in estimating complex models. For models such as those proposed here, we take advantage of the ability of Mplus to fit differing models in each cohort. Essentially, models are fitted in each cohort (treated as a separate group in a multi-group design), in relation to their relative position in the developmental period of interest. In the current research, models were specified such that the first cohort reflected growth over Years 7 and 8, the second Years 8 and 9, the third Years 9 and 10, and the last Years 10 and 11. Through the inclusion of invariance constraints across these multiple groups for the overlapping time points (the cells in boxes in Figure 6.1a), the resulting full model covers 5 years of high school, even though any one participant only has data for 2 years. In Appendices 6.2–6.7, we provide annotated Mplus scripts for the estimation of a variety of models using a cohort-sequential design (see also Brown, Croudace, & Heron, 2011).

# Substantive Application: Physical Self-Concept

Here, we briefly review research literature underpinning the substantive focus of this largely methodological chapter. Physical self-concept is a key construct in sport and exercise psychology. Here, we focus on stability/change over time of perceived body composition (PBC) during the potentially turbulent adolescent period, which is critical for the development of boys and girls and of athletes and nonathletes. An essential underlying assumption in such comparisons is measurement invariance.

Age and gender effects on self-concept have theoretical, practical, and methodological implications. Historically, self-concept researchers have been particularly interested in stability and change in self-concept during the potentially volatile adolescent period (Dusek & Flaherty, 1981; Wylie, 1979, 1989), although most of this research has focused on self-esteem, rather than on physical components of self-concept. Predictions about how self-concept develops with age have been proposed from a variety of theoretical perspectives. Marsh (1989, 1990; Marsh, Craven, & Debus, 1991) proposed that the self-concepts of very young children are consistently high but that with increasing life experience, children learn their relative strengths and weaknesses, so that mean levels of self-concept decline, multiple dimensions of self-concept become more differentiated, and self-concepts become more highly correlated with external indicators of competence (e.g., skills, accomplishments, and self-concepts inferred by significant others). Eccles, Wigfield, Harold, and Blumfeld (1993) similarly proposed that the declines in mean levels of self-concept, particularly during the preadolescent/early adolescent period, reflected an optimistic bias for young children and increased accuracy in responses as they grow older. Based on a large empirical study, Marsh (1989) reported that there was a reasonably consistent pattern of self-concepts declining from a young age through early adolescence, leveling out, and then increasing, at least through to early adulthood.

(a)

| | Year 7 | | Year 8 | | Year 9 | | Year 10 | | Year 11 | |
|---|---|---|---|---|---|---|---|---|---|---|
| | M1 | M2 | M3 | M4 | M5 | M6 | M7 | M8 | M9 | M10 |
| Year 7 cohort 1 | W1 | W2 | W3 | W4 | | | | | | |
| Year 8 cohort 2 | | | W1 | W2 | W3 | W4 | | | | |
| Year 9 cohort 3 | | | | | W1 | W2 | W3 | W4 | | |
| Year 10 cohort 4 | | | | | | | W1 | W2 | W3 | W4 |

*Figure 6.1    (a) Cohort-sequential design with four cohorts and four waves (W1–W4) for each cohort. Light gray squares = collected data. White square = missing by design. M1–M10 are 10 latent means that span the 5-year period. Estimates of M3–M8 are each based on results from two cohorts (i.e., M1 is based on Wave 3 from Year 7, cohort 1, and Wave 1 from Year 8, cohort 2), while those for M1–M2 and M9–M10 are based on a single cohort.*

(b)

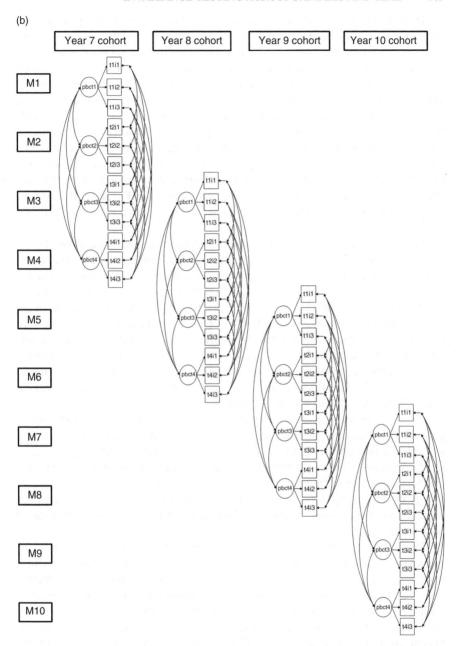

*Figure 6.1    (Continued) (b) Cohort-sequential design with four cohorts and four waves of data for each cohort. M1–M10 represent the 10 latent means that span the 5-year period. Ms in boxes are matching means based on two different cohorts. White square = missing by design. Estimates of M3–M8 are each based on results from two cohorts, while those for M1–M2 and M9–M10 are based on a single cohort.*

Historically, gender differences in self-concept have focused on typically small differences in self-esteem favoring boys (e.g., Feingold, 1994). Marsh (1989), however, demonstrated that these small differences in total scores reflect larger, counterbalancing gender differences in specific components of self-concept. The gender differences in specific scales tended to be consistent with traditional gender stereotypes: (i) boys had higher self-concepts for Physical Ability, Appearance, Math, Emotional Stability, Problem Solving, and Esteem; (ii) girls had higher self-concepts for Verbal/Reading, School, Honesty/Trustworthiness, and Religion/Spiritual Values; and (iii) there were no gender differences for the Parents scale. For all three age ranges, the largest gender differences were the higher scores for boys in Physical Ability and Appearance self-concepts. Whereas the gender differences for preadolescents were larger for Physical Ability than Appearance, the Appearance differences were larger for adolescents and late adolescents.

In this chapter, our focus is on the development/change in self-perception of body composition for adolescent boys and girls ($N = 1268$) attending a prestigious sports high school in Sydney, Australia. Each year, elite athlete students from across the state compete for enrollment in most major sports. However, the school also admits students (62%) from the local catchment area who typically do not participate in the elite athletic program unless they choose to try out for the program. Although we refer to these as the elite athlete and nonathlete groups, respectively, some nonathletes may participate in athletic activities, and all are students in compulsory physical education classes, even though they are not part of the elite athlete program. Hence, we are interested in the development or change in PBC over the adolescent period in relation to gender, athletic group, and their interaction.

Based on previous research, we anticipated that boys would have better PBCs than girls and that athletes would have better PBCs than nonathletes. However, we left as a research question whether gender differences would interact with athlete groups (i.e., whether gender differences in PBC are similar for athlete and nonathlete groups). Of particular relevance to the present investigation is whether there is development and change in these group differences over the adolescent period under consideration— whether gender differences for athletes and nonathletes become larger or smaller during adolescence.

These data also provide a unique opportunity to evaluate how the physical self-concepts of elite athletes develop/change over the 5-year period, starting from the time when they are first selected to participate in this highly selective sporting program. Based on the theoretical self-concept theory underpinning the big-fish–little-pond effect (BFLPE; e.g., Marsh, Abduljabbar, Morin et al., 2015; Marsh, Abduljabbar, Parker et al., 2014; Marsh, Kuyper, Morin, Parker, & Seaton, 2014; Marsh, Seaton et al., 2008), there is a juxtaposition of reflected glory effects (assimilation; "if I am good enough to be selected to be in this program, I must be pretty good"), leading to more positive self-concepts, and social comparison (contrast; "relative to all these other elite athletes, maybe I am not as good as I thought"), leading to more negative effects. Also, there is a temporal aspect to this juxtaposition, wherein positive assimilation effects might dominate when participants are first selected to be in an elite athlete program, but contrast effects become increasingly strong over time as their frame of reference shifts to other elite athletes in the same program. Although there is ample evidence of the negative effects on academic self-concept of attending academically selective high schools and programs, causing long-lasting negative effects on many academic outcomes (e.g., Marsh, 1991; Marsh, Seaton et al., 2008), there is apparently little research in relation to sport and exercise (but see Marsh, Chanal, Sarrazin, & Bois, 2006). Nevertheless, based on research in the academic domain, the athlete/nonathlete difference might be expected to be largest at the start of high school and to decline over this 5-year period.

# Methodology

## The PSDQ Instrument

The short version of the PSDQ (Marsh, Martin, & Jackson, 2010) measures nine specific components and two global components of physical self-concept, based on responses to three or four items for each scale. The theoretical basis of the PSDQ is derived in part from the Shavelson, Hubner, and Stanton (1976) multidimensional, hierarchical model of self-concept but also from Marsh's (1993) CFA of physical fitness indicators, based on Fleishman's (1964) structure of physical fitness. PSDQ research (see reviews by Byrne, 1996; Marsh, 1997; Marsh & Cheng, 2012; Marsh, Martin et al., 2010) has provided good support for the PSDQ factor structure and its generalizability over gender, and different groups of elite and nonelite athletes (Marsh, Perry, Horsely, & Roche, 1995; Marsh, Richards, Johnson, Roche, & Tremayne, 1994), but also for convergent and discriminant validity in relation to a set of external validity criteria, including body composition, physical activity levels, and physical fitness tests of cardiovascular endurance, strength, and flexibility (Marsh, 1996a, 1996b, 1997). For the purposes of the present investigation, we only considered responses to the PBC factor: self-perceptions of body composition measured by a set of three items ("My waist is too large"; "I have too much fat on my body"; "I am overweight").

## Statistical Analyses

Across all models, PBCs were specified as latent variables estimated from multiple items. This requires relatively complex identification constraints. In some models, we used a nonarbitrary metric for factor loadings (which were constrained to average 1 for each factor) and item intercepts (which were constrained to sum to 0 for one factor), allowing results to be interpreted according to the original 6-point Likert scale rather than according to a standardized metric (when the model is identified by constraining factor variances to equal 1 and factor means to equal 0) or as a function of the scale of a referent indicator (when the model is identified by constraining the factor loading of a referent indicator to equal 1 and its intercept to equal 0) (see Little, Slegers, & Card, 2006). The PSDQ was administered on four occasions during a 2-year period of time at approximately 6-month intervals (see Figure 6.1a and b). As is typical in large longitudinal field studies, a substantial portion (23%) of the sample had missing data for at least one of the four occasions, due primarily to absence or the provision of an illegible (or fictitious) name on at least one of the four occasions. All models were fitted using the robust maximum likelihood estimator (MLR) available in Mplus 7.2, which has the advantage of being robust to nonnormality of data and remains equivalent to ML when normality assumptions are met. Multiple imputation was used to handle missing data. The multiple imputation was based on a data file (see Chapter 6 data file in Appendix 6.9, the multiple imputation file used for analyses in the present chapter) in which each student had four waves of data, so that imputation was used to fill in missing values within the four waves actually completed by each cohort of students, but not in the data from waves not completed by the cohort (i.e., imputation for the Year 7 cohort had imputed data for the four waves of data in Years 7 and 8, but not for Years 9 and 10). The analyses were done on five imputed data sets, and the results were combined automatically by Mplus using the Rubin (1987; Schafer, 1997) strategy to obtain unbiased parameter estimates, standard errors, and goodness-of-fit statistics.

Longitudinal models that evaluate development/change of latent means across multiple waves assume strong/scalar invariance in which factor loadings and item intercepts are assumed to be equal across time waves. In a cohort-sequential design, these parameters are thus assumed to be invariant across both time waves and cohorts (thus providing a direct test of possible historical/cohort effects). Furthermore, to estimate the growth trajectories from all time waves and cohorts, cohort-sequential designs also assume that overlapping latent means (e.g., Waves 3 and 4 for the Year 7 cohort, when these students are in Year 8, with Waves 1 and for the Year 8 cohort, when they are also in Year 8; see boxes in Figure 6.1a) are invariant across cohorts. Thus, the model constrains loadings and item intercepts to be invariant over time (strong/scalar invariance), and latent means for overlapping time points to be invariant across time points—providing an additional test of cohort-specific historical effects (see syntax in for Scalar Invariance Model SCl-3d in Appendix 6.5). This is an inherent assumption of cohort-sequential designs for models involving latent means but is rarely tested in applied research.

## Goodness of Fit

Historically, applied SEM researchers sought universal "golden rules" to justify objective interpretations of their data, rather than being forced to defend subjective interpretations (Marsh, Hau, & Wen, 2004). Many fit indices have been proposed (e.g., Marsh, Balla, & McDonald, 1988), but there is even less agreement today than in the past as to what constitutes an acceptable fit. Some still treat the indices and recommended cutoffs as golden rules; others argue that fit indices should be discarded altogether; a few argue that we should rely solely on chi-square goodness-of-fit indices; and many (like us) argue that fit indices should be treated as rough guidelines to be interpreted cautiously in combination with other features of the data. Generally, given the known sensitivity of the chi-square test to sample size, to minor deviations from multivariate normality, and to minor misspecifications, applied SEM research generally focuses on indices that are sample size independent (Hu & Bentler, 1999; Marsh, Balla, & Hau, 1996; Marsh, Hau, & Grayson, 2005; Marsh et al., 2004), such as the root mean square error of approximation (RMSEA), the Tucker–Lewis index (TLI), and the comparative fit index (CFI). Population values of TLI and CFI vary along a 0-to-1 continuum in which values greater than 0.90 and 0.95 typically reflect acceptable and excellent fits to the data, respectively. Values smaller than 0.08 and 0.06 for the RMSEA are typically interpreted as acceptable and good model fits, respectively.

For the comparison of two nested models, the chi-square difference test can be used, but it suffers from even more problems than the chi-square test for single models, which led to the development of other fit indices (see Marsh, Hau, Balla, & Grayson, 1998). Cheung and Rensvold (2002) and Chen (2007) suggested that if the decrease in fit for the more parsimonious model is less than 0.01 for incremental fit indices like the CFI, then there is reasonable support for the more parsimonious model. Chen (2007) suggested that when the RMSEA increases by less than 0.015, there is support for the more constrained model. For indices that incorporate a penalty for lack of parsimony, such as the RMSEA and the TLI, it is also possible for a more restrictive model to result in a better fit than a less restrictive model. However, we emphasize that these cutoff values only constitute rough guidelines.

# Results

## Basic Cohort-Sequence Model: Four Cohort Groups and Four Waves

We begin with the basic cohort-sequence model depicted in Figure 6.1a and b. The critical features of this design are that there are four cohorts (year in school groups) and four waves of data for each cohort. In the first two models (Models Con-1a and Con-1b in Table 6.1; see syntax in Appendix 6.2), we establish that the a priori correlated uniquenesses are required and result in a substantial improvement in fit (Table 6.1). For this reason, correlated uniquenesses are included in all subsequent models. Not surprisingly, given that the PBC scale is brief and has good psychometric properties, the goodness of fit for this model is exceptionally good (e.g., TLI = 1.000; Table 6.1). Inspection of the 48 factor loadings (3 items × 4 waves × 4 cohorts) indicates that all factor loadings are substantial, varying between 0.65 and 0.87 in a standardized metric. In summary, there is good support for configural invariance.

In Models Met-2a–Met-2c (Table 6.1; see Mplus syntax in Appendix 6.3), we demonstrate good support for the invariance of factor loadings over:

- A. Four cohorts (between-group cross-sectional comparisons)

- B. Four waves (within-person longitudinal comparisons)

- C. Four cohorts and four waves (integrating both within and between comparisons; see syntax in Appendix 6.3 along with instructions as to how to alter the syntax to specify Models Met-2a and Met-2b).

Indeed, even constraining factor loadings to be invariant over both the four cohorts and the four waves resulted in almost no decrement of fit (e.g., TLI = 0.998, Model Met-2C). Hence, there is good support for metric invariance.

In Models Scl-3a–Scl-3c (Table 6.1; also see Mplus syntax in Appendix 6.4), we demonstrate good support for the corresponding tests of invariance of intercepts over four cohorts and four waves. Indeed, even constraining item intercepts to be invariant over both the four cohorts and the four waves resulted in almost no decrement of fit (e.g., TLI = 0.997). Hence, there is good support for scalar invariance.

Model Scl-3d (Table 6.1; also see Mplus syntax in Appendix 6.4) is specific to the cohort-sequence design and critical to the interpretation of the results. In particular, it constrains the latent means to be the same with each of the six pairs of matching means (i.e., the matching means in boxes in Figure 6.1a). Thus, for example, the two estimates of M3 based on different cohorts (Wave 3, Year 7 cohort, and Wave 1, Year 8 cohort) are constrained to be equal. The latent mean estimates based on Model Scl-3d are shown in Table 6.2 (with boxes representing the matching means constrained to be equal; Mplus syntax for this model, described in more detail in the results section, is included in Appendix 6.4).

In a supplemental model (Unq-4a), we also tested for the invariance of uniquenesses over cohorts and waves. However, unlike the corresponding tests of the invariance of factor loadings and intercepts, this model resulted in a moderately large decrement in fit (e.g., TLI = 0.971, a $\Delta$TLI = 0.026 compared to Model Scl-3c). We note that this model is borderline in terms of traditional guidelines for testing

Table 6.2    Latent factor means (SEs in parentheses) for Model M4-6b (Table 6.1): complete invariance of factor loadings and intercepts over time and cohort, invariance of matching latent means over cohort (shaded).

| | Cohort 7 | Cohort 8 | Cohort 9 | Cohort 10 |
|---|---|---|---|---|
| M1 | W1 4.602(0.125) | | | |
| M2 | W2 4.448(0.125) | | | |
| M3 | W3 4.477(0.099) | W1 4.477(0.099) | | |
| M4 | W4 4.422(0.101) | W2 4.422(0.101) | | |
| M5 | | W3 4.433(0.094) | W1 4.433(0.094) | |
| M6 | | W4 4.453(0.103) | W2 4.453(0.103) | |
| M7 | | | W3 4.462(0.089) | W1 4.462(0.089) |
| M8 | | | W4 4.395(0.093) | W2 4.395(0.093) |
| M9 | | | | W3 4.395(0.115) |
| M10 | | | | W4 4.485(0.111) |

*Note*: Cohort is the school year group for the first data collection. Wave 1–Wave 4 (W1–W4) are the four waves within each cohort. M1–M10 are the estimated latent means (matching means within boxes are constrained to be equal over cohort). Standard errors (SEs) in parentheses provide a test of significance for each estimate (if the ratio of the estimate/SE is greater than 1.96, the difference is significant at $p < 0.05$).

invariance but also that it might be possible to achieve a more acceptable fit with partial invariance based on ex post facto relaxation of invariance constraints on the uniquenesses (e.g., Byrne, Shavelson, & Muthén, 1989). Instead, we chose to reject this model, because the invariance of uniquenesses is not an assumption underlying the evaluation of latent means. However, strict invariance is a necessary condition for the appropriate evaluation of manifest means (i.e., means-based scale scores formed from the average or sum of items and not corrected for measurement errors). Indeed, this is an important advantage of the latent variable models, in that they do not require uniquenesses to be invariant over groups and occasions.

Finally, in Model M4-5a, we test a model in which the latent means are constrained to be equal across all four waves and four groups—in addition to constraints on factor loadings and intercepts (Model Scl-3c). The fit for Model Ngr-5a was very good (e.g., TLI=0.995), indicating that latent means are very stable when averaged across gender and athlete groups. Were our primary interest in stability/change over this 5-year period, it might be reasonable simply to stop at this point and to conclude that mean levels of PBC are stable over this potentially turbulent adolescent period. However, because our primary interest is on stability/change in relation to gender, athlete group, and their interaction, we now extend the analyses to focus on these issues.

# Cohort-Sequence Design of Multiple Indicators, Multiple Causes Models

A unique aspect of these data is that 38% of the adolescents are elite athletes selected through a highly competitive process, whereas the remaining 62% are nonathletes of similar ages attending the same school and taking mostly the same classes. From this perspective, it is of substantive interest to compare developmental stability/change in PBC over time as a function of gender for these two groups of students.

In the first multiple indicators, multiple causes (MIMIC) model (Mim-6a, Table 6.1), we simply added the three MIMIC variables to the final cohort sequence (Scl-3c with invariance of factor loadings and item intercepts and matching means for overlapping time points), in which the latent factors (PBC) are predicted by the three covariates (gender, boys vs. girls; athlete group, athletes vs. nonathletes; and the gender-by-athlete-group interaction). In this model, no constraints were placed on the effects of the MIMIC variables, which were freely estimated, and the fit was very good (e.g., TLI=0.984). In the next model (Mim-6b, Table 6.1; also Mplus syntax in Appendix 6.7), the effects of the MIMIC variables were constrained to be the same within each of the six pairs of matching means (i.e., the matching means in boxes in Figure 6.1a). Thus, for example, the two estimates of gender differences for cell M3, based on different cohorts (e.g., Wave 3, Year 7 cohort, and Wave 1, Year 8 cohort) were constrained to be equal. The imposition of this set of 18 constraints (three MIMIC variables across six pairs of cells) resulted in nearly no decrement in fit (e.g., TLI=0.988). In the next model (Mim-6c, Table 6.1), we constrained the effects of all the MIMIC variables to be zero (i.e., no differences associated with group or gender over the four waves and four cohorts). The results of this model showed a substantial decrement in fit (e.g., TLI=0.960, ΔTLI=0.028 compared to

Model Mim-6b), indicating that there are gender and group differences. (Mplus syntax for this model, described in more detail in the results section, is included in Appendix 6.7.)

An important feature of the MIMIC model is parsimony, especially when compared to the corresponding multigroup approach. Thus, for example, the 2 (athlete group)×2 (gender)×4 (cohort) design would require testing over 16 groups in the multigroup approach. In the 16-multigroup design, it would be very complicated to disentangle invariance associated with each of the three facets (group, gender, and cohort) and their combinations. Furthermore, in the present investigation, the sample sizes of some of the groups would be so small as to make the analyses dubious. Nevertheless, there were critical drawbacks to the use of the MIMIC model, in that researchers cannot easily test the invariance of factor loadings. However, in the MIMIC model, it is possible to test the invariance of items' intercepts by freely estimating the effects of the MIMIC variables on all items' intercepts and constraining their effects on the latent means to be zero. Comparison of this model (Mim-6d in Table 6.1) with the corresponding model, with the effects of the MIMIC variables on the items' intercepts constrained to be zero and their effects on the latent means freely estimated (Mim-6a in Table 6.1; see syntax in Appendix 6.7), provides a test of intercept invariance across the set of MIMIC variables. If all intercept differences can be explained in terms of a much smaller number of latent means, then there is support for intercept invariance. Results support the invariance of the intercepts, in that Mim-6a fits the data very well (e.g., CFI = 0.989) and that the difference between the two models is smaller than the typically recommended guidelines ($\Delta$CFI $\le$ 0.010; $\Delta$RMSEA $\le$ 0.015). Had there been a lack of invariance of intercepts over the MIMIC variables, it might have been appropriate to evaluate invariance for each of the MIMIC variables separately or, perhaps, to explore the possibility of partial invariance. We note, however, that the post hoc models of partial invariance are typically more defensible when there is a larger number of indicators per factor (there are only three in our example) and intercept invariance holds for all but one (or a small proportion) of a larger number of indicators.

## Use of Model Constraint with Orthogonal Polynomial Contrasts to Evaluate Cohort Sequence and MIMIC Latent Means

Based on the cohort-sequence model of these longitudinal data, we estimated 10 latent means (i.e., 2 means per year for each of the 5 years covered by this design). In order to evaluate the nature of change over time, we then fitted a latent growth model based on traditional orthogonal polynomial contrasts (e.g., Cohen, Cohen, West, & Aiken, 2003) to estimate polynomial (i.e., linear, quadratic, cubic, etc.) components. Orthogonal polynomials have two defining characteristics: they sum to 0 for each component and are mutually independent for pairs of components (Cohen et al., 2003). The coefficients used to define the polynomial contrasts (e.g., linear, quadratic, and cubic components) will vary depending on the number of means (i.e., M1–M10) but are readily available from most textbooks that discuss contrast coding and can be generated from statistical packages such as R (see Appendix 6.6 for the coefficients and Mplus syntax used here). Although familiar to most researchers who use contrasts in analyses of manifest models (e.g., polynomial contrasts with ANOVA or multiple regression) using standard statistical packages such as SPSS (where polynomial contrasts are the default for repeated measures ANOVAs), here the polynomial functions are fitted to latent means as part of the same analyses used to estimate the latent factor structure. In combination with grouping variables (gender, male vs. female; athlete group, elite athlete vs. nonathlete), it is then possible to test interactions between each of the growth curve components and various combinations of these grouping variables (e.g., does change over time differ for males and females). Although orthogonal polynomial contrast codes are often defined in terms of integer values, it is also possible to normalize them, such that the sum of squared coefficients for each contrast sums to 1.0.

We began with the total effects for each wave, averaged across gender and group. These are presented in the form of a table (Table 6.2) that highlights the cohort-sequence design underpinning these data. In Table 6.3, the same values are presented as a single column of means, along with tests of the orthogonal polynomial contrasts. These results show that there are few or no linear or quadratic effects in the longitudinal data represented by the 10 cells. Indeed, not even the mean squared differences between values of the 10 latent means (MSqDiff in Table 6.3) are statistically significant (see Mplus syntax in Appendix 6.7 for the computation of this value using model constraints). This suggests that PBC is highly stable over this adolescent period—at least when averaged across gender and athlete groups. These results are of course consistent with those based on Model Scl-3d. Again, we note that because our primary interest is in stability/change in relation to gender, athlete group, and their interaction, we now look to extend the analyses to focus on these issues.

In Table 6.3, the next three columns represent the MIMIC variables: the main effects of gender, athletic group, and gender-by-group interaction. The "grand mean" effects represent the main effects of each MIMIC variable averaged across the 10 cells in our longitudinal design. The results show that there are substantial main effects, due both to gender (higher values for boys) and group (higher values for athletes). However, the gender-by-group interaction is not statistically significant, suggesting that gender differences are similar across the two groups (or that group differences are similar for boys and girls) averaged over time and cohort (see Mplus syntax in Appendix 6.7 for the computation of this value using model constraints).

Next, we evaluate developmental stability/change in these main effects: whether gender and group effects are longitudinally consistent across the 10 cells of our cohort-sequence design. In the language of ANOVA, we are testing the time-by-gender, time-by-group, and time-by-gender-by-group interactions. Here, we evaluate these effects using traditional polynomial contrasts typically used in ANOVAs, but keeping in mind that these contrasts are applied to latent means based on our cohort-sequence design.

For gender, there is a significant negative linear effect, but a significantly positive quadratic effect; cubic and quartic components are nonsignificant. Inspection of the means (Table 6.3) demonstrates that gender differences in favor of boys were

Table 6.3   Development as a function of athlete/nonathlete group and gender: multigroup (4 cohorts) cohort-sequence analysis with gender, group, and their interaction as MIMIC variables with orthogonal contrasts of time evaluated with orthogonal (model constraint) contrasts.

| Group | Main effects | | | Interaction |
|---|---|---|---|---|
| | Total | Gender (M–F) | Group(E–N) | Gender by group |
| M1 | 4.602(0.125) | −0.257(0.142) | 0.740(0.128) | −0.055(0.264) |
| M2 | 4.448(0.125) | −0.563(0.148) | 0.491(0.137) | 0.274(0.305) |
| M3 | 4.477(0.099) | −0.462(0.102) | 0.351(0.099) | −0.055(0.206) |
| M4 | 4.422(0.101) | −0.619(0.104) | 0.461(0.101) | 0.218(0.203) |
| M5 | 4.433(0.094) | −0.701(0.099) | 0.340(0.096) | 0.184(0.201) |
| M6 | 4.453(0.103) | −0.731(0.105) | 0.293(0.099) | 0.292(0.211) |
| M7 | 4.462(0.089) | −0.752(0.105) | 0.146(0.105) | 0.009(0.211) |
| M8 | 4.395(0.093) | −0.753(0.120) | 0.099(0.112) | −0.148(0.225) |
| M9 | 4.395(0.115) | −0.569(0.167) | 0.024(0.158) | 0.179(0.288) |
| M10 | 4.485(0.111) | −0.349(0.144) | 0.010(0.155) | −0.018(0.336) |
| Summary | | | | |
| Model contrast (orthogonal polynomial contrasts) | | | | |
| Grand mean | 4.457(0.090) | −0.576(0.064) | 0.296(0.057) | 0.088(0.130) |
| Linear | 0.916(1.205) | −2.759(3.330) | −12.092(3.061) | −1.309(6.297) |
| Quadratic | 1.143(0.886) | 5.157(1.451) | 0.729(1.430) | −1.910(2.949) |
| Cubic | −2.798(5.640) | 10.864(9.541) | −4.948(10.176) | 11.292(19.448) |
| Quartic | 4.811(3.124) | 4.770(5.411) | 7.739(6.504) | 1.414(11.789) |
| MSqDiff | 0.003(0.002) | 0.029(0.013) | 0.050(0.023) | 0.026(0.023) |

*Note*: M1–M10 are the estimated latent means (see Figure 6.1a). Standard errors (SEs) in parentheses provide a test of significance for each estimate (if the ratio of the estimate/SE is greater than 1.96 the difference is significant at $p < 0.05$). For each of the covariates (MIMIC variables: female, elite, and their interaction), the corresponding tests evaluate the grand mean and the nature of growth. The grand means are the mean of M1–M10 and provide an overall test of each covariate. MSqDiff is the mean squared difference among M1–M10; this provides a test of no growth (i.e., no significant differences between M1 and M10). Polynomial components test the nature of growth. Results are based on Model Mim-6b in Table 6.1 (also see Appendix 6.7 for Mplus syntax).

smallest at the start of high school (−0.257 for M1; Wave 1, Year 7 cohort), increase over time, level out, and then became smaller (−0.349 for M10; Wave 4, Year 10 cohort).

For the athlete group, there is a significant negative linear effect: quadratic, cubic, and quartic components are nonsignificant. Inspection of the 10 cells across our cohort-sequence design suggests that group differences in favor of elite athletes are substantial at the start of high school (−0.740 for M1) but decline rapidly, so that group differences are not even statistically significant for the last four cells (Years 10 and 11).

However, there are no significant differences over time for the gender-by-group interaction. The time-by-gender-by-group interactions are nonsignificant for all polynomial components.

# Use of Latent Growth Curve Models to Evaluate Stability/Change over Time

When researchers have longitudinal data, growth curve models aim to model trait trajectories in a variable or set of variables over time (see Chapter 7 in this book). Typically, the aim is to find a smoothed line through noisy longitudinal data that provides a test of a hypothesized trajectory. Example hypotheses may include the prediction that (i) a variable shows linear improvement (or decline) across the course of a training program, (ii) a variable has a U-shaped or inverted U-shaped trajectory as individuals transition from a lower to higher competitive levels in football, or (iii) a given training program dramatically lifts performance from the previous trend, prior to introduction of the intervention, and that the improvement is maintained over subsequent time waves. Growth curves can be estimated within a number of frameworks, including structural equation models, multilevel models, and hierarchical Bayes models (Diallo, Morin, & Parker, 2014). In many cases where data are balanced, trends are estimated from complete observed data, and the Bayes priors are uninformative (see Chapter 8), the models provide very similar information. In all cases, latent growth curve (LGC) models provide considerable flexibility in estimating a range of trends, and a means of estimating models with missing data treated via full information maximum likelihood or multiple imputation, and allow for the estimation of growth trends from latent variables with various invariance constraints (see Diallo & Morin, 2015; Diallo et al., 2014; Ram & Gerstorf, 2009; Ram & Grimm, 2007).

LGC models decompose variance in the repeated measures of a variable into intercept and slope components reflecting the initial level and growth trajectories (see Duncan, Duncan, & Strycker, 2006; also see Chapter 7 in this book). Typically, tests of significance for both the mean and the variance of the intercept and slope components are provided as an indication of the significance of the observed growth component (mean) and of the presence of interindividual variability on this growth component (variance) present within the sample. Additionally, comparisons of trajectories can be tested via either multigroup models or within an MIMIC framework. Here, we apply this LGC approach to our cohort-sequence design, as shown in Figure 6.1a (see Brodbeck et al., 2012, for an example; also see Appendix 6.8: Mplus Syntax for Latent Growth Curve Model LGC-7b1) (Figure 6.2).

## Coding the Intercept in LGC Models

A potential complication in applications of latent growth modeling is the question of how to code time. Historically, orthogonal polynomial contrasts (like those presented earlier) have been used, but these complicate interpretations in that it is difficult to graph the results in relation to a metric that is common to different growth components.

(a)

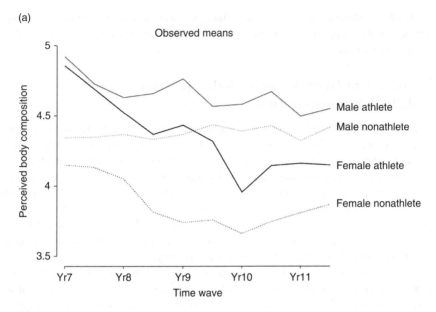

(b)

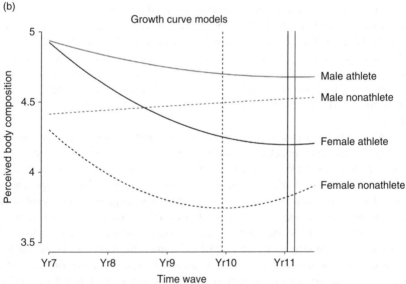

*Figure 6.2    Graphs of results for (a) latent growth curve models based on Model M4-7b1 (see Tables 6.1 and 6.4). (b) Observed means based on model of orthogonal polynomial contrasts Model M4-6b (Tables 6.1 and 6.3). Time waves 0–9 represent Waves 1–10 (see Figure 6.1a), spanning the 5-year period (with two waves per year) from the start of high school (Year 7) to near the end of Year 11. Vertical lines represent turning points for the quadratic functions. The dependent variable is body composition, in which low scores reflect an overly fat body.*

However, in LGC models, estimates of the growth components and tests of their statistical significance are idiosyncratic to the placement of the intercept, which is a function of how time is coded. Thus, for example, the intercept (and all but the highest-order growth component) will vary according to the point in the temporal sequence (or outside the sequence) coded to be zero (i.e., the intercept). Importantly, however, the different codings result in equivalent models. In particular, coefficients based on models that differ only in terms of the intercept are merely transformations of each other so that they all result in the same graphs (Biesanz, Deeb-Sossa, Papadakis, Bollen, & Curran, 2004; also see Mehta & West, 2000). For this reason, it is critical to actually plot the polynomial function as the basis of interpretation of the results.

In some applications, there might be a "logical" coding that is based on the experimental design and on research questions. Thus, for example, in experimental designs where there is an intervention introduced within the temporal sequence, it might be logical to code the intercept to be zero immediately prior to the intervention. In the present investigation, we are interested in stability/change over the high school years, so it is reasonable to code the intercept to be at the start of high school (Year 7, Wave 1) or, perhaps, the end of the temporal sequence (Year 10, Wave 4). However, in some applications which do not involve an intervention (or a critical transition experienced by all participants, such as moving from primary to secondary school), the placement of the intercept might be arbitrary. It is also important to emphasize that typically, interpretation of the growth coefficients (for all but the highest-order component) is highly dependent upon the placement of the intercept. For the present purposes, we illustrate this by considering three different codings of the data, placing the intercept at the:

- Start of the temporal sequence (e.g., M1 (Yr7, Wave 1)=0; M2 (Yr7, Wave 2) = 1; ... M10 (Yr10, Wave 4)=9; Model LGC-7b1a in Table 6.4) (see Appendix 6.7: Mplus Syntax for Latent Growth Curve Model LGC-7b1)

- Midpoint of the temporal sequence (e.g., M1 (Yr7, Wave 1)=−4.5; ... M4 (Yr7, Wave 4, and Yr8, Wave 2)=−0.5; M5 (Yr8, Wave 3 and Yr9, Wave1)=+0.5; ... M10 (Yr10, Wave 4)=+4.5; Model LGCMb2 in Table 6.4)

- End of the temporal sequence (e.g., M1 (Yr7, Wave 1)=−9; M2 (Yr7, Wave 2) =−8; ... M10 (Yr10, Wave 4)=0; Model LGCMb3 in Table 6.4)

Inspection of the results based on these three intercepts results in highly different growth coefficients (Table 6.4), even though the three models are equivalent and merely represent transformations of each other. Thus, for example, the intercept for the group contrast is highly significant (in favor of athletes) when the intercept is placed at the start of the time sequence, much smaller but still significant when the intercept is placed in the middle of the time sequence, and not statistically significant when placed at the end of the time sequence. These results demonstrate that the group differences vary systematically in relation to time (a similar pattern of results was demonstrated with the estimated means using the polynomial contrast approach in Table 6.3, in which group differences started out large in the first wave, gradually declined, and were nonsignificant for the last waves). Because the growth coefficients

Table 6.4 Adolescent development as a function of athlete group (elite vs. nonelite athletes) and gender (male vs. female): multigroup (4 cohorts) cohort-sequence analysis with gender, group, and their interaction as MIMIC variables.

| Group | Main effects | | Interaction | | Residual | Covariances | |
|---|---|---|---|---|---|---|---|
| | Total | Gender (M–F) | Group(E–N) | Gender×group | Variances | Intercept | Linear |
| Latent growth modeling (intercept at first time point) | | | | | | | |
| Intercept | 4.889(0.076) | −0.273(0.133) | 0.672(0.125) | −0.040(0.259) | 0.924(0.189) | | |
| Linear | −0.084(0.034) | −0.199(0.055) | −0.081(0.053) | 0.103(0.110) | 0.037(0.059) | 0.065(0.111) | |
| Quadratic | 0.007(0.003) | 0.020(0.006) | 0.001(0.006) | −0.011(0.012) | 0.000(0.001) | −0.032(0.020) | 0.000(0.008) |
| Latent growth modeling (intercept at midpoint) | | | | | | | |
| Intercept | 4.656(0.038) | −0.756(0.133) | 0.334(0.073) | 0.204(0.152) | 1.021(0.079) | | |
| Linear | −0.020(0.010) | −0.020(0.021) | −0.070(0.019) | 0.006(0.041) | 0.044(0.020) | −0.034(0.015) | |
| Quadratic | 0.007(0.003) | 0.020(0.006) | 0.001(0.006) | −0.011(0.012) | 0.000(0.001) | −0.030(0.007) | 0.001(0.001) |
| Latent growth modeling (intercept at last time point) | | | | | | | |
| Intercept | 4.710(0.080) | −0.451(0.149) | 0.046(0.134) | 0.011(0.310) | 0.489(0.206) | | |
| Linear | −0.044(0.034) | −0.159(0.058) | 0.058(0.057) | 0.091(0.121) | 0.055(0.067) | 0.072(0.135) | |
| Quadratic | 0.007(0.003) | 0.020(0.006) | 0.001(0.006) | −0.011(0.012) | 0.000(0.001) | −0.027(0.022) | −0.001(0.008) |

*Note:* Results based on three equivalent latent growth models (intercept, linear, and quadratic components) that differ in terms of the placement of the intercept. For each of the covariates (MIMIC variables: female, elite, and their interaction), the corresponding tests evaluate the effect at the intercept and the linear and quadratic trend components (i.e., the extent to which the effect of the covariate varies with time). Standard errors (SEs) in parentheses provide a test of significance for each estimate (see Appendix 6.8: Mplus Syntax for Latent Growth Curve Model LGC-7b1).

are so heavily dependent on the placement of the intercept, it is absolutely essential that interpretations are based on a graph of the LGC results.

## LGC Results

Preliminary results presented for the model constraint approach showed significant linear and quadratic effects (but nonsignificant cubic or quartic components; see tests of orthogonal polynomial contrasts in Table 6.3). Hence, for LGC models, we limited consideration to linear and quadratic growth components. The fit for this model was very good (e.g., RMSEA=0.031, CFI=0.981, TLI=0.978). As noted earlier, all three codings (intercept at the start, middle, or end of the temporal sequence) necessarily result in the same goodness of fit and graph of the data, but different growth coefficient estimates for all but the highest-order growth component (quadratic in this application). Hence, the graph of the results is essential for interpretation.

When the intercept is placed at the start of the temporal sequence, overall there are small but significant linear (negative) and quadratic (positive) trends. Although there is substantial variation in the intercepts for different participants (residual variance component=0.924), these residual variance components are not statistically significant for the linear and quadratic growth components. While boys start off with much higher scores than girls (gender effect=−0.273), there is a substantial linear decline in the size of the gender differences over time, as well as a small quadratic component. The athlete/nonathlete group difference is substantial at the start of the time sequence (group effect=0.672), but linear and quadratic trends in this difference are not significant.

However, these estimates were systematically different for different codings of time. Thus, for example, compared to the start of the temporal sequence, the gender difference was substantially larger (−0.756) at the midpoint and, to a lesser extent, at the end of the sequence (−0.451). The athlete/nonathlete differences were even more dramatic, in that the very large difference at the start of high school (0.672) was much smaller at the middle of the time sequence (0.334), but not even statistically significant at the end of the time sequence (0.046, SE=0.134).

# Summary, Implications, and Further Directions

In this chapter, we have outlined a substantive-methodological synergy applying new and evolving statistical methodology to address substantively important issues with theoretical and practical implications. Our primary focus has been on methodological tests of invariance based on a cohort-sequence design (Figure 6.1a and b). Substantively, we have evaluated stability/change in PBC over the potentially turbulent adolescent period as a function of gender, group, and their interaction.

## Methodological Implications, Limitations, and Further Directions

We have presented a multigroup approach to testing invariance in a cohort sequence. We began by demonstrating good support for the invariance of factor loadings and item intercepts across the four cohort groups and four occasions, spanning five school years. Critically, we then demonstrated support for invariance constraints in latent means across these multiple groups for the overlapping time points (the cells in boxes in Figure 6.1a), resulting in a full model covering 5 years of high school, even though any one participant only completed data across 2 years.

Next, we extended the typical cohort-sequence design by integrating it with an MIMIC model of the effects of three covariates (gender, athlete group, and their interaction). The effects of these covariates and their interaction with time were explored by two complementary approaches, one based on the traditional orthogonal polynomial contrasts traditionally applied in ANOVAs (but here based on latent rather than manifest means) and the other based on LGC models. Not surprisingly, both approaches resulted in similar interpretations, but each has potentially complementary advantages. In order to illustrate the differences, we present graphs of the results based on both approaches. The LGC graph is smoothed, in that estimated points are only based on the linear and quadratic growth components. In the ANOVA approach, the means are freely estimated so that the graph does not represent smoothed polynomial plots. Nevertheless, the interpretation of both graphs is similar, as will typically be the case.

A potentially important advantage of the orthogonal polynomial approach is that it results in reasonably independent estimates of each polynomial component so that the convergence problems that plague LGC models are not so likely to occur— particularly for models estimating more than two or three growth components. Here, for example, we were able to show, with the orthogonal polynomial approach, that cubic and quartic growth components—and their interactions with the three covariates—were all nonsignificant. This provided a good rationale for limiting LCG models to linear and quadratic growth components. However, the estimated trajectories based on LGC models that are so critical in the interpretation of the results are not easily derived from estimates based on the orthogonal model. Also, there was considerable recent development in the application of LGC models, which is likely to provide new and evolving advantages to this approach (e.g., Biesanz et al., 2004; Bollen & Curran, 2006; Morin, Maïano, Marsh, Janosz, & Nagengast, 2011; Morin, Maïano, Marsh, Nagengast, & Janosz, 2013). Although a detailed juxtaposition of the two approaches is beyond the scope of this chapter, we suggest that they should be viewed as complementary rather than alternative approaches to describing growth trajectories and how they vary as a function of other variables.

In this chapter, we relied heavily on MIMIC models that implicitly assume that factor loadings and intercepts are invariant over these grouping variables as well as over cohort and occasion. Although it is possible to test the invariance of intercepts with the MIMIC model, the invariance of factor loadings is not readily testable. An alternative in the present investigation might have been to test invariance over 16 groups (2 gender × 2 athlete groups × 4 cohorts) and four occasions, but sample sizes in many of the groups were too small for this to be reasonable. Furthermore, the multigroup approach to testing the invariance of estimates based on the MIMIC variable is only viable in applications such as the present one, in which the covariates are categorical, with relatively few discrete categories. For reasonably continuous covariates, Marsh, Nagengast et al. (2013) proposed a hybrid MIMIC model in which the same continuous variable (e.g., age) is included as a multigroup variable that allows more rigorous tests of invariance and a continuous variable to determine how much explained variance is lost by categorizing a continuous model. Interestingly, Mehta and West (2000) had previously proposed a similar solution to evaluating age effects in a cohort-sequence design. We could have included age as a covariate, in addition to the implicit effect of age represented by the age cohort. Although this was beyond the scope of the present analysis, these possibilities offer potentially important areas for further development.

In this chapter, the factor structure was very simple, based on only three items with strong psychometric properties, and the fit of invariance models was always very good. However, this will not always be the case, particularly for models based on a large number of items for each construct and, perhaps, multiple latent constructs. When misfit is due to lack of invariance, it might be possible to fit partial invariance models. However, these should be used with appropriate caution, particularly when based on ex post facto model modifications. Nevertheless, when there is substantial misfit, even in the configural model with no invariance constraints, the use of growth curve models is problematic. In the past, applied researchers have sometimes resorted to typically dubious practices such as the use of item parcels, which camouflages misfit rather than resolving the problem (see discussion by Marsh, Lüdtke, Nagengast, Morin, & Von Davier, 2013). Nevertheless, there are new and evolving approaches that do not require applied researchers to evaluate potentially overly restrictive models that preclude item loading on more than one factor. These include exploratory structural equation models that integrate most of the advantages of CFA with the flexibility of EFA structures and evolving Bayesian approaches (e.g., Marsh, Morin, et al., 2014; Morin, Marsh, & Nagengast, 2013; see also Chapter 8 in this book). Although these approaches typically have not been applied to growth modeling, their application provides an important direction for further research.

# References

Bell, R. Q. (1953). Convergence: An accelerated longitudinal approach. *Child Development, 24*, 145–152.

Biesanz, J. C., Deeb-Sossa, N., Papadakis, A. A., Bollen, K. A., & Curran, P. J. (2004). The role of coding time in estimating and interpreting growth curve models. *Psychological Methods, 9*(1), 30.

Bollen, K. A., & Curran, P. J. (2006). *Latent curve models: A structural equation perspective.* Hoboken, NJ: John Wiley & Sons.

Brodbeck, J., Bachmann, M. S., Croudace, T. J., & Brown, A. (2012). Comparing growth trajectories of risk behaviors from late adolescence through young adulthood: An accelerated design. *Developmental Psychology, 49*, 1732–1738.

Brown, A., Croudace, T., & Heron, J. (2011). Longitudinal data modelling: Sequential cohort design [Course handout]. Retrieved from http://www.restore.ac.uk/appliedpsychometrics/Tutorial.materials/Intro.to.longitudinal.modelling/

Byrne, B. M. (1996). *Measuring self-concept across the life span: Issues and instrumentation.* Washington, DC: American Psychological Association.

Byrne, B. M., Shavelson, R. J., & Muthén, B. (1989). Testing for the equivalence of factor covariance and mean structures: The issue of partial measurement invariance. *Psychological Bulletin, 105*, 456–466.

Chen, F. F. (2007). Sensitivity of goodness of fit indices to lack of measurement invariance. *Structural Equation Modeling, 14*, 464–504.

Cheung, G. W., & Rensvold, R. B. (2002). Evaluating goodness-of-fit indexes for testing measurement invariance. *Structural Equation Modeling, 9*, 233–255. doi:10.1207/ S15328007SEM0902_5

Cohen, J., Cohen, P., West, S. G., & Aiken, L. S. (2003). *Applied multiple regression/correlation analysis for the behavioral sciences* (3rd ed.). Mahwah, NJ: Lawrence Erlbaum Associates.

Diallo, T. M. O., & Morin, A. J. S. (2015). Power of latent growth curve models to detect piecewise linear trajectories. *Structural Equation Modeling, 22*(3), 449–460.

Diallo, T. M. O., Morin, A. J. S., & Parker, P. D. (2014). Statistical power of latent growth curve models to detect quadratic growth. *Behavioural Research Methods, 46*(2), 357–371.

Duncan, T. E., Duncan, S. C., & Strycker, L. A. (2006). *An introduction to latent variable growth curve modeling: Concepts, issues, and applications.* New York, NY: Lawrence Erlbaum.

Dusek, J. B., & Flaherty, J. F. (1981). *The development of self-concept during adolescent years*, Monographs of the Society for Research in Child Development, Vol. *46* No. 4, Serial No. 191. Chicago, IL: University of Chicago Press.

Eccles, J., Wigfield, A., Harold, R. D., & Blumfeld, P. (1993). Age and gender differences in children's self- and task-perceptions during elementary school. *Child Development, 64*, 830–847.

Enders, C. (2010). *Applied missing data analysis.* New York, NY: Guilford Press.

Feingold, A. (1994). Gender differences in personality: A meta-analysis. *Psychological Bulletin, 116*, 429–456.

Fleishman, F. A. (1964). *The structure and measurement of physical fitness.* Englewood Cliffs, NJ: Prentice-Hall.

Graham, J. W. (2012). *Missing data: Analysis and design.* New York, NY: Springer.

Hu, L., & Bentler, P. M. (1999). Cut-off criteria for fit indexes in covariance structure analysis: Conventional criteria versus new alternatives. *Structural Equation Modeling, 6*(1), 1–55.

Jöreskog, K. G. (1979). Statistical estimation of structural models in longitudinal investigations. In J. R. Nesselroade & B. Baltes (Eds.), *Longitudinal research in the study of behavior and development* (pp. 303–351). New York, NY: Academic Press.

Jöreskog, K. G., & Sörbom, D. (1988). *LISREL 7: A guide to the program and applications* (2nd ed.). Chicago, IL: SPSS.

Jöreskog, K. G., & Sörbom, D. (1993). *LISREL 8: Structural equation modeling with the SIMPLIS command language.* Chicago, IL: Scientific Software International.

Little, T. D., Slegers, D. W., & Card, N. A. (2006). A non-arbitrary method of identifying and scaling latent variables in SEM and MACS models. *Structural Equation Modeling, 13*, 59–72.

Marsh, H. W. (1989). Age and sex effects in multiple dimensions of self-concept: Preadolescence to early-adulthood. *Journal of Educational Psychology, 81*, 417–430.

Marsh, H. W. (1990). A multidimensional, hierarchical self-concept: Theoretical and empirical justification. *Educational Psychology Review, 2*, 77–172.

Marsh, H. W. (1991). The failure of high ability high schools to deliver academic benefits: The importance of academic self-concept and educational aspirations. *American Educational Research Journal, 28*, 445–480.

Marsh, H. W. (1994). Confirmatory factor analysis models of factorial invariance: A multifaceted approach. *Structural Equation Modeling, 1*, 5–34.

Marsh, H. W. (1996a). Construct validity of physical self-description questionnaire responses: Relations to external criteria. *Journal of Sport & Exercise Psychology, 18*, 111–131.

Marsh, H. W. (1996b). Physical self description questionnaire: Stability and discriminant validity. *Research Quarterly for Exercise and Sport, 67*, 249–264.

Marsh, H. W. (1997). The measurement of physical self-concept: A construct validation approach. In K. Fox (Ed.), *The physical self: From motivation to well-being* (pp. 27–58). Champaign, IL: Human Kinetics.

Marsh, H. W. (1998). Age and gender effects in physical self-concepts for adolescent elite-athletes and non-athletes: A multi-cohort-multi-occasion design. *Journal of Sport & Exercise Psychology, 20*(3), 237–259.

Marsh, H. W. (2007). Application of confirmatory factor analysis and structural equation modeling in sport/exercise psychology. In G. Tenenbaum & R. C. Eklund (Eds.), *Handbook of sport psychology* (3rd ed., pp. 774–798). New York, NY: John Wiley & Sons.

Marsh, H. W. (1993). The multidimensional structure of physical fitness: Invariance over gender and age. *Research Quarterly for Exercise and Sport, 64*, 256–273.

Marsh, H. W., Abduljabbar, A. S., Morin, A. J. S., Parker, P., Abdelfattah, F., Nagengast, B., & Abu-Hilal, M. M. (2015). The big-fish-little-pond effect: Generalizability of social comparison processes over two age cohorts from Western, Asian and Middle-Eastern Islamic countries. *Journal of Educational Psychology, 107*, 258–271.

Marsh, H. W., Abduljabbar, A. S., Parker, P. D., Morin, A. J. S., Abdelfattah, F., & Nagengast, B. (2014). The big-fish-little-pond effect in mathematics: A cross-cultural comparison of U.S. and Saudi Arabian TIMSS responses. *Journal of Cross-Cultural Psychology, 45*(5), 777–804. doi:10.1177/0022022113519858

Marsh, H. W., Abduljabbar, A. S., Parker, P. D., Morin, A. J., Abdelfattah, F., Nagengast, B., Möller, J., & Abu-Hilal, M. M. (2015). The internal/external frame of reference model: Age-cohort and cross-national differences in paradoxical relations between TIMSS math and science achievement, self-concept and intrinsic motivation. *American Educational Research Journal, 52*, 168–202.

Marsh, H. W., Balla, J. R., & Hau, K. T. (1996). An evaluation of incremental fit indices: A clarification of mathematical and empirical processes. In G. A. Marcoulides & R. E. Schumacker (Eds.), *Advanced structural equation modeling: Issues and techniques* (pp. 315–353). Hillsdale, NJ: Erlbaum.

Marsh, H. W., Balla, J., & McDonald, R. P. (1988). Goodness of fit in confirmatory factor analysis: The effect of sample size. *Psychological Bulletin, 103*, 391–410.

Marsh, H. W., Chanal, J. P., Sarrazin, P. G., & Bois, J. E. (2006). Self-belief does make a difference: A reciprocal effects model of the causal ordering of physical self-concept and gymnastics performance. *Journal of Sports Sciences, 24*, 101–111.

Marsh, H. W., & Cheng, J. H. S. (2012). Physical self-concept. In G. Tenenbaum, R. C. Eklund, & A. Kamata (Eds.), *Measurement in sport and exercise psychology* (pp. 215–226). Champaign, IL: Human Kinetics.

Marsh, H. W., Craven, R. G., & Debus, R. (1991). Self-concepts of young children aged 5 to 8: Their measurement and multidimensional structure. *Journal of Educational Psychology, 83*, 377–392.

Marsh, H. W., Craven, R. G., & Debus, R. (1998). Structure, stability, and development of young children's self-concepts: A multicohort-multioccasion study. *Child Development, 69*(4), 1030–1053.

Marsh, H. W., Craven, R. G., & Debus, R. (1999). Separation of competency and affect components of multiple dimensions of academic self-concept: A developmental perspective. *Merrill–Palmer Quarterly–Journal of Developmental Psychology, 45*, 567–601.

Marsh, H. W., & Grayson, D. (1994). Longitudinal confirmatory factor analysis: Common, time-specific, item-specific, and residual-error components of variance. *Structural Equation Modeling, 1*, 116–146.

Marsh, H. W., & Hau, K.-T. (1996). Assessing goodness of fit: Is parsimony always desirable? *Journal of Experimental Education, 64*, 364–390.

Marsh, H. W., & Hau, K. T. (2007). Applications of latent-variable models in educational psychology: The need for methodological-substantive synergies. *Contemporary Educational Psychology, 32*, 151–170.

Marsh, H. W., Hau, K.-T., Balla, J. R., & Grayson, D. (1998). Is more ever too much? The number of indicators per factor in confirmatory factor analysis. *Multivariate Behavioral Research, 33*, 181–220.

Marsh, H. W., Hau, K.-T., & Grayson, D. (2005). Goodness of fit evaluation in structural equation modeling. In A. Maydeu-Olivares & J. McArdle (Eds.), *Contemporary psychometrics. A festschrift for Roderick P. McDonald* (pp. 275–340). Mahwah, NJ: Erlbaum.

Marsh, H. W., Hau, K. T., & Wen, Z. (2004). In search of golden rules: Comment on hypothesis testing approaches to setting cutoff values for fit indexes and dangers in overgeneralising Hu & Bentler's (1999) findings. *Structural Equation Modelling, 11*, 320–341.

Marsh, H. W., Kuyper, H., Morin, A. J. S., Parker, P. D., & Seaton, M. (2014). Big-fish-little-pond social comparison and local dominance effects: Integrating new statistical models, methodology, design, theory and substantive implications. *Learning and Instruction, 33*, 50–66. http://dx.doi.org/ 10.1016/j.learninstruc.2014.04.0020959-4752/

Marsh, H. W., Liem, G. A. D., Martin, A. J., Morin, A. J. S., & Nagengast, B. (2011). Methodological measurement fruitfulness of exploratory structural equation modeling (ESEM): New approaches to key substantive issues in motivation and engagement. *Journal of Psychoeducational Assessment, 29*(4), 322–346. doi:10.1177/0734282911406657

Marsh, H. W., Lüdtke, O., Muthén, B., Asparouhov, T., Morin, A. J. S., Trautwein, U., & Nagengast, B. (2010). A new look at the big-five factor structure through exploratory structural equation modeling. *Psychological Assessment, 22*, 471–491. doi:10.1037/a0019227

Marsh, H. W., Lüdtke, O., Nagengast, B., Morin, A. J. S., & Von Davier, M. (2013). Why item parcels are (almost) never appropriate: Two wrongs do not make a right—Camouflaging misspecification with item parcels in CFA models. *Psychological Methods, 18*(3), 257–284. doi:10.1037/a0032773

Marsh, H. W., Martin, A. J., & Jackson, S. (2010). Introducing a short version of the physical self description questionnaire: New strategies, short-form evaluative criteria, and applications of factor analyses. *Journal of Sport & Exercise Psychology, 32*, 438–482.

Marsh, H. W., Morin, A. J. S., Parker, P., & Kaur, G. (2014). Exploratory structural equation modeling: An integration of the best features of exploratory and confirmatory factor analysis. *Annual Review of Clinical Psychology, 10*, 85–110. Retrieved from http://dx.doi. org/ 10.1146/annurev-clinpsy-032813-153700

Marsh, H. W., Muthén, B., Asparouhov, T., Lüdtke, O., Robitzsch, A., Morin, A. J. S., & Trautwein, U. (2009). Exploratory structural equation modeling, integrating CFA and EFA: Application to students' evaluations of university teaching. *Structural Equation Modeling, 16*(3), 439–476. doi:10.1080/10705510903008220

Marsh, H. W., Nagengast, B., & Morin, A. J. S. (2013). Measurement invariance of big-five factors over the life span: ESEM tests of gender, age, plasticity, maturity, and la dolce vita effects. *Developmental Psychology, 49*(6), 1194–1218. doi:10.1037/a0026913

Marsh, H. W., Nagengast, B., Morin, A. J. S., Parada, R. H., Craven, R. G., & Hamilton, L. R. (2011). Construct validity of the multidimensional structure of bullying and victimization: An application of exploratory structural equation modeling. *Journal of Educational Psychology, 103*(3), 701–732. doi:10.1037/a0024122

Marsh, H. W., Perry, C., Horsely, C., & Roche, L. (1995). Multidimensional self-concepts of elite athletes: How do they differ from the general population? *Journal of Sport & Exercise Psychology, 17*, 70–83.

Marsh, H. W., Richards, G. E., Johnson, S., Roche, L., & Tremayne, P. (1994). Physical self description questionnaire: Psychometric properties and a multitrait-multimethod analysis of relations to existing instruments. *Sport and Exercise Psychology, 16*, 270–305.

Marsh, H. W., Seaton, M., Trautwein, U., Lüdtke, O., Hau, K. T., O'Mara, A. J., & Craven, R. G. (2008). The big-fish-little-pond-effect stands up to critical scrutiny: Implications for theory, methodology, and future research. *Educational Psychology Review, 20*, 319–350. doi:10.1007/s10648-008-9075-6

Mehta, P. D., & West, S. G. (2000). Putting the individual back into individual growth curves. *Psychological Methods, 5*(1), 23. doi:I0.1037//10S2–989X.5.I.23

Meredith, W. (1964). Rotation to achieve factorial invariance. *Psychometrika, 29*, 187–206.

Meredith, W. (1993). Measurement invariance, factor analysis and factorial invariance. *Psychometrika, 58*(4), 525–543.

Millsap, R. E. (2011). *Statistical approaches to measurement invariance.* New York, NY: Routledge.

Morin, A. J., Maïano, C., Marsh, H. W., Janosz, M., & Nagengast, B. (2011). The longitudinal interplay of adolescents' self-esteem and body image: A conditional autoregressive latent trajectory analysis. *Multivariate Behavioral Research, 46*, 157–201.

Morin, A. J. S., Maïano, C., Marsh, H. W., Nagengast, B., & Janosz, M. (2013). School life and adolescents' self-esteem trajectories. *Child Development, 84*, 1967–1988.

Morin, A. J. S., Marsh, H. W., & Nagengast, B. (2013). Exploratory structural equation modeling: An introduction. In G. R. Hancock & R. O. Mueller (Eds.), *Structural equation modeling: A second course* (2nd ed., pp. 395–436). Greenwich, CT: IAP.

Nesselroade, J. R., & Baltes, P. B. (1979). *Longitudinal research in the study of behavior and development.* San Diego, CA: Academic Press.

Parker, P. D., Marsh, H. W., Seaton, M., & Van Zanden, B (2015). If one goes up the other must come down: Examining ipsative relationships between mathematics and English self-concept trajectories across high school. *British Journal of Educational Psychology, 85*(2), 172–191.

Ram, N., & Gerstorf, D. (2009). Time-structured and net intraindividual variability: Tools for examining the development of dynamic characteristics and processes. *Psychology & Aging, 24*, 778–791.

Ram, N., & Grimm, K. J. (2007). Using simple and complex growth models to articulate developmental change: Matching theory to method. *International Journal of Behavioral Development, 31*, 303–316.

Rubin, D. B. (1987). *Multiple imputation for nonresponse in surveys.* New York, NY: John Wiley & Sons.

Schafer, J. L. (1997). *Analysis of incomplete multivariate data.* New York, NY: Chapman & Hall.

Schutz, R. W., & Gessaroli, M. E. (1993). Use, misuse and disuse of psychometrics in sport psychology research. In R. N. Singer, M. Murphy, & L. K. Tennant (Eds.), *Handbook of research on sport psychology* (pp. 901–917). New York, NY: Macmillan.

Shavelson, R. J., Hubner, J. J., & Stanton, G. C. (1976). Validation of construct interpretations. *Review of Educational Research, 46*, 407–441.

Vandenberg, R. J., & Lance, C. E. (2000). A review and synthesis of the measurement invariance literature: Suggestions, practices, and recommendations for organizational research. *Organizational Research Methods, 3*(1), 4–69.

Wylie, R. C. (1979). *The self-concept* (Vol. 2). Lincoln, NE: University of Nebraska Press.

Wylie, R. C. (1989). *Measures of self-concept.* Lincoln, NE: University of Nebraska Press.

# 7

# Cross-lagged structural equation modeling and latent growth modeling

## Andreas Stenling[1], Andreas Ivarsson[2], and Magnus Lindwall[3]

[1] *Department of Psychology, Umeå University, Umeå, Sweden*
[2] *Center of Research on Welfare, Health and Sport, Halmstad University, Halmstad, Sweden*
[3] *Department of Food and Nutrition, and Sport Science, Department of Psychology, University of Gothenburg, Gothenburg, Sweden*

## General Introduction

Most of the theories that researchers use to explain human behavior in sport and exercise psychology are process-based (Sliwinski & Mogle, 2008), highlighting the concept and dynamics of change. Therefore, one of the most essential aims in sport and exercise psychology research is to study how single variables change and how changes in different variables are associated. Despite the process-based nature of most theories underlying research in sport and exercise psychology, a considerable amount of the current research is cross-sectional and correlational in nature (Hagger & Chatzisarantis, 2009) and is thereby ill-suited to address questions about change. The problems of "snapshot" cross-sectional research are well known, and the most serious problem relates to the limited capacity of drawing causal inferences. In addition,

*An Introduction to Intermediate and Advanced Statistical Analyses for Sport and Exercise Scientists*, First Edition.
Edited by Nikos Ntoumanis and Nicholas D. Myers.
© 2016 John Wiley & Sons, Ltd. Published 2016 by John Wiley & Sons, Ltd.
Companion website: www.wiley.com/go/ntoumanis/sport

many of the theories used to explain human behavior in sport and exercise psychology contain causal processes by including explanatory variables, mediators, and outcome variables. The use of these chains of events to explain human behavior implies that the processes involved take time to unfold. In cross-sectional data, however, these processes are assumed to be instantaneous (Selig & Preacher, 2009). More specifically, when applying models to cross-sectional data, researchers assume that the effects are instantaneous and that the magnitude of the effect is not dependent on the length of time between the measurements of the variables.

Studies using longitudinal data with multiple measurements and appropriate analytical frameworks and tools, on the other hand, have a much stronger platform for enhancing our understanding of the temporal and causal processes related to human behavior. Acknowledging the time aspect and the fact that most phenomena in psychological research (e.g., emotions, behaviors, and motivation) can and frequently do change (e.g., Schack & Hackfort, 2007), it should be of central interest to study the dynamics of change.

# A Theoretical Framework for the Study of Change

Baltes and Nesselroade (1979) proposed a framework for the study of change in human behavior and development. More specifically, they proposed five central aims with longitudinal research: (i) direct identification of within-person change, (ii) direct identification of between-person differences of within-person change, (iii) analysis of interrelationships of change, (iv) analysis of causes (determinants) of within-person change, and (v) analysis of causes (determinants) of between-person differences in within-person change. Together, these five aims illustrate the complexity of longitudinal research and particularly the necessity of measuring and modeling change at two distinct levels: the within-person and between-person levels (Hofer & Sliwinski, 2006). Whereas between-person refers to differences between persons, within-person refers to change within persons, how the individual changes, and in later steps, when and why the individual changes over time (Nesselroade & Ram, 2004). The distinction between within-person change and between-person differences is important, as it provides an opportunity to more fully understand how people change over time.

# Utility of the Method in Sport and Exercise Science

## Analysis of Change

Researchers have typically analyzed longitudinal data in sport and exercise psychology research with a variety of methods, such as analysis of variance (repeated measures ANOVA), multivariate analysis of variance (MANOVA), cross-lagged panel models (CLPM), multilevel modeling (MLM), and latent growth modeling (LGM). Longitudinal analyses can be categorized into three different groups based on the questions they can answer (Little, Bovaird, & Slegers, 2006). One group contains analyses that focus on differences between group means (e.g., repeated measures ANOVA).

A second group contains analyses that address change in between-person differences (i.e., reshuffling of individuals, e.g., CLPM). The third group includes analyses that can address true within-person changes (e.g., LGM). A recent review (Stenling, Ivarsson, & Lindwall, 2015) of analytical procedures used in sport and exercise psychology research (based on studies with longitudinal designs that were published in the 2010–2014 volumes of *Psychology of Sport and Exercise* and *Journal of Sport and Exercise Psychology*) showed that the most common analysis was repeated measures ANOVA, almost twice as common as any other statistical analysis.

Given that repeated measures ANOVA still appears to be the most common technique for analyzing longitudinal data in sport and exercise psychology, it is important to highlight that this procedure only lets us investigate differences between group means. An important note is that the investigation of differences between group means is not included in the framework of Baltes and Nesselroade (1979) for the study of change because researchers are often interested in more than just differences between group means. Another potential shortcoming is that ANOVA tests are based on an assumption of an equal variance and an equal correlation over time (McCall & Appelbaum, 1973). These assumptions are, however, highly unlikely to be met in empirical longitudinal data (McArdle, 2009).

To be able to analyze the data in a more extended way, a number of different structural equation modeling (SEM) techniques have been suggested (e.g., McArdle & Nesselroade, 2014). Two of them, which we will focus on in this chapter, are CLPM and LGM. In comparison to the repeated measures ANOVA, in a CLPM, the data do not need to fulfill the assumption of equal variance and equal correlation over time. Instead, by using a CLPM, it is possible to investigate between-person differences or covariance stability over time (McArdle, 2009).

Hertzog and Nesselroade (2003) highlighted some key limitations of the CLPM, which it shares with the repeated measures ANOVA: (i) it does not address two fundamental issues related to longitudinal research (within-person change and between-person differences in within-person change), (ii) it does not allow the researcher to use change in a construct as a cause or outcome variable in the model, and (iii) it does not explicitly target change (at least not within-person change) but rather predictions or between-person differences across time (controlling for baseline value) that may be seen as an indirect measure of change. Therefore, the CLPM is likely most useful when the variables under study do not exhibit large within-person change over time (Selig & Preacher, 2009). In a CLPM, the researcher assumes that the previous behavior is the best predictor of the present behavior, and therefore, the goal is to explain the leftover variability not explained by the autoregressive effects (Geiser, 2013).

When within-person change and between-person differences in within-person change are of primary interest, LGM should be used (cf. Baltes & Nesselroade, 1979). With LGM, it is possible to both estimate between-person variation in within-person change (slope variance) and average change (slope mean). Moreover, LGM provides several attractive features (Park & Schutz, 2005). First, the change can be modeled to take on several different forms, such as linear, quadratic, or cubic trajectories. Second, the model can account for measurement error. Third, the occasions of measurement do not need to be equally spaced. Fourth, predictors of change and/or correlates of change are easily implemented into the model. Fifth, partially missing data can be estimated, for example, with the full information maximum likelihood (FIML) function (Enders, 2010). Sixth, because SEM-based LGM have the same flexibility as other SEM models, a variety of extensions of the basic LGM are possible, such as multigroup analysis (see Chapter 6, this volume), change in multivariate latent factors, analysis with dichotomous or ordinal variables (Bollen & Curran, 2006), and growth mixture modeling (see Chapter 9, this volume).

# The Substantive Example

## Theoretical Background

In the substantive example, we highlight (i) the longitudinal associations of perceived sport competence (PSC) and general/global self-esteem (SE) in adolescents, (ii) within-person change in SE, and (iii) associations of within-person change in PSC and SE. Previous research in sport and exercise psychology has frequently highlighted the question of how individuals' levels of SE are associated with their perceived competence in specific domains (e.g., sport; Fox & Corbin, 1989; Lindwall & Aşçı, 2014; Lindwall, Aşçı, Palmeira, Fox, & Hagger, 2011). Also, a number of theoretical frameworks and models have been developed and examined that are linked to SE and PSC. For example, based on the structure of the proposed hierarchical models of the self (Shavelson, Hubner, & Stanton, 1976), it is hypothesized that involvement in specific behavior (such as sport) will influence general SE (at the apex) through PSC at the midlevel (e.g., Fox & Corbin, 1989). However, the opposite direction of effects is also possible (Harter, 2012); that is, a higher SE will lead to more positive perceptions of specific subdomains (e.g., sport competence), which will result in a greater likelihood of engaging in specific behavior (i.e., sport) that targets the specific self-perception (sport competence). Although previous work has demonstrated a clear link between SE and PSC, the majority of previous research has used cross-sectional data. Therefore, it is unclear up to this point whether the theoretically derived, and in previous work empirically supported, associations between SE and PSC also hold longitudinally. Linked to CLPM discussed previously, the question of direction of effects (what drives what) is relevant to pursue, as it is very much at the center of some of the theoretical models, frameworks, and hypotheses.

## The Data: Participants and Measurement

To examine the longitudinal associations of SE and PSC in the substantive example, we use data from a longitudinal cohort design study in Swedish adolescents. The main focus of the study was to examine psychosocial development in youths, with an emphasis on sport involvement (see Wagnsson, Augustsson, & Patriksson, 2013). Three waves of measurement ($T1$ = year 1, $T2$ = year 2, $T3$ = year 3) were used in the study, and the measurements were separated by 1 year. Data were collected each spring (2005–2007). The sample was based on a three-step randomly stratified sampling procedure. The total sample consisted of 1358 pupils, distributed almost equally over primary school ($n$ = 465), lower secondary school ($n$ = 439), and upper secondary school ($n$ = 454).

Informed consent was obtained from parents, teachers, and study participants. The participation rate was high, including 1174 participants at $T1$ (85%), 1152 at $T2$ (80%), and 1164 at $T3$ (80%). The mean baseline age of participants was 13.78 years (±2.40 years). Approximately 59% of the study participants were male and 41% were female (52% vs. 48% at 10–12 years, 55% vs. 45% at 13–15 years, and 66% vs. 34% at 16–18 years).

The main focus of the substantive example is to examine change in one of the variables in the study, SE, and the longitudinal relationships between two variables in the data, SE and PSC. A shortened six-item and a one-item-one-pole format of Harter's (1985) Self-Perception Profile for Children (SPPC) was used to assess SE (three items) (e.g., "I am happy with the way I am") and PSC (three items) (e.g., "I am very good at sports"). Participants responded on a five-point Likert scale, ranging from *I strongly disagree* (1) to *I strongly agree* (5).

All analyses were conducted with Mplus version 7.3 (Muthén & Muthén, 1998–2012), and we used the robust FIML estimator (MLR in Mplus).[1] Missing data were assumed to be missing at random (MAR), and therefore, we used the FIML estimation (Enders, 2010; see also Graham, 2009). In the longitudinal CFAs, in the CLPM, and in the second-order LGM, we used the default scale setting method in Mplus, the marker variable method, which fixes the loading of the first indicator of each latent factor to 1.0. There are other methods for scale setting available, such as the fixed factor method and the effects coding method, and these various scale setting methods are covered extensively in Little (2013). Model fit in SEM can be evaluated by looking at a combination of fit indices, and in the examples provided in this chapter, we present commonly used model fit measures. In Table 7.1, the chi-square ($\chi^2$), the comparative fit index (CFI), the root mean square error of approximation (RMSEA), and the standardized root mean square residual (SRMR) are presented for each model. All models in these examples displayed acceptable model fit; hence, we will not comment further on each model's fit. For elaborate discussions about model fit and model selection procedures (e.g., nested model comparisons), we refer readers to Little (2013), Marsh (2007), and West, Taylor, and Wu (2012). The Mplus data and input files (see Appendices 7.1–7.11) for all the estimated models can be found in the online supplemental material. Although Mplus was used to estimate these models, they can easily be estimated with other SEM software, such as R, AMOS, EQS, or LISREL (e.g., Byrne, 2012; Fox, Byrnes, Boker, & Neale, 2012).

# The Synergy

## CLPM

The CLPM or the autoregressive model is a popular method for analyzing longitudinal data (Little, Preacher, Selig, & Card, 2007). A simple path diagram of a two-wave CLPM is depicted in Figure 7.1. The main parameters of interest in the CLPM are the

---

[1] A variety of estimators is possible depending on the nature of the data. Besides the maximum likelihood-based estimators (such as the robust maximum likelihood estimator used in this chapter), weighted least squares and Bayesian estimation can, for example, also be applied.

Table 7.1 Model fit of the CLPM and LGM.

| CLPM | N | $\chi^{2a}$ | df | p value | CFI | RMSEA [LL, UL] | SRMR |
|---|---|---|---|---|---|---|---|
| 1a. Configural invariance | 1322 | 120.321 | 42 | 0.000 | 0.984 | 0.038 [0.030, 0.046] | 0.031 |
| 1b. Metric invariance | 1322 | 121.743 | 46 | 0.000 | 0.984 | 0.035 [0.028, 0.043] | 0.031 |
| 1c. Scalar invariance | 1322 | 129.619 | 50 | 0.000 | 0.983 | 0.035 [0.027, 0.042] | 0.032 |
| 1d. Cross-lagged panel model | 1322 | 129.618 | 50 | 0.000 | 0.983 | 0.035 [0.027, 0.042] | 0.032 |
| First-order LGM | | | | | | | |
| 2a. Unconditional | 1357 | 0.004 | 1 | 0.947 | 1.00 | 0.000 [0.000, 0.010] | 0.000 |
| 2b. Conditional, sex as TIC | 1350[b] | 1.336 | 2 | 0.513 | 1.00 | 0.000 [0.000, 0.048] | 0.008 |
| 2c. Unconditional, PSC as TVC | 1357 | 2.627 | 1 | 0.105 | 0.999 | 0.035 [0.000, 0.089] | 0.014 |
| 3. Parallel process model | 1357 | 17.940 | 4 | 0.001 | 0.995 | 0.051 [0.028, 0.076] | 0.013 |
| Second-order LGM | | | | | | | |
| 4a. Unconditional, configural invariance | 1357 | 14.443 | 16 | 0.566 | 1.00 | 0.000 [0.000, 0.023] | 0.012 |
| 4b. Unconditional, metric invariance | 1357 | 18.287 | 20 | 0.569 | 1.00 | 0.000 [0.000, 0.021] | 0.018 |
| 4c. Unconditional, scalar invariance | 1357 | 43.612 | 24 | 0.009 | 0.994 | 0.025 [0.012, 0.036] | 0.017 |

CLPM, cross-lagged panel model; LGM, latent growth model; SE, general/global self-esteem; PSC, perceived sport competence; TIC, time-invariant covariate; TVC, time-varying covariate.

[a] This is the scaled chi-square, which is the normal-theory chi-square statistic divided by a scaling correction to better approximate chi-square under nonnormality.

[b] Seven participants did not report sex and were therefore excluded from this analysis.

autoregressive and cross-lagged parameters. The autoregressive paths ($\beta_{3,1}$ and $\beta_{4,2}$ in Figure 7.1) are illustrated by the paths connecting a variable at time point 1 ($T1$) with itself at time point 2 ($T2$). The cross-lagged paths ($\beta_{3,2}$ and $\beta_{4,1}$ in Figure 7.1) are cross-time linkages connecting one construct with another construct over time. Any other effects leading to the same construct are controlled for; for example, the cross-lagged effect between variable $X$ at $T1$ and $Y$ at $T2$ is the unique effect of $X$ at $T1$ on $Y$ at $T2$ while controlling for the autoregressive effect between variable $Y$ at $T1$ and variable $Y$ at $T2$ (Little, 2013).

Different types of effects can be examined in a CLPM, such as stability, stationary effects, temporal causality, and reciprocal effects (Cole & Maxwell, 2003). Stability refers to the autoregressive effects, that is, how much change in individual differences occurs within a construct from one time point to another. Another way to explain the stability coefficient is "the degree to which there is a reshuffling of individuals standing on the measured construct" (Selig & Preacher, 2009, p. 149). A large coefficient indicates a small change in individual differences (i.e., small change in rank order). Stationary effects refer to the stability in the effect one variable has on another variable between different time points (e.g., $T1 \rightarrow T2$ vs. $T2 \rightarrow T3$). If the two effects are similar, the overall effect is referred to as stationary. However, the effect can also become larger or more pronounced over time or decrease or diminish over time. Temporal causality (i.e., the cross-lagged effect) refers to the effect of one variable at $T1$ on another variable at $T2$ and corresponds to the question of direction of effects (what drives what). In Figure 7.1, this would, for example, refer to the effect of SE at $T1$ on PSC at $T2$ ($\beta_{3,2}$). Finally, reciprocal effects refer to the effect of variable $X$ at $T1$ on $Y$ at $T2$ in combination with the effect of $Y$ at $T1$ on $X$ at $T2$. This could be illustrated in Figure 7.1 by the effect of SE at $T1$ on PSC at $T2$ ($\beta_{3,2}$) and the effect of PSC at $T1$ on SE at $T2$ ($\beta_{4,1}$).

## CLPM Example

In the substantive example, we examined the relationship between PSC and SE across two time points ($T1$ and $T2$) separated by 1 year. This example illustrates a multiple indicator latent variable approach.[2] As seen in Figure 7.1, each variable at $T1$ was allowed to predict itself (autoregressive effect/stability) and the other variable at $T2$ (cross-lagged effect). The model in Figure 7.1 consists of two exogenous variables (independent variables explained by variables not included in the model), PSC at $T1$ and SE at $T1$, and two endogenous variables (dependent variables predicted by

---

[2] One option is to use a manifest path model without multiple indicators; and although these are quite common in psychology, they have been criticized due to the lack of correction for measurement error (Cole & Preacher, 2014). Cole and Preacher showed that uncorrected measurement error in manifest path analysis can lead to several problems: (i) most path coefficients will be over- or underestimated when measurement error is present in the data; (ii) power is diminished and invalid models may not be rejected when extensive measurement error is present; (iii) valid models can appear invalid even when small measurement error is present in the data; (iv) when different parts of the model contain differential measurement error, it can change the substantive conclusions derived from the manifest path analysis; and (v) all of these problems become more severe in complex models.

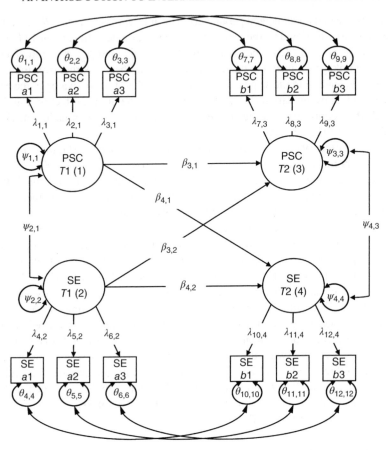

*Figure 7.1   A two-wave CLPM linking PSC and SE across time. The $\beta$ symbol represents regression coefficients and the $\psi$ symbol represents the (residual) variance of a latent construct or the (residual) covariance between two latent constructs. The $\lambda$ symbol is the estimated loading of an indicator on a latent construct, and the $\theta$ symbol is the (residual) variance or (residual) covariance between two indicators.*

other variables in the model), PSC at $T2$ and SE at $T2$. Each latent variable consists of three observed indicators measured at two time points. We also hypothesized occasion-specific associations as illustrated by the covariance/correlation ($\psi_{2,1}$ and $\psi_{4,3}$ in Figure 7.1) between variables at each time point (this covariance is channeled through the residual variances at $T2$). The interpretation of a positive occasion-specific association is that adolescents reporting higher levels of PSC also reports higher levels of SE at the same time point. A negative association would indicate that adolescents with higher levels of PSC report lower levels of SE and vice versa. Prior to specifying the structural model, we established strong/scalar measurement invariance in the measurement model by imposing equality constraints over time on the factor loadings and indicator intercepts. We retained the imposed equality constraints

Table 7.2    Estimates from the CLPM.

| | Model 1d: CLPM | | |
| --- | --- | --- | --- |
| | Estimate | SE | p value |
| Autoregressive paths[a] | | | |
| SET1 → SET2 | 0.643 | 0.041 | 0.000 |
| PSCT1 → PSCT2 | 0.884 | 0.025 | 0.000 |
| Cross-lagged paths[a] | | | |
| SET1 → PSCT2 | −0.042 | 0.034 | 0.220 |
| PSCT1 → SET2 | 0.131 | 0.039 | 0.001 |
| Correlations | | | |
| SET1 ↔ PSCT1 | 0.511 | 0.030 | 0.000 |
| SET2 ↔ PSCT2 | 0.468 | 0.059 | 0.000 |
| | $R^2$ | | |
| SET2 | 0.516 | | |
| PSCT2 | 0.744 | | |

[a] Standardized coefficients.

on factor loadings and intercepts in the structural model. Establishing measurement invariance across time is important because it demonstrates that the participants interpret the individual questions and the underlying latent construct in the same way at each time point (see Chapter 6, this volume, for more information on invariance testing).[3] Furthermore, to account for indicator-specific effects over time, each indictor was allowed to correlate over time. Little (2013) argued that these correlations are always justifiable and should only be excluded after careful consideration. The reason is that indicator-specific variance that is reliable is likely to correlate with itself over time.

As displayed in Table 7.2, the autoregressive effect was statistically significant and quite strong for PSC ($\beta = 0.884$), indicating a relatively small degree of reshuffling of individuals' rank order on that variable from $T1$ to $T2$. The autoregressive effect for SE was also statistically significant but somewhat weaker ($\beta = 0.643$) compared to PSC, indicating a higher degree of reshuffling of individuals' rank order on this variable from $T1$ to $T2$. These results indicate that between-person differences in these two variables were quite stable over 1 year, but there was additional variance to be explained by other variables. This additional variance could, at least partially, be explained by the cross-lagged effects included in the model. As displayed in Table 7.2, SE at $T1$ had a nonsignificant negative effect on PSC at $T2$ ($\beta = -0.042$), and PSC at

[3] A key feature of latent variable analysis is the possibility to examine measurement invariance of parameters across groups and/or time (Meredith, 1993; Widaman, Ferrer, & Conger, 2010). An elaborate discussion about the various levels of measurement invariance is beyond the scope of this chapter (see Chapter 6 this volume; Little, 2013); generally, strong/scalar invariance (invariant factor loadings and item intercepts) is recommended for group or time comparisons. However, the required level of measurement invariance may differ depending on the research question.

*T*1 had a statistically significant and positive effect on SE at *T*2 ($\beta$ = 0.131). These effects were relatively small compared to the autoregressive effects and only explained a small amount of the between-person differences at *T*2. This trend, with the autoregressive effects explaining the majority of the variance and the cross-lagged effects explaining only a small part, seems to be a common finding in CLPM papers. The interpretation of the latter cross-lagged effect is that adolescents who reported higher levels of PSC at *T*1 (compared to others) also reported higher SE at *T*2 1 year later (compared to others), even when prior level of SE is controlled for. The occasion-specific associations indicate that participants reporting higher levels of PSC at each time point also reported higher levels of SE at each time point. The model explained 51.6% of the variance in SE at *T*2 and 74.4% of the variance in PSC at *T*2.

Although in this example we only included two time points, the CLPM can easily be extended in a variety of ways, for example, with additional time points (McArdle, 2009) or multiple groups (see Chapter 6 this volume) or can be used to examine longitudinal mediation processes (Cole & Maxwell, 2003; Selig & Preacher, 2009).

## Latent Growth Modeling

When faced with data measured on at least three repeated occasions, the researcher's options for studying true individual change increases. One useful and very flexible approach for the study of change over time is the LGM.[4] With LGM, it is possible to examine individuals' growth trajectories where the latent growth factors are interpreted as individual differences in attributes of growth trajectories over time (McArdle, 1988). Two interesting attributes of growth trajectories are rates of change, referred to as the *slope*, and initial status, called the *intercept*. The slope and intercept each have mean and variance values that correspond to different levels of analysis. The means correspond to group-level information, and the variances correspond to individual differences (Duncan & Duncan, 2004). The means can be viewed as fixed effects where all individuals' trajectories in the sample have been pooled together and the variances can be seen as random effects representing the individual trajectories around the group mean (Chou, Bentler, & Pentz, 1998).

The intercept and slope factors are latent factors (i.e., are not directly observed) in the LGM. An important advantage of LGM in SEM is that the slope and intercept can be used not only as primary outcome variables but also as any other latent variables in SEM, for example, as predictors or can be predicted by other variables (Duncan & Duncan, 2004). The intercept mean can be defined as the average initial status of the outcome variable, and the intercept variance corresponds to individual differences around the mean. Important to note is that what is defined as initial status is often an arbitrary choice made by the researcher (Preacher, Wichman, MacCallum, & Briggs, 2008). Initial status is often defined as the first measurement point in the

---

study. However, the placement of the intercept can be at any of the measurement points and should be placed on a meaningful occasion of measurement (Biesanz, Deeb-Sossa, Papadakis, Bollen, & Curran, 2004). The placement of the intercept partly determines the choice in time where the intercept mean, variance, and the intercept–slope covariance are interpreted (Rogosa & Willett, 1985), and the placement may also influence estimates in LGM, for example, the covariance between the intercept and slope (Biesanz et al., 2004). As Little (2013, p. 256) pointed out, it is important to keep in mind "that the intercept is defined by the location of the 0 in the specification of the slope factor."

The slope mean can be defined as the average rate of change in the outcome variable per unit change in time, and the slope variance corresponds to individual deviations from the group mean (i.e., heterogeneity in growth trajectories). The scaling of time (i.e., parameterization of the slope) should, as the placement of the intercept, be chosen based on interpretability and substantive meaning (Biesanz et al., 2004). For example, data collected yearly can be defined as 0, 1, and 2, where 0 represents the first occasion, 1 represents the second occasion, and 2 represents the third occasion. We could, however, choose to define the slope as 0, 12, and 24, if it made more sense to code in months than years; or, if data were collected in uneven intervals, we could code time according to that—for example, 0, 1, 2, 4, and 8—if data were collected over 8 months with an increasing interval between occasions. Alternatively, if our primary interest was to understand effects and relationships at the end of the assessed growth process (e.g., the end of an intervention period), we could place the origin of time (i.e., the intercept) at the last measurement point (e.g., define the slope as −8, −4, −2, −1, and 0). For more elaborate discussions about time scaling and examples of various ways to code time, see Biesanz et al. (2004), Bollen and Curran (2006), and Little (2013).

## LGM Example

The same dataset utilized in the CLPM example was used to illustrate an unconditional linear LGM and various extensions thereof. In this example, we will illustrate analyses that correspond to the following questions: (i) What is the mean rate of change in SE (model 2a)? The slope's mean is used to determine the mean rate of change. (ii) Does significant between-person variability exist around the mean rate of change in SE (model 2a)? This is examined with the variance of the slope. (iii) Does sex, as a time-invariant covariate, predict/account for the between-person variability in mean rate of change in SE (model 2b)? This is illustrated by sex as a predictor of the slope factor (coefficient $\beta_2$ in Figure 7.2b). (iv) Does PSC, as a time-varying covariate (TVC), have occasion-specific effects on SE (model 2c)? These occasion-specific effects are illustrated by the coefficients $\beta_1$, $\beta_2$, and $\beta_3$ in Figure 7.2c. (v) Does change over time in SE relate to change over time in PSC (model 3)? This is determined by the covariance/correlation between the slope factors ($\psi_{4,2}$ in Figure 7.3). We will estimate a series of LGM that corresponds to each of these research questions and also illustrate how to estimate a multiple indicator LGM, also known as a second-order LGM (model 4).

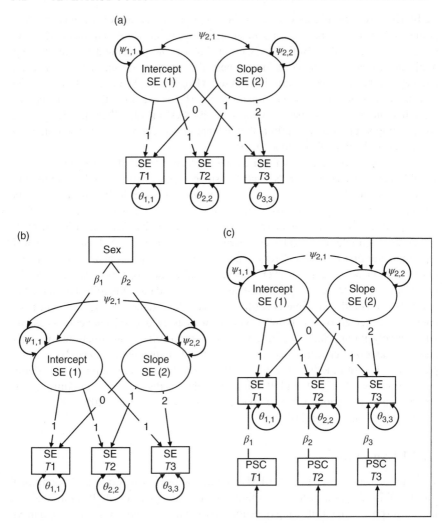

*Figure 7.2   (a) Unconditional LGM, (b) conditional LGM with sex as predictor of the intercept and slope factors, and (c) unconditional LGM with PSC as time-varying covariate (TVC) at each time point. All covariances between slope factors, intercept factors, and TVC variables were estimated in model 2c. The β symbol represents regression coefficients, and the ψ symbol represents the (residual) variance of a latent construct or the (residual) covariance between two latent constructs. The θ symbol is the (residual) variance or (residual) covariance between two indicators.*

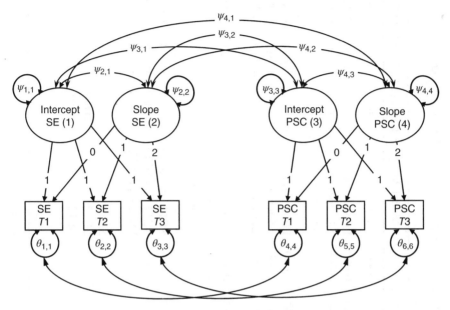

*Figure 7.3    Parallel process LGM. The ψ symbol represents the (residual) variance of a latent construct or the (residual) covariance between two latent constructs. The θ symbol is the (residual) variance or (residual) covariance between two indicators.*

## Model 2a: Unconditional LGM

As a first step, we estimated an unconditional LGM[5] for SE. The basic setup for the unconditional LGM is depicted in Figure 7.2a. Manifest subscale scores were used as indicators at each time point, and we estimated a linear growth process[6] across the 3 years. We also estimated a slope factor and an intercept factor. The covariance/correlation between the intercept and slope factors represents the relationship between initial status and rate of change in SE. The results of the unconditional LGM are summarized in Table 7.3. There was a negative nonsignificant average rate of change in SE (−0.014) across the 3 years, and there were between-person differences in the rate of change, as indicated by the statistically significant slope variance in SE (0.060). The

---

[5] The unconditional LGM was specified as a linear growth process (slope specified as 0, 1, and 2). Other specifications are possible for the unconditional LGM when examining the growth process. Besides the commonly used linear and quadratic specifications, the researcher can, for example, specify the first and second time point as 0 and 1 and freely estimate the remaining time points (referred to as the latent basis model), which would scale the slope factor as the amount of change between time point 1 and time point 2. See Little (2013) and Ram and Grimm (2007) for more information about LGM specifications.

[6] It is possible to examine different shapes of the growth processes in LGM. Four time points allow for estimation of a quadratic curve and five time points a cubic curve, and various types of nonlinear and piecewise trajectories are also possible to estimate. These different shapes of growth trajectories are extensively covered in Bollen and Curran (2006), Little (2013), and Ram and Grimm (2007).

Table 7.3 Estimates from the unconditional LGM (2a), conditional LGM (2b), and unconditional LGM with time-varying covariate (2c).

| | Model 2a: unconditional LGM | | | | Model 2b: conditional LGM | | | | Model 2c: unconditional LGM (PSC TVC) | | |
|---|---|---|---|---|---|---|---|---|---|---|---|
| | Estimate | SE | p value | | Estimate | SE | p value | | Estimate | SE | p value |
| Means | | | | Intercepts | | | | Means | | | |
| I (intercept) | 3.751 | 0.023 | 0.000 | I (intercept) | 3.377 | 0.080 | 0.000 | I (intercept) | 3.126 | 0.166 | 0.000 |
| S (slope) | −0.014 | 0.012 | 0.253 | S (slope) | −0.143 | 0.043 | 0.001 | S (slope) | −0.143 | 0.139 | 0.304 |
| Variances | | | | Residual variances | | | | Variances | | | |
| I (intercept) | 0.439 | 0.037 | 0.000 | I (intercept) | 0.430 | 0.037 | 0.000 | I (intercept) | 0.347 | 0.034 | 0.000 |
| S (slope) | 0.060 | 0.017 | 0.001 | S (slope) | 0.062 | 0.017 | 0.000 | S (slope) | 0.047 | 0.016 | 0.003 |
| Covariance of I and S | −0.028 | 0.019 | 0.145 | Covariance of I and S | −0.036 | 0.019 | 0.057 | Covariance of I and S | −0.031 | 0.019 | 0.098 |
| Correlation of I and S | −0.172 | 0.094 | 0.067 | Correlation of I and S | −0.220 | 0.087 | 0.011 | Correlation of I and S | −0.241 | 0.107 | 0.024 |
| | | | | Covariate regressions[a] | | | | Covariate regressions[a] | | | |
| | | | | I on sex | 0.176 | 0.034 | 0.000 | SET1 on PSCT1 | 0.279 | 0.074 | 0.000 |
| | | | | S on sex | 0.161 | 0.052 | 0.002 | SET2 on PSCT2 | 0.342 | 0.046 | 0.000 |
| | | | | | | | | SET3 on PSCT3 | 0.407 | 0.083 | 0.000 |
| | $R^2$ | | | | $R^2$ | | | | $R^2$ | | |
| SET1 | 0.643 | | | SET1 | 0.651 | | | SET1 | 0.641 | | |
| SET2 | 0.632 | | | SET2 | 0.629 | | | SET2 | 0.661 | | |
| SET3 | 0.756 | | | SET3 | 0.767 | | | SET3 | 0.759 | | |
| | | | | I (intercept) | 0.031 | | | | | | |
| | | | | S (slope) | 0.026 | | | | | | |

*Note:* All covariances between slope factors, intercept factors, and TVC variables were estimated in model 2c.

[a] Standardized coefficients.

between-person differences in the rate of change indicate that there was heterogeneity in the sample in regard to how the adolescents in the sample changed over time. The variance of the intercept indicates that there were statistically significant between-person differences in the initial status of SE (0.439). The correlation between the intercept and slope was nonsignificant and negative (−0.172). The negative slope means that a higher initial status of SE was weakly related to a larger decrease over time. The intercept and slope factors explained 64.3, 63.2, and 75.6% of the variance in SE across $T1$, $T2$, and $T3$, respectively. The interpretation of the small average rate of change is that the participants' SE remained relatively stable across the three years. However, the statistically significant variance for both intercept and slope suggests that there are between-person differences in terms of initial status SE as well as in change in SE.

## Model 2b: Conditional LGM

In the unconditional model (2a), we discovered that there were between-person differences in the participating adolescents' initial status and rate of change in SE. The between-person variance in the intercept and slope can be interpreted as unexplained variance. To examine this unexplained variance further, we can include predictors that may account for the unexplained variance in the random variables (Preacher et al., 2008). When predictors are introduced in a LGM, the model is sometimes referred to as a conditional LGM (Bollen & Curran, 2006). In this example, we only included one variable, sex, as a predictor of the between-person differences. However, any number of variables could be included as predictors to explain between-person variability. Such variables are referred to as time-invariant covariates because they are assumed to remain constant over time (Bollen & Curran, 2006). The setup for this model is depicted in Figure 7.2b. The conditional LGM is identical to the unconditional model, with the exception that sex is included as an exogenous variable that predicts the intercept and slope factors. The results are summarized in Table 7.3. Sex was a positive predictor of the intercept ($\beta = 0.176$) and slope ($\beta = 0.161$) factors for SE. Sex was coded as 1 = female and 2 = male. Consequently, the interpretation of the positive coefficients is that males reported higher initial status of SE and that they also reported a smaller decline over time compared to females. The positive effect of sex on the slope indicates that higher values in sex (2 instead of 1) are related to higher values in the slope. As the average slope (change) factor was negative (−0.014), indicating an average weak decline in the sample, higher slope values, in this case, refer to less decline (which, from a substantive point of view, is positive for males, who were coded as 2).

The intercept and slope factors explained 64.3, 63.2, and 75.6% of the variance in SE across $T1$, $T2$, and $T3$, respectively, whereas sex explained 3.1 and 2.6% of the variance in the intercept and slope factors, respectively.

## Model 2c: Unconditional LGM with TVCs

It is also possible to include TVCs in an LGM. TVCs can be used to examine occasion-specific effects on the outcome variable (Bollen & Curran, 2006). The

LGM with a TVC is depicted in Figure 7.2c. We used PSC as an exogenous TVC that predicts SE at each time point to illustrate this analytical approach. In this example, PSC is used to predict occasion-specific deviations in the outcome variables, in this case SE, and the effect of PSC may differ across time, but not across individuals (Preacher et al., 2008). This model reflects the growth in the outcome variable while controlling for the occasion-specific effect of the TVC or the opposite, the time-specific effect of the TVC on the outcome variable while controlling for the influence of the growth process (Bollen & Curran, 2006). The results for this model are summarized in Table 7.3. The occasion-specific effects are displayed at the bottom of Table 7.3, and these ranged from 0.279 to 0.407, indicating that PSC was positively related to SE at each time point after controlling for the between-person differences accounted for by the intercept and slope factors. The positive occasion-specific effects indicate that participants reporting higher levels of PSC at each time point also reported higher levels of SE at each time point. The intercept factor, slope factor, and the TVC explained 64.1, 66.1, and 75.9% of the variance in SE across $T1$, $T2$, and $T3$, respectively.

## Model 3: Parallel Process LGM

Models 2a–2c have included a single growth process, but it is also possible to estimate several growth processes simultaneously and examine if and how these change processes are related over time. This type of model is sometime referred to as a parallel process LGM (Cheong, MacKinnon, & Khoo, 2003), a multivariate LGM (Bollen & Curran, 2006), or an associative LGM (Duncan & Duncan, 2004). A simple parallel process model consists of two LGMs simultaneously estimated in a single model (Figure 7.3). Covariances/correlations are estimated between the intercept and slope factors, and residual covariances/correlations are estimated between the occasion-specific indicators. As seen in Table 7.4, there was a statistically significant and positive correlation between initial status in PSC and SE (0.478), meaning that those reporting higher levels of PSC at $T1$ also reported higher levels of SE at $T1$. The slope–slope correlation between PSC and SE was positive (0.407) and statistically significant. In this example, with negative mean slopes, the interpretation is that adolescents with a larger decrease in PSC over time also had a larger decrease in SE over time. In this model, we also estimated correlations between the occasion-specific item residuals of PSC and SE. These are correlations between occasion-specific deviations from the expected curve and reflect whether PSC and SE travel together over time (Sliwinski & Mogle, 2008). The within-person correlations were all weak and positive, indicating that persons above the expected level on PSC at each time point were also above the expected level on SE at each time point. The intercept and slope factors explained between 63.8 and 85.5% of the variance in SE and PSC across $T1$, $T2$, and $T3$.

The parallel process model can be extended in various ways. We could, for example, specify the slope of PSC as a predictor of the slope of SE. Such specification does, however, imply a hypothesis about a causal relationship between these variables, not merely a relationship (Preacher et al., 2008). The basic parallel process

Table 7.4    Estimates from the parallel process LGM.

| Model 3: parallel process model | | | |
|---|---|---|---|
| Means | Estimate | SE | $p$ value |
| IPSC (intercept) | 2.979 | 0.031 | 0.000 |
| SPSC (slope) | −0.011 | 0.013 | 0.408 |
| ISE (intercept) | 3.747 | 0.023 | 0.000 |
| SSE (slope) | −0.011 | 0.012 | 0.356 |
| Variances | | | |
| IPSC (intercept) | 0.983 | 0.049 | 0.000 |
| SPSC (slope) | 0.081 | 0.023 | 0.000 |
| ISE (intercept) | 0.437 | 0.037 | 0.000 |
| SSE (slope) | 0.057 | 0.017 | 0.001 |
| Covariances | | | |
| IPSC ↔ SPSC | −0.031 | 0.025 | 0.213 |
| ISE ↔ SSE | −0.026 | 0.019 | 0.166 |
| IPSC ↔ ISE | 0.313 | 0.035 | 0.000 |
| SPSC ↔ SSE | 0.028 | 0.014 | 0.053 |
| IPSC ↔ SSE | 0.012 | 0.019 | 0.535 |
| ISE ↔ SPSC | −0.012 | 0.017 | 0.499 |
| Correlations | | | |
| IPSC ↔ SPSC | −0.061 | 0.086 | 0.478 |
| ISE ↔ SSE | −0.166 | 0.096 | 0.085 |
| IPSC ↔ ISE | 0.478 | 0.043 | 0.000 |
| SPSC ↔ SSE | 0.407 | 0.176 | 0.021 |
| IPSC ↔ SSE | 0.050 | 0.082 | 0.544 |
| ISE ↔ SPSC | −0.061 | 0.086 | 0.478 |
| Within-person residual covariances | | | |
| PSCT1 ↔ SET1 | 0.032 | 0.029 | 0.264 |
| PSCT2 ↔ SET2 | 0.075 | 0.014 | 0.000 |
| PSCT3 ↔ SET3 | 0.043 | 0.028 | 0.123 |
| Within-person residual correlations | | | |
| PSCT1 ↔ SET1 | 0.132 | 0.109 | 0.228 |
| PSCT2 ↔ SET2 | 0.287 | 0.047 | 0.000 |
| PSCT3 ↔ SET3 | 0.221 | 0.126 | 0.080 |
| | $R^2$ | | |
| SET1 | 0.638 | | |
| SET2 | 0.634 | | |
| SET3 | 0.748 | | |
| PSCT1 | 0.807 | | |
| PSCT2 | 0.789 | | |
| PSCT3 | 0.855 | | |

model could also be extended by including time-invariant covariates or TVCs (as described in model 2b and model 2c), mediational processes (e.g., Selig & Preacher, 2009), or more than two growth processes.

## Model 4: Second-Order LGM

Models 2 and 3 have been first-order LGM and have not taken advantage of one of the most useful features of SEM, namely, the use of multiple indicators (Preacher et al., 2008). To account for measurement error in LGM, multiple indicators can be included in the model, and a second-order LGM can be specified (Bollen & Curran, 2006; Geiser, Keller, & Lockhart, 2013; McArdle, 1988). Applications of second-order LGMs are not very common, despite many known advantages over first-order LGMs. Geiser et al. (2013) summarized some of the most important strengths of second-order LGMs: (i) they allow for a proper separation of measurement error from true trait change and reliable time-specific variance, (ii) they allow for testing invariance over time, (iii) they have greater statistical power to detect between-person differences in change, and (iv) their use of multiple indicators allows for the isolation of indicator-specific effects from shared construct variance.

Figure 7.4 illustrates an unconditional second-order LGM for SE; the estimates for this model are presented in Table 7.5. We examined measurement invariance (see Chapter 6 in this volume) over time by comparing increasingly restricted models (see Table 7.5; models 4a–4c), where equality constraints were imposed on the factor loadings (model 4b) and the indicator intercepts (model 4c). The interpretation of the parameters is the same as for the first-order LGM. In model 4c, we found a statistically significant between-person intercept variance (0.506); that is, adolescents vary in their initial status of SE at $T1$. In comparison to the first-order LGM (model 2a), the intercept variance is slightly larger in the second-order LGM. This illustrates why separating measurement error from the true score is beneficial. The slope mean was nonsignificant and negative (−0.023), and there were between-person differences in the individual trajectories over time as indicated by the statistically significant slope variance (0.063). The intercept and slope factors explained 76.8, 74.0, and 81.7% of the variance in the latent SE variables across $T1$, $T2$, and $T3$, respectively.

In the synergy, we provided examples of CLPM and LGM and variations of these models. An important issue for the applied researcher is how to write up the results from a CLPM and LGM in a research report. To our knowledge, there are no established standards for this. There are, however, several sources that offer useful guidelines regarding how to write up results from more specific applications of SEM, such as the CLPM and LGM. Boomsma, Hoyle, and Panter (2012) provide an overview of important considerations when writing up the results from various SEM applications, and Jackson (2010) provides guidelines specifically for LGM. These two sources and other references in this chapter, particularly those given in the summary, provide a good starting point for the applied researcher.

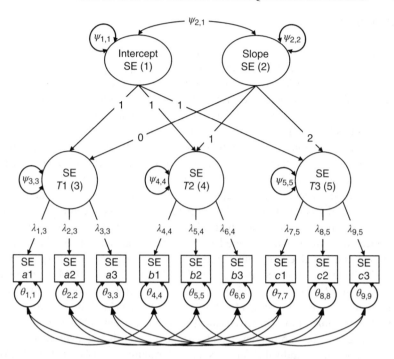

*Figure 7.4   Unconditional second-order LGM. The $\psi$ symbol represents the (resid-ual) variance of a latent construct or the (residual) covariance between two latent constructs. The $\lambda$ symbol represents the estimated loading of an indicator on a latent construct, and the $\theta$ symbol is the (residual) variance or (residual) covariance between two indicators.*

Table 7.5     Estimates from the second-order unconditional LGM.

| Model 4c: unconditional second-order LGM | | | |
|---|---|---|---|
| Means | Estimate | SE | $p$ value |
| I (intercept) | 3.823 | 0.026 | 0.000 |
| S (slope) | −0.011 | 0.014 | 0.449 |
| Variances | | | |
| I (intercept) | 0.506 | 0.049 | 0.000 |
| S (slope) | 0.063 | 0.022 | 0.005 |
| Covariance of I and S | −0.023 | 0.024 | 0.335 |
| Correlation of I and S | −0.126 | 0.115 | 0.273 |
| | $R^2$ | | |
| SET1 | 0.768 | | |
| SET2 | 0.740 | | |
| SET3 | 0.817 | | |

# Summary

In this chapter, we have described the basics of CLPM and LGM and illustrated how to perform and interpret these analyses with an example from the domain of sport and exercise psychology. Despite the usefulness of these models, they appear to be underutilized tools in sport and exercise psychology (Stenling et al., 2015). When it comes to analyses of longitudinal data, SEM-based approaches, such as those presented in this chapter, are powerful tools that can provide researchers with answers to interesting questions regarding between-person differences and within-person changes. Examples of studies in sport and exercise psychology utilizing the CLPM can be found in Marsh, Chanal, and Sarrazin (2006), who examined the reciprocal effects between physical self-concept and gymnastics performance in adolescents, and the study of Gerber et al. (2015) on the relationships between perceived stress, vigorous exercise, and exercise self-regulation. Gerber et al. also specified a latent difference score model (not covered in the present chapter; see McArdle, 2009), which makes it possible to examine correlations of within-person changes over time even when only two time points are available. An example of LGM is provided in Ivarsson et al. (2015), who examined well-being trajectories among Swedish youth academy football players using a factor-of-curves model (McArdle, 1988). Ivarsson et al. also examined how perceived talent development environment could predict these young athletes' initial level and change in well-being over time. Finally, Ivarsson, Johnson, Lindwall, Gustafsson, and Altemyr (2014) used an LGM to examine how initial level and change in psychosocial stress, measured weekly for 10 weeks, predicted injury occurrence among elite junior football players.

These aforementioned studies illustrate the utility of CLPM and LGM in sport and exercise psychology, various extensions of these methods, and how they can be used to address interesting research questions. There are also other extensions of these models not covered in the present chapter, for example, the autoregressive latent trajectory (ALT) model, which is a combination of the CLPM and LGM (Bollen & Curran, 2006). The ALT model makes it possible to simultaneously estimate autoregressive paths and cross-lagged paths from the CLPM along with intercept and slope factors from the LGM. Further extensions of these models are SEM-based models with latent change scores (McArdle, 2009; McArdle & Nesselroade, 2014). These newer SEM-based latent change score models open up possibilities to address questions regarding dynamic changes over time that correspond nicely to the original aims of longitudinal research, as posed by Baltes and Nesselroade (1979) regarding within-person changes.

Although these methods can aid researchers when addressing complex questions, it is important to remember that they are statistical tools that help us understand empirical phenomenon. To interpret and discuss the meaningfulness of the results provided by these tools is, therefore, always in the hand of the researcher. Related to this, we want to highlight important, but often overlooked, components when conducting longitudinal research, namely, the integration of the theoretical model of change, temporal design, and statistical model (Collins, 2006; see also Timmons & Preacher, 2015). In this chapter, we assumed that the models we estimated were correctly specified in terms of the change processes and temporal design (i.e., spacing of measurement intervals). It is rare, however, that researchers justify the choice of change process (e.g., linear, quadratic, cubic, irregular up and down) and particularly the spacing of measurement intervals (Timmons & Preacher, 2015). Whether the chosen interval is correct or the theoretically justified is seldom discussed; the chosen intervals are often derived from practical reasons rather than theoretical reasons. An elaborate discussion about these issues is beyond the scope of this chapter. However, we encourage researchers who engage in longitudinal research to pay as much attention to these aspects (theory of change and temporal design) as they do to other design issues and choice of statistical model. Collins (2006) and Timmons and Preacher (2015) illustrate the importance of these issues, and McArdle (2009, p. 601) argued that any repeated measures analysis should start by asking "What is your model for change?" and not "What is your data collection design?" or "What computer program can you use?"

Statistical models are simplified representations of a very complex reality, and we as researchers try to capture highly complex phenomenon with these models (e.g., Kass, 2011). As previously mentioned, repeated measures ANOVA seems to be the most utilized statistical tool in sport and exercise psychology for analyzing longitudinal data. ANOVAs, however, do not address even the most basic aim (direct identification of within-person change) in Baltes and Nesselroade's (1979) framework for longitudinal research. ANOVAs rely on certain statistical assumptions, and the inferences from such analyses are limited by the accuracy of those statistical assumptions (McArdle, 2009). In addition, SEM offers a powerful tool that researchers can use to obtain results typically captured through ANOVA/MANOVA/ANCOVA, for example, via multigroup analyses (see Chapter 6, this volume; McArdle, 2009). Finally, a useful model can be defined as a model that makes sense, both from a statistical and a substantive point of view. The development of SEM-based approaches for analyzing longitudinal data (e.g., McArdle, 2009) provides exciting possibilities for researchers to directly address questions of (within-person) change that more accurately reflect the process-based theories used to explain human behavior.

# References

Baltes, P. B., & Nesselroade, J. R. (1979). History and rationale of longitudinal research. In J. R. Nesselroade & P. B. Baltes (Eds.), *Longitudinal research in the study of behavior and development* (pp. 1–39). New York, NY: Academic Press.

Biesanz, J. C., Deeb-Sossa, N., Papadakis, A. A., Bollen, K. A., & Curran, P. J. (2004). The role of coding time in estimating and interpreting growth curve models. *Psychological Methods, 9*, 30–52.

Bollen, K. A., & Curran, P. J. (2006). *Latent curve models: A structural equation perspective.* Hoboken, NJ: John Wiley & Sons, Inc.

Boomsma, A., Hoyle, R. H., & Panter, A. T. (2012). The structural equation modeling research report. In R. H. Hoyle (Ed.), *Handbook of structural equation modeling* (pp. 341–360). New York, NY: Guilford Press.

Byrne, B. (2012). Choosing structural equation modeling computer software: Snapshots of LISREL, EQS, Amos, and Mplus. In R. H. Hoyle (Ed.), *Handbook of structural equation modeling* (pp. 307–324). New York, NY: Guilford Press.

Cheong, J., MacKinnon, D. P., & Khoo, S. T. (2003). Investigation of mediational processes using parallel process latent growth curve modeling. *Structural Equation Modeling: A Multidisciplinary Journal, 10,* 238–262.

Chou, C. P., Bentler, P. M., & Pentz, M. A. (1998). Comparisons of two statistical approaches to study growth curves: The multilevel model and the latent curve analysis. *Structural Equation Modeling: A Multidisciplinary Journal, 5,* 247–266.

Cole, D. A., & Maxwell, S. E. (2003). Testing mediational models with longitudinal data: Questions and tips in the use of structural equation modeling. *Journal of Abnormal Psychology, 112,* 558–577.

Cole, D. A., & Preacher, K. J. (2014). Manifest variable path analysis: Potentially serious and misleading consequences due to uncorrected measurement error. *Psychological Methods, 19,* 300–315.

Collins, L. M. (2006). Analysis of longitudinal data: The integration of theoretical model, temporal design, and statistical model. *Annual Review of Psychology, 57,* 505–528.

Duncan, T. E., & Duncan, S. C. (2004). An introduction to latent growth curve modeling. *Behavior Therapy, 35,* 333–363.

Enders, C. K. (2010). *Applied missing data analysis.* New York, NY: Guilford Press.

Fox, J., Byrnes, J. E., Boker, S, & Neale, M. C. (2012). Structural equation modeling in R with the sem and OpenMx package. In R. H. Hoyle (Ed.), *Handbook of structural equation modeling* (pp. 325–340). New York, NY: Guilford Press.

Fox, K. R., & Corbin, C. B. (1989). The physical self-perception profile: Development and preliminary validation. *Journal of Sport and Exercise Psychology, 11,* 408–430.

Geiser, C. (2013). *Data analysis with Mplus.* New York, NY: Guilford Press.

Geiser, C., Keller, B. T., & Lockhart, G. (2013). First-versus second-order latent growth curve models: Some insights from latent state-trait theory. *Structural Equation Modeling: A Multidisciplinary Journal, 20,* 479–503.

Gerber, M., Lindwall, M., Brand, S., Lang, C., Elliot, C., & Pühse, U. (2015). Longitudinal relationships between perceived stress, exercise self-regulation and exercise involvement among physically active adolescents. *Journal of Sports Sciences, 33,* 368–380.

Graham, J. W. (2009). Missing data analysis: Making it work in the real world. *Annual Review of Psychology, 60,* 549–576.

Hagger, M. S., & Chatzisarantis, N. L. (2009). Assumptions in research in sport and exercise psychology. *Psychology of Sport and Exercise, 10,* 511–519.

Harter, S. (1985). *Manual for the self-perception profile for children.* Denver, CO: University of Denver.

Harter, S. (2012). *Construction of the self: Developmental and sociocultural foundations.* New York, NY: Guilford.

Hertzog, C., & Nesselroade, J. R. (2003). Assessing psychological change in adulthood: An overview of methodological issues. *Psychology and Aging, 18,* 639–657.

Hofer, S. M., & Sliwinski, M. J. (2006). Design and analysis of longitudinal studies of aging. In J. E. Birren & K. W. Schaie (Eds.), *Handbook of the psychology of aging* (6th ed., pp. 15–37). San Diego, CA: Academic Press.

Ivarsson, A., Johnson, U., Lindwall, M., Gustafsson, H., & Altemyr, M. (2014). Psychosocial stress as a predictor of sport injuries in elite junior soccer: A latent growth curve analysis. *Journal of Science and Medicine in Sport, 17*, 366–370.

Ivarsson, A., Stenling, A., Fallby, J., Johnson, U., Borg, E., & Johansson, G. (2015). The predictive ability of the talent development environment on youth elite football players' well-being: A person-centered approach. *Psychology of Sport and Exercise, 16*, 15–23.

Jackson, D. L. (2010). Reporting results of latent growth modeling and multilevel modeling analyses: Some recommendations for Rehabilitation Psychology. *Rehabilitation Psychology, 55*, 272–285.

Kass, R. E. (2011). Statistical inference: The big picture. *Statistical Science, 26*, 1–9.

Lindwall, M., & Aşçı, F. H. (2014). Physical activity and self-esteem. In A. Clow & S. Edmunds (Eds.), *Physical activity and mental health* (pp. 83–103). Champaign, IL: Human Kinetics.

Lindwall, M., Aşçı, F. H., Palmeira, A., Fox, K. R., & Hagger, M. S. (2011). The Importance of importance in the physical self: Support for the theoretically appealing but empirically elusive model of James. *Journal of Personality, 79*, 303–333.

Little, T. D. (2013). *Longitudinal structural equation modeling.* New York, NY: Guilford Press.

Little, T. D., Bovaird, J. A., & Slegers, D. (2006). Methods for the analysis of change. In D. Mroczek & T. D. Little (Eds.), *Handbook of personality development* (pp. 181–211). Mahwah, NJ: Erlbaum.

Little, T. D., Preacher, K. J., Selig, J. P., & Card, N. A. (2007). New developments in latent variable panel analyses of longitudinal data. *International Journal of Behavioral Development, 31*, 357–365.

Marsh, H. W. (2007). Application of confirmatory factor analysis and structural equation modeling in sport and exercise psychology. In G. Tenenbaum & R. C. Eklund (Eds.), *Handbook of sport psychology* (3rd ed., pp. 774–798). Hoboken, NJ: John Wiley & Sons, Inc.

Marsh, H. W., Chanal, J. P., & Sarrazin, P. G. (2006). Self-belief does make a difference: A reciprocal effects model of the causal ordering of physical self-concept and gymnastics performance. *Journal of Sports Sciences, 24*, 101–111.

McArdle, J. J. (1988). Dynamic but structural equation modeling of repeated measures data. In J. R. Nesselroade, & R. B. Cattell (Eds.), *Handbook of multivariate experimental psychology* (pp. 561–614). New York, NY: Plenum Press.

McArdle, J. J. (2009). Latent variable modeling of differences and changes with longitudinal data. *Annual Review of Psychology, 60*, 577–605.

McArdle, J. J., & Nesselroade, J. R. (2014). *Longitudinal data analysis using structural equation models.* Washington, DC: American Psychological Association.

McCall, R. B., & Appelbaum, M. I. (1973). Bias in the analysis of repeated-measures designs: Some alternative approaches. *Child Development, 44*, 401–415.

Meredith, W. (1993). Measurement invariance, factor analysis and factorial invariance. *Psychometrika, 58*, 525–543.

Muthén, L. K., & Muthén, B. O. (1998–2012). *Mplus user's guide.* (7th ed.). Los Angeles, CA: Muthén & Muthén.

Nesselroade, J. R., & Ram, N. (2004). Studying intraindividual variability: What we have learned that will help us understand lives in context. *Research in Human Development, 1*, 9–29.

Park, I., & Schutz, R. W. (2005). An introduction to latent growth model: Analysis of repeated measures physical performance data. *Research Quarterly for Exercise and Sport, 76,* 176–192.

Preacher, K. J., Wichman, A. L., MacCallum, R. C., & Briggs, N. E. (2008). *Latent growth curve modeling.* Thousand Oaks, CA: Sage Publications.

Ram, N., & Grimm, K. (2007). Using simple and complex growth models to articulate developmental change: Matching theory to method. *International Journal of Behavioral Development, 31,* 303–316.

Rogosa, D. R., & Willett, J. B. (1985). Understanding correlates of change by modeling individual differences in growth. *Psychometrika, 50,* 203–228.

Schack, T., & Hackfort, D. (2007). An action theory approach to applied sport psychology. In G. Tenenbaum & R. C. Eklund (Eds.), *Handbook of sport psychology* (3rd ed., pp. 332–351). New York, NY: John Wiley & Sons, Inc.

Selig, J. P., & Preacher, K. J. (2009). Mediation models for longitudinal data in developmental research. *Research in Human Development, 6,* 144–164.

Shavelson, R. J., Hubner, J. J., & Stanton, G. C. (1976). Self-concept: Validation of construct interpretations. *Review of Educational Research, 46,* 407–441.

Sliwinski, M. J., & Mogle, J. A. (2008). Time-based and process-based approaches to analysis of longitudinal data. In D. Alwin & S. Hofer (Eds.), *The handbook of cognitive aging* (pp. 477–491). Thousand Oaks, CA: Sage Publications.

Stenling, A., Ivarsson, A., & Lindwall, M. (2015, July). Longitudinal data analysis in sport and exercise psychology: Exploring new horizons, paper presented at the 14th European Congress of Sport Psychology, Bern, Switzerland.

Timmons, A. C., & Preacher, K. J. (2015). The importance of temporal design: How do measurement intervals affect the accuracy and efficiency of parameter estimates in longitudinal research?. *Multivariate Behavioral Research, 50,* 41–55.

Wagnsson, S, Augustsson, C., & Patriksson, G. (2013). Associations between sport involvement and youth psychosocial development in Sweden: A longitudinal study. *Journal of Sport for Development, 1,* 37–47.

West, S. G., Taylor, A. B., & Wu, W. (2012). Model fit and model selection in structural equation modeling. In R. H. Hoyle (Ed.), *Handbook of structural equation modeling* (pp. 209–231). New York, NY: Guilford Press.

Widaman, K. F., Ferrer, E., & Conger, R. D. (2010). Factorial invariance within longitudinal structural equation models: Measuring the same construct across time. *Child Development Perspectives, 4,* 10–18.

# 8

# Exploratory structural equation modeling and Bayesian estimation

## Daniel F. Gucciardi[1] and Michael J. Zyphur[2]

[1] *School of Physiotherapy and Exercise Science, Curtin University, Perth, WA, Australia*
[2] *Department of Management and Marketing, The University of Melbourne, Parkville, VIC, Australia*

## General Introduction

Scholars typically strive for theoretical precision. Yet, our models rarely embody perfectly specified relations among (un)observable concepts, or the operationalization of our constructs is imperfect. In these instances, highly restrictive analytical approaches that assume measures of constructs are perfect indicators may be inappropriate (Marsh, Morin, Parker, & Kaur, 2014; Morin, Arens, & Marsh, in press). Beyond the issue of measurement, scientists also aim to build upon existing knowledge, showing that new data replicate and extend what is already known about a phenomenon. Often, however, these prior expectations or beliefs are not explicitly integrated into statistical analyses, thereby limiting the extent to which knowledge is formally accumulated over time by synthesizing prior knowledge and the information from a particular dataset. Cognizant of these issues, scholars require flexible statistical approaches that maximize the synergy between substance and method

*An Introduction to Intermediate and Advanced Statistical Analyses for Sport and Exercise Scientists*, First Edition.
Edited by Nikos Ntoumanis and Nicholas D. Myers.
© 2016 John Wiley & Sons, Ltd. Published 2016 by John Wiley & Sons, Ltd.
Companion website: www.wiley.com/go/ntoumanis/sport

(Marsh & Hau, 2007), accommodating the increasingly complex topics examined in sport and exercise science. Exploratory structural equation modeling (ESEM; Asparouhov & Muthén, 2009; for a review, see Marsh et al., 2014) and Bayesian estimation (for reviews, see Kaplan & Depaoli, 2012; Levy & Choi, 2013; van de Schoot & Depaoli, 2014; van de Schoot et al., 2014; Zyphur & Oswald, 2015) are two such approaches that have the potential to offer flexibility in the representation of complex models when compared with alternative approaches that typically rely on unrealistic assumptions.

Our aims in this chapter are twofold. First, we will highlight the usefulness of ESEM and Bayesian estimation for sport and exercise science. To date, ESEM has been primarily employed in the field to test the psychometric properties of items that form instruments designed to capture psychosocial concepts such as mental toughness, motivation, and coaching efficacy (see Appendix 8.1). Bayesian estimation has been applied with greater diversity than ESEM, including psychometric evaluations as well as tests of theoretical sequences and multilevel structural equation modeling (SEM) (see Appendix 8.2). Second, to illustrate the usefulness and practical application of ESEM and Bayesian estimation, we will reanalyze published research on mental toughness (Gucciardi, Jackson, Hanton, & Reid, 2015) to enable a comparison of ESEM and Bayesian estimation with a common analytical approach. In so doing, our aim is to familiarize readers with the procedural aspects of ESEM and Bayesian analysis. From the outset, it is important to recognize that ESEM and our Bayesian approach involve not merely different model specifications, but fundamentally different estimation methods. ESEM is an extension of the traditional latent variable framework that incorporates exploratory factor analysis (EFA) factors. Conversely, Bayesian estimation uses a fundamentally different probability calculus (see Table 8.1).

# Utility of the Methods in Sport and Exercise Science

The reliable and valid measurement of psychosocial concepts is central to the progression of scientific knowledge in the psychological sciences, as well as to multidisciplinary efforts in sport and exercise science (e.g., overtraining, talent development). As most psychosocial concepts are not directly observable, they are often modeled as latent variables and inferred from indicators hypothesized to represent a latent construct. In most cases, several items are developed to capture the breadth of a construct, which is often regarded as causing data along the indicators. For example, *intentions* to continue participating in organized sport may be captured by items such as "I intend on continuing my participation in sport next season" (1 = extremely unlikely to 7 = extremely likely) or "Will you continue to participate in your sport next season" (1 = definitely plan not to do so to 7 = definitely plan to do so). Responses to these two items would provide insight into individuals' strength of behavioral intentions, such that the variance in responses to the items captures individual differences in behavioral intentions. Because latent variable indicators are not perfectly reliable, both systematic and random errors are incorporated into the model in the form of residual variance—a graphical display of a measurement model is displayed in Appendix 8.3. A latent

Table 8.1   Overview of the similarities and differences between frequentist and Bayesian statistics.

| | Frequentist statistics | Bayesian statistics |
|---|---|---|
| Definition of the $p$ value | The probability of observing the same or more extreme data assuming that the null hypothesis is true in the population | The probability of the (null) hypothesis |
| Large samples needed? | Usually, when normal theory-based methods are used | Not necessarily |
| Inclusion of prior knowledge possible? | No | Yes |
| Nature of the parameters in the model | Unknown but fixed | Unknown and therefore random |
| Population parameter | One true value | A distribution of values reflecting uncertainty |
| Uncertainty is defined by | The sampling distribution based on the idea of infinite repeated sampling | Probability distribution for the population parameter |
| Estimated intervals | Confidence interval: over an infinity of samples taken from the population, 95% of these contain the true population value | Credibility interval: a 95% probability that the population value is within the limits of the interval |

Reproduced with permission from van de Schoot et al. (2014).

variable approach is useful because it accounts for measurement error, permitting less inflated parameter estimations of structural relations among constructs.

It is important that the dimensionality of a scale (e.g., number of latent factors) and the nature of its dimensions (e.g., strength and direction of factor loadings) are established before one proceeds to other forms of analyses, such as predictive validity or group differences. Often referred to as factorial validity, accurate dimensionality is essential for developing or supporting theoretical models and therefore facilitates interpretations of target constructs with external variables such as performance, injury rehabilitation adherence, and exercise levels. For example, if one has used a four-factor measure of mental toughness but the hypothesized multidimensional structure is not supported in a specific sample, it would be erroneous to subsequently examine antecedents (e.g., coaching climate, stress inoculation training) or outcomes (e.g., performance, adherence to rehabilitation program) of the multiple facets of this concept.

As confirmatory factor analysis (CFA) allows one to test an a priori representation of a psychological concept with new data, it has played an important role in the measurement of latent variables across many disciplines of psychology. However, the independent clusters model is central to confirmatory factor analysis (ICM-CFA) such that one freely estimates intended factor loadings (e.g., intention items load on latent intention factor) yet constrains cross-loadings between items and nonintended latent factors to be zero (e.g., intention items load on a latent subjective norm factor@0). Although EFA is often considered less useful than CFA because of the "semantically based misconception that it is purely an 'exploratory' method that should be used only when the researcher has no a priori assumption regarding factor structure," the key difference between the two approaches pertains to the modeling of cross-loadings (Marsh et al., 2014, p. 87). In other words, in EFA, cross-loadings on unintended factors are freely estimated, whereas in CFA, they are constrained to zero. The highly restrictive nature of the ICM-CFA approach means that it is often difficult for measurement models to achieve sound fit with data (for a review, see Marsh et al., 2014). Both ESEM and Bayesian estimation can alleviate concerns associated with the ICM-CFA approach (e.g., cross-loadings encompass method effects, and items are imperfect indicators).

Equally important is the need for scholars to integrate or update existing beliefs with new data—this might be said to be the point of science. Researchers conduct studies in the context of previous theory and research, enabling the generation of expectations in the form of hypotheses to be tested based on observed data. However, degrees of (un)certainty associated with prior expectations are often ignored in conventional frequentist approaches to estimation and testing (e.g., maximum likelihood, null hypothesis significance testing with $p$ values). Put differently, existing knowledge is not integrated into analyses, meaning that researchers essentially test "the same null hypothesis over and over again, ignoring the lessons of previous studies" (van de Schoot et al., 2014, p. 843). Bayesian estimation provides an alternative to this conventional frequentist approach by allowing probabilistic information about parameters of interest to be formally incorporated into analyses so that results reflect a cumulative progression of knowledge gained across studies (Muthén & Muthén, 2012; van de Schoot et al., 2014; Zyphur & Oswald, 2015). For example, despite its focus on the null hypothesis, frequentist methods do not enable researchers to directly test the null if the alternate hypothesis is that an effect or correlation is zero, which can be achieved with Bayesian estimation (Zyphur & Oswald, 2015). In so doing, Bayesian estimation is concerned with the probability that a hypothesis is true given the data, rather than the probability of obtaining one's observed or more extreme results given the null hypothesis as in frequentist approaches (i.e., $p < 0.05$ signal extreme data for frequentists).

Bayesian tools also allow for intuitive interpretations of a hypothesized model (or prior beliefs), "given" or "conditional on" an observed dataset. Consider an example wherein athletes self-report their mental toughness prior to performing a task that is a proxy for behavioral perseverance (e.g., a "beep test"). If the combination of prior knowledge (e.g., similar previous studies and/or experts' beliefs) with new data indicates that the association between mental toughness and behavioral perseverance is centered on $\beta = 0.24$, with some uncertainty around this value (95%

CI=0.14, 0.34), this finding means that there is a 95% chance that the relation between mental toughness and behavioral perseverance ranges between 0.14 and 0.34. In other words, Bayesian models provide a distribution of possible values for a parameter, rather than a single true value. In frequentist statistics, this interpretation of confidence intervals does not mean the same thing. Instead, it serves as a tool for estimating a range of estimates wherein one true parameter would appear 95% of the time if a study were to be conducted an infinite number of times. Thus, values outside of the 95% confidence interval provide information on what the parameter is not "in the long run," with probabilistic information on plausible estimates of the one true value contained within this range "in the long run." This less intuitive piece of information is of questionable use and is hard to teach to students and explain to practitioners because of the reliance on a hypothetical infinity of repetitions of a study. A summary of other key differences between frequentist and Bayesian statistics is detailed in Table 8.1. We now offer examples of ESEM and Bayesian estimation to illustrate our points thus far.

# The Substantive Example(s)

Scholars have compared the usefulness of ESEM with the traditional ICM-CFA approach for the assessment of psychosocial concepts in sport and exercise contexts such as motivation, physical self-concept, mental toughness, coaching efficacy, referee self-efficacy, and impression motivation (for an overview, see Appendix 8.1). As the majority of research to date has focused on the dimensionality of psychological tools, we have purposefully chosen an example to illustrate the flexibility of ESEM for the examination of theoretical sequences that encompass causal paths between latent variables in measurement models. As the ICM-CFA approach was adopted in the published paper of our example, it offers an opportunity to compare these results with those obtained using ESEM.

Empirical demonstrations of Bayesian estimation in sport and exercise settings include the development and validation of psychological tools, analyses of theoretical sequences or models, assessments of referee bias, psychological performance crisis in competition, and psychological processes associated with winning and losing streaks in fencing (for an overview, see Appendix 8.2). Given the popularity of structural equation models in sport and exercise science, the target example also afforded an opportunity to demonstrate how readers can apply Bayesian estimation to the examination of theoretical sequences.

# The Motivational Correlates of Mentally Tough Behavior

Mental toughness is a term that often captures peoples' attention in contexts such as sport, wherein innovation, success, and competitive advantage are driven by high performance. Initial work in this area was founded on professional practice knowledge, with the past decade characterized by systematic attempts to generate and understand peoples' perceptions of key features of mental toughness, predominantly using qualitative methods (for a review, see Gucciardi & Hanton, in press). Collectively, the evidence generated thus far suggests that mental toughness represents a psychological capacity for high performance on a regular basis despite varying degrees of situational demands. As this area of research has progressed over the past decade, alternative ways of studying the concept have emerged. One approach is to identify observable behaviors that are characteristic of mentally tough individuals and the key correlates or antecedents of the behaviors, rather than infer the importance of specific thoughts, feelings, and attitudes for mental toughness in the absence of data (e.g., performance data). Accordingly, the substantive focus of the example in this chapter is on mentally tough behavior.

A two-phase research project was implemented by Gucciardi et al. (2015) to examine the motivational correlates of mentally tough behavior. The aim of the first phase of the study was to generate a brief checklist of mentally tough behaviors, with a focus on content and face validity. Coaches who worked with elite tennis players ($n = 17$) and adolescent players involved in Tennis Australia's elite development pathway ($n = 20$; $M_{age} = 14.80$, SD = 2.31) participated in focus group interviews. In two separate focus groups, coaches ($n_{group1} = 10$, $n_{group2} = 7$) and scholarship athletes ($n_{group1} = 3$, $n_{group2} = 4$) first generated an initial pool of behavioral descriptors guided by the question, "what does mental toughness look like?" This initial item pool ($n = 12$) was subsequently assessed for comprehensibility by two separate groups of adolescent tennis players ($n_{group3} = 7$, $n_{group4} = 6$). Finally, the 12 behavioral descriptors were assessed for their representativeness by academics with expertise in mental toughness and/or questionnaire development ($1 = poor$, $3 = good$, $5 = excellent$). This three-step process in phase 1 of the project resulted in the generation of 10 mentally tough behaviors (see Appendix 8.4).

The aim of the second phase of the study was to examine the relations between motivational orientations and mentally tough behavior. A total of 347 adolescent tennis players ($n_{males} = 184$; $n_{females} = 163$) aged 12–18 years ($M = 13.93$, SD = 1.47) and one respective parent took part in this phase. Gucciardi et al. (2015) examined adaptive and maladaptive motivational orientations that provided insight into different layers of one's personality (McAdams & Pals, 2006), including fear of failure (dispositional layer), inspiration (characteristic adaptations layer), and passion (identity layer). Using a cross-sectional design, athletes self-reported their motivational orientations, whereas parents provided an assessment of their child's mentally tough behaviors. The associations among the study variables were examined within an SEM framework whereby mentally tough behaviors were regressed on the motivational orientations. It was hypothesized that fear of failure and obsessive passion would be inversely related to mentally tough behaviors, whereas harmonious passion and both frequency and intensity of inspiration would be positively associated with mentally tough behaviors. SEM using a robust maximum likelihood estimator (MLR) provided support for these expectations.

# Developing Synergies through Statistical Modeling

For the purposes of this chapter, the illustrations of ESEM and Bayesian estimation are presented in separate sections. First, we compare ESEM with the commonly used ICM-CFA approach for assessing structural equation models that encompass latent variables (which is consistent with the original paper by Gucciardi et al. (2015). Here, ESEM is used in a "confirmatory" manner in that we have a priori expectations regarding the measurement model of the latent constructs in the theoretical sequence, although the technique can be applied for exploratory investigations to identify an optimal factorial solution (see Morin, Marsh, & Nagengast, 2013). Second, we use Bayesian estimation to show readers how they can incorporate prior knowledge into their analyses and thereby formally update their beliefs about parameters of interest. All output files are included in the online supplementary material, including extensive annotations to help readers understand features of the model syntax and interpret the results (see M*plus* output file "bayes_model 2(informative substantive paths).out" in the online supplementary material).

## ESEM

### Statistical Analyses

We implemented both ESEM and ICM-CFA in M*plus* 7.2 (Muthén & Muthén, 2012) with a robust MLR that produces standard errors and model-data fit indices that are robust against violations of normality assumptions and the use of categorical variables when there are at least five response categories (Bandalos, 2014; Rhemtulla, Brosseau-Laird, & Savalei, 2012). The robust variance-adjusted weighted least squares estimator (WLSMV) can be used when there are fewer than five responses categories (for an example including annotated inputs, see Guay, Morin, Litalien, Valois, & Vallerand, 2015). Graphical representations of the ESEM and ICM-CFA approaches are presented in Figures 8.1 and 8.2, respectively. In the ICM-CFA approach, item indicators were allowed to load only on their intended latent factor (i.e., nonzero loading, represented by the → from the latent factor to the item), with no cross-loadings on unintended factors (i.e., zero loading). For example, the factor loadings of items fof1, fof2 … fof5 on the latent factor "fof" (fear of failure) were freely estimated, whereas their loading on all other latent factors (e.g., ps_harm, ins_fre) were forced to be zero as indicated by the lack of path from the latent factor to the item (see Figure 8.1). With the exception of inspiration items (i.e., insp1, insp2 … insp8), residual variances (represented by the → on each item) were specified as uncorrelated. We modeled correlated residuals among inspiration items wherein the same statement (e.g., "As a tennis player, I feel inspired") was rated twice using a frequency ("how often?") and intensity stem ("how deeply or strongly") to represent a method effect. The ESEM model differed from the ICM-CFA approach in that item indicators were allowed to cross-load on unintended factors (see Figure 8.2). Rather than rely on an exploratory rotation technique (e.g., geomin), we used the TARGET

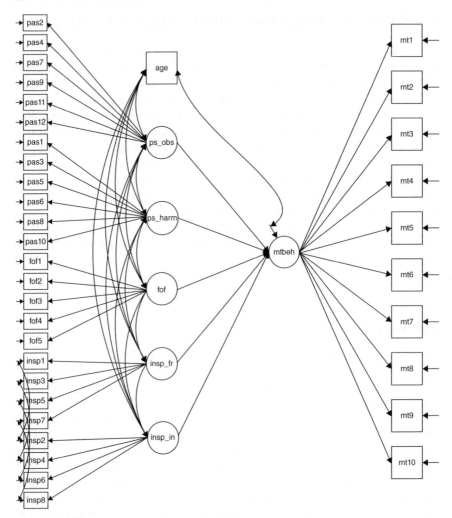

*Figure 8.1    Schematic overview of the theoretical sequence that encompasses ICM-CFA factors.*

rotation setting to guide cross-loadings with a target value close to zero (Browne, 2001), which is consistent with a confirmatory approach but does not impose the highly restrictive feature of exactly zero loadings (Asparouhov & Muthén, 2009). The M*plus* syntax for both the ICM-CFA and ESEM approaches are detailed in Appendices 8.5 and 8.6, respectively.

As the $\chi^2$ test of model-data fit is sensitive to sample size and model misspecifications (Marsh, Hau, & Grayson, 2005), we adopted a multifaceted approach to gauge model fit and comparisons between the ICM-CFA and ESEM approaches. Alongside the $\chi^2$ goodness-of-fit index, we considered the comparative fit index (CFI), Tucker–Lewis index (TLI), and root mean square error of approximation (RMSEA) for

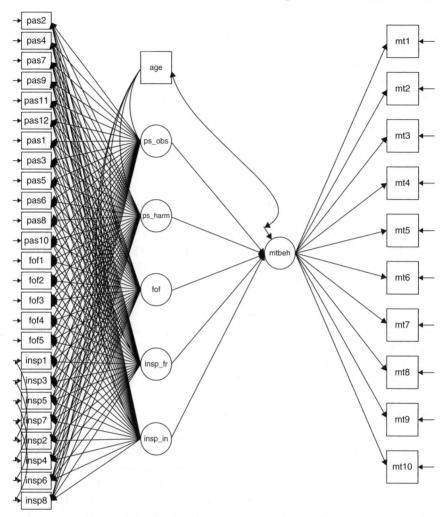

*Figure 8.2    Schematic overview of the theoretical sequence that encompasses ESEM (fear of failure, inspiration, passion) with ICM-CFA factors (mentally tough behavior).*

assessing model fit. Based on commonly adopted recommendations (Marsh et al., 2005), CFI and TLI values ≥0.90 and RMSEA values under 0.08 are considered to indicate acceptable fit.[1] The Satorra–Bentler scaled $\chi^2$ difference test (SBS$\Delta\chi^2$; Satorra & Bentler, 1999) was employed to statistically examine the difference between the ICM-CFA and ESEM approaches, alongside information criteria, including

---

[1] It is important to note that these model-data fit recommendations are based on guidelines drawn from the ICM-CFA approach and therefore their appropriateness for ESEM remains unknown.

Akaike's information criterion (AIC), consistent AIC (CAIC), Bayesian information criterion (BIC), and the sample size-adjusted BIC ($BIC_{SSA}$)—smaller values along these information criteria indicate better model fit (i.e., losing less information when moving from observed data to an estimated model). It is also important to consider changes in fit indices when comparing alternative models, particularly TLI and RMSEA, as they are corrected for model parsimony (Marsh et al., 2014). Support for the more parsimonious model is provided when the decrease in CFI/TLI is less than 0.01 and the increase in RMSEA is no greater than 0.015 (Chen, 2007). Latent factor reliability estimates are computed using McDonald's (1970) omega coefficient ($\omega$).

## Comparison of Model Fit Indices

The fit statistics indicated acceptable model-data fit with ESEM, $\chi^2(490)=909.09$, $p<0.001$, CFI=0.934, TLI=0.915, RMSEA=0.050 (90% CI=0.045–0.055), AIC=36456.15, CAIC=37484.21, BIC=37272.21, $BIC_{SSA}$ = 36598.32, and the ICM-CFA approach, $\chi^2(570)=1108.60$, $p<0.001$, CFI=0.915, TLI=0.906, RMSEA= 0.052 (90% CI=0.048–0.057), AIC=36535.96, CAIC=37176.07, BIC=37044.07, $BIC_{SSA}$ = 36625.33. The ESEM solution provided a significantly better fit than the alternative ICM-CFA model, $SBS\Delta\chi^2$ (80)=193.99, $p<0.001$. Both the $BIC_{SSA}$ and AIC and the changes in TLI ($\Delta=0.09$) and RMSEA ($\Delta=0.002$) supported this interpretation; however, the penalty for increased model parameters inherent in the BIC and CAIC favored the simpler ICM-CFA model. Scale reliability estimates, which ranged from 0.79 to 0.91, were similar for both ESEM and the ICM-CFA approach (see Table 8.2).

## Comparison of Measurement Model Estimates

An overview of standardized factor loadings is detailed in Table 8.2. All items loaded strongly on their intended factor in both analytical approaches: harmonious passion ($M_{cfa}=0.66$, $SD_{cfa}=0.05$; $M_{esem}=0.57$, $SD_{esem}=0.29$), obsessive passion ($M_{cfa}=0.70$, $SD_{cfa}=0.10$; $M_{esem}=0.68$, $SD_{esem}=0.14$), fear of failure ($M_{cfa}=0.70$, $SD_{cfa}=0.11$; $M_{esem}=0.70$, $SD_{esem}=0.11$), inspiration frequency ($M_{cfa}=0.83$, $SD_{cfa}=0.02$; $M_{esem}=0.75$, $SD_{esem}=0.09$), and inspiration intensity ($M_{cfa}=0.85$, $SD_{cfa}=0.01$; $M_{esem}=0.77$, $SD_{esem}=0.02$). For the ESEM model, cross-loadings were small and primarily nonsignificant (ranging from −0.18 to 0.28, $M=0.07$, SD=0.06), with the exception of two items of harmonious passion that evidenced similar loadings on the intended factor and obsessive passion (item 3, $\lambda_{harmonious}=0.29$ and $\lambda_{obsessive}=0.22$; item 5, $\lambda_{harmonious}=0.28$ and $\lambda_{obsessive}=0.28$). The $R^2$ estimates of communalities were comparable for the ESEM ($M=0.54$, SD=0.13) and ICM-CFA solutions ($M=0.56$, SD=0.13).

## Comparison of Factor Correlations and Structural Paths

An overview of standardized factor correlations and structural paths is provided in Table 8.3. Overall, the factor correlations among the hypothesized motivational correlates were higher for the ICM-CFA model (−0.16 to 0.86; $M=0.44$, SD=0.28) when compared with the ESEM solution (−0.17 to 0.79; $M=0.39$, SD=0.23). An inspection

Table 8.2 Standardized parameter estimates and score reliabilities ($\omega$) for the ICM-CFA and ESEM approaches to the structural analysis of Gucciardi et al. (2015).

| | Mentally tough behavior | | Obsessive passion | | Harmonious passion | | Fear of failure | | Inspiration frequency | | Inspiration intensity | | $R^2$ | |
| --- | --- | --- | --- | --- | --- | --- | --- | --- | --- | --- | --- | --- | --- | --- |
| | CFA | ESEM | CFA | ESEM | CFA | ESEM | CFA | ESEM | CFA | ESEM | CFA | ESEM | CFA | ESEM |
| mt1 | 0.64* | 0.64* | — | — | — | — | — | — | — | — | — | — | 0.41 | 0.41 |
| mt2 | 0.69* | 0.69* | — | — | — | — | — | — | — | — | — | — | 0.47 | 0.47 |
| mt3 | 0.79* | 0.79* | — | — | — | — | — | — | — | — | — | — | 0.62 | 0.62 |
| mt4 | 0.75* | 0.75* | — | — | — | — | — | — | — | — | — | — | 0.56 | 0.56 |
| mt5 | 0.74* | 0.74* | — | — | — | — | — | — | — | — | — | — | 0.54 | 0.54 |
| mt6 | 0.77* | 0.76* | — | — | — | — | — | — | — | — | — | — | 0.59 | 0.58 |
| mt7 | 0.76* | 0.76* | — | — | — | — | — | — | — | — | — | — | 0.57 | 0.57 |
| mt8 | 0.75* | 0.75* | — | — | — | — | — | — | — | — | — | — | 0.57 | 0.56 |
| mt9 | 0.60* | 0.60* | — | — | — | — | — | — | — | — | — | — | 0.36 | 0.36 |
| mt10 | 0.66* | 0.66* | — | — | — | — | — | — | — | — | — | — | 0.44 | 0.44 |
| pas2 | — | — | 0.54* | 0.47* | — | -0.02 | — | 0.06 | — | 0.11 | — | 0.02 | 0.31 | 0.52 |
| pas4 | — | — | 0.75* | 0.62* | — | 0.06 | — | -0.06 | — | 0.22* | — | -0.02 | 0.29 | 0.29 |
| pas7 | — | — | 0.79* | 0.90* | — | 0.01 | — | -0.06 | — | -0.11 | — | -0.06 | 0.54 | 0.49 |
| pas9 | — | — | 0.70* | 0.68* | — | 0.10 | — | 0.01 | — | 0.05 | — | -0.09 | 0.56 | 0.59 |
| pas11 | — | — | 0.80* | 0.76* | — | 0.01 | — | 0.02 | — | 0.03 | — | 0.04 | 0.41 | 0.38 |
| pas12 | — | — | 0.63* | 0.65* | — | -0.01 | — | 0.17* | — | -0.16* | — | 0.11 | 0.44 | 0.37 |
| pas1 | — | — | — | -0.12* | 0.56* | 0.83* | — | 0.03 | — | 0.06 | — | -0.18* | 0.62 | 0.70 |
| pas3 | — | — | — | 0.22* | 0.73* | 0.29* | — | -0.07 | — | 0.11 | — | 0.22* | 0.45 | 0.44 |
| pas5 | — | — | — | 0.28* | 0.65* | 0.28* | — | -0.08 | — | 0.06 | — | 0.12 | 0.49 | 0.50 |

(*Continued*)

Table 8.2 (Continued)

| | Mentally tough behavior | | Obsessive passion | | Harmonious passion | | Fear of failure | | Inspiration frequency | | Inspiration intensity | | $R^2$ | |
|---|---|---|---|---|---|---|---|---|---|---|---|---|---|---|
| | CFA | ESEM | CFA | ESEM | CFA | ESEM | CFA | ESEM | CFA | ESEM | CFA | ESEM | CFA | ESEM |
| pas6 | — | — | — | −0.01 | 0.67* | 0.45* | — | −0.10 | — | 0.05 | — | 0.16 | 0.47 | 0.78 |
| pas8 | — | — | — | 0.13* | 0.67* | 0.55* | — | −0.03 | — | −0.01 | — | 0.07 | 0.64 | 0.63 |
| pas10 | — | — | — | −0.098 | 0.69* | 1.00* | — | 0.08* | — | −0.11 | — | −0.04 | 0.40 | 0.45 |
| fof1 | — | — | — | −0.10* | — | 0.03 | 0.73* | 0.76* | — | 0.01 | — | 0.05 | 0.53 | 0.67 |
| fof2 | — | — | — | 0.09* | — | −0.06 | 0.81* | 0.80* | — | 0.16* | — | −0.16* | 0.66 | 0.73 |
| fof3 | — | — | — | 0.07 | — | 0.03 | 0.78* | 0.77* | — | −0.01 | — | 0.03 | 0.61 | 0.64 |
| fof4 | — | — | — | 0.01 | — | −0.01 | 0.62* | 0.62* | — | −0.04 | — | 0.09 | 0.38 | 0.72 |
| fof5 | — | — | — | −0.01 | — | 0.01 | 0.55* | 0.55* | — | −0.12 | — | 0.07 | 0.31 | 0.74 |
| ins1 | — | — | — | −0.01 | — | 0.05 | — | 0.06 | 0.82* | 0.67* | — | 0.13 | 0.67 | 0.71 |
| ins3 | — | — | — | 0.04 | — | 0.04 | — | −0.06 | 0.81* | 0.71* | — | 0.06 | 0.73 | 0.74 |
| ins5 | — | — | — | −0.02 | — | 0.05 | — | −0.06 | 0.84* | 0.88* | — | −0.05 | 0.66 | 0.71 |
| ins7 | — | — | — | 0.03 | — | −0.01 | — | 0.01 | 0.86* | 0.75* | — | 0.13 | 0.72 | 0.55 |
| ins2 | — | — | — | 0.06 | — | 0.03 | — | 0.02 | — | 0.06 | 0.85* | 0.76* | 0.71 | 0.69 |
| ins4 | — | — | — | −0.01 | — | 0.07 | — | 0.17 | — | 0.02 | 0.85* | 0.80* | 0.72 | 0.61 |
| ins6 | — | — | — | −0.04 | — | 0.06 | — | 0.03 | — | 0.11 | 0.85* | 0.74* | 0.73 | 0.39 |
| ins8 | — | — | — | −0.01 | — | 0.01 | — | −0.07 | — | 0.09 | 0.84* | 0.76* | 0.70 | 0.32 |
| ω | 0.91 | 0.91 | 0.85 | 0.85 | 0.82 | 0.79 | 0.83 | 0.83 | 0.90 | 0.88 | 0.91 | 0.89 | | |

*$p < 0.05$.

Table 8.3 Standardized latent variable correlations and structural paths for both ICM-CFA and ESEM approaches to the analysis of Gucciardi et al.'s (2015) model of the motivational correlates of mentally tough behavior.

| | Latent variable correlations | | | | | MT behavior | |
| | 1 | 2 | 3 | 4 | 5 | CFA | ESEM |
|---|---|---|---|---|---|---|---|
| 1 Obsessive passion | — | 0.44 [0.34, 0.54] | 0.44 [0.34, 0.53] | 0.46 [0.37, 0.56] | 0.09 [−0.03, 0.21] | −0.15 [−0.27, −0.04] | −0.12 [−0.22, −0.01] |
| 2 Harmonious passion | 0.57 [0.46, 0.69] | — | 0.58 [0.46, 0.68] | 0.59 [0.48, 0.70] | −0.16 [−0.28, −0.04] | 0.26 [0.09, 0.43] | 0.19 [0.04, 0.35] |
| 3 Inspiration frequency | 0.50 [0.40, 0.60] | 0.70 [0.60, 0.80] | — | 0.79 [0.69, 0.88] | −0.17 [−0.28, −0.06] | 0.32 [0.14, 0.49] | 0.29 [0.13, 0.46] |
| 4 Inspiration intensity | 0.50 [0.41, 0.60] | 0.72 [0.63, 0.82] | 0.86 [0.81, 0.90] | — | −0.15 [−0.26, −0.03] | 0.13 [−0.07, 0.34] | 0.20 [0.02, 0.38] |
| 5 Fear of failure | 0.13 [−0.01, 0.27] | −0.16 [−0.29, −0.02] | −0.12 [−0.24, −0.01] | −0.13 [−0.25, −0.01] | — | −0.32 [−0.43, −0.21] | −0.33 [−0.44, −0.22] |

*Note*: CFA and ESEM correlations below and above the diagonal, respectively; confidence intervals presented in brackets.

of the confidence intervals indicated that the ESEM ($M_{ci} = 0.24$, $Mdn_{ci} = 0.22$, $SD_{ci} = 0.06$) and the ICM-CFA ($M_{ci} = 0.22$, $Mdn_{ci} = 0.22$, $SD_{ci} = 0.06$) were comparable in their precision in the estimation of the latent factor correlations. In contrast, the ESEM solution ($M_{ci} = 0.45$, $Mdn_{ci} = 0.40$, $SD_{ci} = 0.17$) provided greater precision in the estimation of the structural paths between the motivational correlates and mentally tough behavior when compared with the ICM-CFA model ($M_{ci} = 0.50$, $Mdn_{ci} = 0.52$, $SD_{ci} = 0.14$). Consistent with previous research, these findings indicated that ESEM resulted in better model-data fit and less inflated correlations among latent factors than the traditional ICM-CFA approach (Marsh et al., 2014). Further, they illustrate the explicit attempt to relax the largely unreasonable assumptions of ICM-CFA models—namely, the assumption of no cross-loadings (even if small).

## Bayesian Estimation

### Statistical Analyses

We implemented Bayesian structural equation modeling (BSEM; Muthén & Asparouhov, 2012) in M*plus* 7.2 (Muthén & Muthén, 2012) using Markov chain Monte Carlo (MCMC) simulation procedures with a Gibbs sampler and four chains. Briefly, MCMC algorithms "mix" prior beliefs with observed data to produce "an approximation of the joint distribution of all parameters" in a model (Muthén & Asparouhov, 2012, p. 334; for a technical discussion, see Gelman et al., 2013). Owing to convergence issues (e.g., slow mixing and >800 free parameters), a process called "thinning" the Markov chains was used to minimize the influence of high autocorrelation among the MCMC estimates with every 10th iteration—with a total of 50000 iterations used to describe the posterior distribution. Our decision here is practical; nevertheless, it is important to recognize that in some cases thinning can produce results that differ from those when the full chain is used (Link & Eaton, 2012). We used "posterior predictive checking" to assess model-data fit, such that the posterior distribution generated by a model is compared with the observed data; if the replicated data closely matches the observed data, one can conclude acceptable model-data fit (Muthén & Asparouhov, 2012). M*plus* produces the posterior predictive *p* value (*PPP*-value), which provides an indication of the degree to which the posterior distribution—obtained from the mixing of prior beliefs and new data—is similar to the observed data. Values around 0.50 indicate a well-fitting model, whereas small values (e.g., <0.05) suggests poor model-data fit (Muthén & Asparouhov, 2012; Zyphur & Oswald, 2015). Nevertheless, it is important to recognize that these proposed values have not yet been empirically validated. Bayesian model comparisons were aided by the deviance information criterion (DIC), BIC, and $BIC_{SSA}$. Further information on the analytical strategy is detailed in the following sections (see also Appendix 8.7 for a 10-point diagnostic checklist for Bayesian analysis).

### Description and Justification of Priors

It is important for researchers to describe and justify where their priors came from and why it is appropriate to mix them with the data to make inferences with posteriors (van de Schoot & Depaoli, 2014; Zyphur & Oswald, 2015). Priors represent background knowledge that can be derived from theoretical expectations, pilot research, expert knowledge, or meta-analyses and other forms of previous empirical research (for examples, see van de Schoot et al., 2014; Zyphur & Oswald, 2015; or Appendix 8.2). There are three broad categories of priors (van de Schoot & Depaoli, 2014): (i) noninformative priors reflect substantial uncertainty in one's expectations about the nature of a parameter (e.g., equal probability of every parameter value between minus and plus infinity), (ii) weakly informative priors incorporate some prior knowledge regarding the population parameter (e.g., specific value of the mean most likely, though every parameter value between minus and plus infinity is plausible), and (iii) informative priors reflect a great deal of certainty in the population parameter (i.e., small variance around a specific value of the mean). Noninformative priors do not influence the final results (i.e., posterior distributions are data driven), weakly informative priors do not substantially influence the final parameter estimate in the posterior distribution once combined with the data, and informative priors are highly influential for final estimates (van de Schoot et al., 2014).

For the purposes of this chapter, two Bayesian models were tested to compare results when noninformative or informative priors are specified for substantive parameters, namely, the intended factor loadings and structural paths between the motivational correlates and mentally tough behavior (for an overview, see Appendix 8.8). In Model 1, we applied noninformative priors for all parameters of the model except for the item cross-loadings among the motivational correlates. As the items captured unique concepts within a broad motivational framework, we expected items to have small associations with nonintended latent factors (Asparouhov & Muthén, 2009). We did not expand these cross-loadings to include items for mentally tough behaviors as they were rated by a parent and therefore did not share the same method or substantive content. In Model 2, we applied informative priors for item factor loadings and structural paths between the motivational correlates and mentally tough behavior. Item factor loadings were guided by statistical recommendations for the quality of factor loadings, whereas structural paths were informed by theoretical expectations of a small-to-moderate association among the motivational correlates and mentally tough behavior.

The M*plus* syntax for Models 1 and 2 are detailed in Appendices 8.9 and 8.10, respectively. In all models, factor loadings and structural paths between the motivational correlates and mentally tough behavior were specified with a normal prior, whereas latent factor correlations, residual variances, and correlated residuals were reflected by an inverse-Wishart distribution because it results in a positive definite matrix (for further information, see Muthén & Asparouhov, 2012). We chose to model correlated residuals for both theoretical and analytical considerations. From a theoretical perspective, we expected that residual variances for observed variables not explained by the target latent variable (e.g., inspiration) might be correlated with other indicators because they each capture slightly different but potentially related aspects of one's personality; of course, we cannot ever be certain as to the exact causes of residual covariances (e.g., method effects or a general personality construct). Given the teaching goals of this chapter, we also wanted to provide an example of how Bayesian analysis can facilitate the examination of new types of models. In this instance, Bayesian analysis allows accommodating all correlations among residual variances, something that often results in identification issues with maximum likelihood estimation (see Cole, Ciesla, & Steiger, 2007).[2]

## Chain Convergence

We specified a fixed number of 100 000 iterations for each MCMC chain using the FBITERATIONS function so that we could examine "potential scale reduction" (PSR) development over iterations beyond the point at which M*plus* deemed our model to converge. The PSR uses variation in parameter estimates over multiple iterations between chains versus total parameter variation over multiple iterations (between/total) to assess convergence based on the idea that convergence is achieved when multiple chains agree on parameter estimates (default convergence criterion is PSR=0.05). In addition to this statistical diagnostic criterion, we visually inspected trace plots for stability in the mean and variance of each chain (van de Schoot et al., 2014).

## Sensitivity Analysis

In instances where there is some degree of subjectivity in the choice of priors or when sample size is small, researchers are encouraged to perform a sensitivity analysis to understand the influence of priors on posterior distributions (van de Schoot et al., 2014; Zyphur & Oswald, 2015). By adjusting the level of (un)certainty in the priors, one can examine whether or not these fluctuations in background knowledge influence the stability of substantive conclusions. For the purposes of this chapter, two sensitivity analyses were performed to illustrate this process. In Model 3a, we altered the informative prior for the structural paths such that we retained the original mean from Model 2 but specified less variance, whereas for Model 3b the mean was increased yet the direction of the hypothesized association was retained with greater variance (see Appendices 8.11 and 8.12, respectively).

## Convergence and Model Fit

Given our a priori focus on Model 2, we report convergence information for this model only. Trace plots of parameter estimates were visually inspected to examine whether or not there was stability in the mean and variance in each chain in the post-burn-in portion (i.e., last 50 000 iterations). Example trace plots from Model 2 are detailed in Appendices 8.13 and 8.14. As can be seen in these figures, all four chains were stable and appeared to converge to a similar target distribution. Statistical criteria also revealed that convergence was obtained with the fixed number of 100 000 iterations. There was a decrease in the PSR value until 48 000 iterations where it remained at or below 1.05. The first 50 000 iterations are discarded as part of the

---

[2] The results do not substantially differ when correlations among residual variances are included or excluded; model fit is primarily affected.

"burn-in" period. Collectively, visual inspections and statistical criteria indicated that the posterior distribution was based on a model that achieved convergence. Just as with frequentist analyses, this finding motivates examining model-fit indices, and these, if acceptable, in turn prompt examining specific parameter estimates and their associated posterior distributions for hypothesis testing.

For Model 1, the probability of the hypothesized theoretical model, given the data, was excellent (PPP=0.639, $\Delta$observed and replicated $\times 2$ 95% CI [−123.30, 86.14], DIC = 36 389.96, BIC = 39 942.74, $BIC_{SSA}$ = 37 331.95). Only 25 of 595 of the correlated residuals (4.20%) seemed of a magnitude that was relevant (based on examining the posterior distributions for their exclusion of zero residual covariation in a 95% credibility interval). For Model 2, the probability of the hypothesized theoretical model, given the data, was excellent (PPP=0.647, $\Delta$observed and replicated $\times 2$ 95% CI [−125.29, 85.59], DIC = 36 396.73, BIC = 39 934.72, $BIC_{SSA}$ = 37 323.91). Only 25 of 595 of the correlated residuals (4.20%) seemed of a magnitude that was relevant. For Model 3a, the probability of the hypothesized theoretical model, given the data, was excellent (PPP=0.648, $\Delta$observed and replicated $\times 2$ 95% CI [−125.38, 85.67], DIC = 36 396.31, BIC = 39 934.87, $BIC_{SSA}$ = 37 324.07). Only 25 of 595 of the correlated residuals (4.20%) were of a magnitude that was important. For Model 3b, the probability of the hypothesized theoretical model, given the data, was excellent (PPP=0.646, $\Delta$observed and replicated $\times 2$ 95% CI [−124.97, 85.86], DIC = 36 397.32, BIC = 39 934.46, $BIC_{SSA}$ = 37 323.65). Only 25 of 595 of the correlated residuals (4.20%) seemed of a magnitude that was relevant. BIC and $BIC_{SSA}$ values indicated that the models using informative priors (Models 2, 3a, and 3b) provided a better fit with the data when compared with the model using noninformative priors (Model 1).

## Comparison of Substantive Interpretations

An overview of the standardized parameter estimates for the measurement and structural components of all models tested are detailed in Tables 8.4, 8.5, 8.6, and 8.7. First, to understand the influence of our theoretically informed priors (Model 2), we compared these prior beliefs with a noninformative prior model (Model 1). Both intended and nonintended factor loadings were comparable in their strength and direction, with the exception of passion items where there were some minor differences in the strength of loadings (see Table 8.4). Most latent variable correlations and structural paths (see Table 8.7) were also comparable in their strength and direction, although there were some minor differences in the size of the associations (e.g., fear of failure). However, the structural path from obsessive passion to mentally tough behavior was of a magnitude that is relevant for the informative prior model ($\beta$=−0.12, 95% CI =−24, −0.01) but not for the noninformative prior model ($\beta$=−0.09, 95% CI =−22, 0.03). Second, we conducted a sensitivity analysis to ascertain the influence of prior knowledge on the posterior distributions when the prior was varied by precision (Model 3a) or by its mean with a more disperse variance (Model 3b). There were minimal differences in the direction and strength of factor loadings between the original model (Model 2) and the two variations (see Tables 8.5 and 8.6), as well as the latent variable correlations and structural paths (see Table 8.7).

Table 8.4  Standardized parameter estimates and score reliabilities ($\omega$) for Bayesian structural equation modeling (Models 1 and 2) analyses of Gucciardi et al.'s (2015) model.

| | Mentally tough behavior | | Obsessive passion | | Harmonious passion | | Fear of failure | | Inspiration frequency | | Inspiration intensity | | $R^2$ | |
|---|---|---|---|---|---|---|---|---|---|---|---|---|---|---|
| | M1 | M2 | M1 | M2 | M1 | M2 | M1 | M2 | M1 | M2 | M1 | M2 | M1 | M2 |
| mt1 | 0.66* | 0.67* | — | — | — | — | — | — | — | — | — | — | 0.45 | 0.44 |
| mt2 | 0.72* | 0.71* | — | — | — | — | — | — | — | — | — | — | 0.51 | 0.51 |
| mt3 | 0.78* | 0.78* | — | — | — | — | — | — | — | — | — | — | 0.61 | 0.61 |
| mt4 | 0.75* | 0.75* | — | — | — | — | — | — | — | — | — | — | 0.57 | 0.57 |
| mt5 | 0.75* | 0.75* | — | — | — | — | — | — | — | — | — | — | 0.56 | 0.56 |
| mt6 | 0.76* | 0.76* | — | — | — | — | — | — | — | — | — | — | 0.58 | 0.58 |
| mt7 | 0.75* | 0.74* | — | — | — | — | — | — | — | — | — | — | 0.55 | 0.55 |
| mt8 | 0.77* | 0.77* | — | — | — | — | — | — | — | — | — | — | 0.60 | 0.60 |
| mt9 | 0.67* | 0.67* | — | — | — | — | — | — | — | — | — | — | 0.45 | 0.45 |
| mt10 | 0.70* | 0.70* | — | — | — | — | — | — | — | — | — | — | 0.49 | 0.49 |
| pas2 | — | — | 0.57* | 0.69* | 0.01 | 0.00 | 0.02 | 0.02 | 0.00 | −0.02 | 0.01 | −0.01 | 0.47 | 0.48 |
| pas4 | — | — | 0.62* | 0.63* | 0.09 | 0.09 | −0.05 | −0.05 | 0.07 | 0.06 | 0.08 | 0.08 | 0.57 | 0.57 |
| pas7 | — | — | 0.88* | 0.59* | −0.02 | 0.04 | −0.02 | 0.00 | −0.05 | −0.01 | −0.03 | 0.01 | 0.41 | 0.40 |
| pas9 | — | — | 0.81* | 0.57* | −0.01 | 0.02 | 0.03 | 0.06 | 0.00 | 0.03 | −0.02 | 0.02 | 0.39 | 0.39 |
| pas11 | — | — | 0.77* | 0.69* | 0.00 | 0.02 | −0.04 | −0.04 | 0.05 | 0.07 | 0.02 | 0.03 | 0.57 | 0.56 |
| pas12 | — | — | 0.72* | 0.59* | −0.02 | 0.01 | 0.06 | 0.05 | −0.03 | 0.00 | −0.02 | 0.00 | 0.37 | 0.38 |
| pas1 | — | — | −0.08 | −0.02 | 0.85* | 0.66* | −0.02 | −0.04 | −0.03 | −0.01 | −0.08 | −0.04 | 0.41 | 0.41 |
| pas3 | — | — | 0.13 | 0.01 | 0.44* | 0.63* | −0.04 | −0.03 | 0.14 | 0.08 | 0.12 | 0.05 | 0.54 | 0.54 |

|  |  |  |  |  |  |  |  |  |  |  |  |  |  |  |
|---|---|---|---|---|---|---|---|---|---|---|---|---|---|---|
| pas5 | — | — | 0.14 | 0.04 | 0.56* | 0.70* | -0.02 | -0.01 | 0.02 | -0.02 | 0.03 | -0.02 | 0.59 | 0.50 |
| pas6 | — | — | -0.09 | -0.19 | 0.63* | 0.79* | -0.04 | -0.03 | 0.07 | 0.00 | 0.05 | 0.00 | 0.52 | 0.52 |
| pas8 | — | — | 0.08 | -0.01 | 0.64* | 0.71* | 0.02 | 0.02 | 0.01 | -0.02 | 0.03 | -0.01 | 0.47 | 0.48 |
| pas10 | — | — | -0.03 | -0.03 | 0.88* | 0.78* | 0.05 | 0.03 | -0.06 | -0.05 | -0.02 | 0.00 | 0.54 | 0.54 |
| fof1 | — | — | -0.10 | -0.09 | 0.03 | 0.01 | 0.77* | 0.74* | 0.02 | 0.00 | 0.01 | -0.01 | 0.54 | 0.54 |
| fof2 | — | — | 0.09 | 0.09 | -0.06 | -0.09 | 0.78* | 0.75* | 0.02 | -0.01 | -0.05 | -0.07 | 0.63 | 0.62 |
| fof3 | — | — | 0.04 | -0.02 | 0.04 | 0.04 | 0.82* | 0.80* | -0.03 | -0.05 | 0.03 | 0.01 | 0.63 | 0.63 |
| fof4 | — | — | 0.00 | -0.01 | -0.01 | -0.03 | 0.69* | 0.69* | 0.02 | 0.02 | 0.04 | 0.02 | 0.47 | 0.47 |
| fof5 | — | — | -0.04 | -0.08 | 0.01 | -0.01 | 0.65* | 0.64* | 0.00 | -0.01 | 0.00 | 0.00 | 0.41 | 0.41 |
| ins1 | — | — | 0.00 | -0.04 | 0.02 | 0.01 | -0.05 | -0.05 | 0.76* | 0.78* | 0.06 | 0.05 | 0.66 | 0.66 |
| ins3 | — | — | 0.01 | -0.01 | 0.01 | 0.01 | 0.05 | 0.04 | 0.87* | 0.84* | -0.04 | -0.03 | 0.68 | 0.68 |
| ins5 | — | — | -0.03 | -0.05 | 0.01 | 0.01 | 0.02 | 0.02 | 0.90* | 0.87* | -0.04 | -0.02 | 0.71 | 0.70 |
| ins7 | — | — | 0.02 | -0.01 | -0.01 | 0.00 | -0.02 | -0.03 | 0.78* | 0.79* | 0.08 | 0.07 | 0.71 | 0.71 |
| ins2 | — | — | 0.05 | 0.03 | 0.03 | 0.03 | -0.01 | -0.01 | 0.01 | 0.01 | 0.80* | 0.80* | 0.70 | 0.70 |
| ins4 | — | — | 0.00 | -0.02 | 0.01 | 0.01 | 0.03 | 0.03 | 0.00 | 0.00 | 0.86* | 0.84* | 0.71 | 0.71 |
| ins6 | — | — | -0.03 | -0.03 | 0.01 | 0.01 | 0.01 | 0.01 | 0.03 | 0.02 | 0.84* | 0.84* | 0.72 | 0.72 |
| ins8 | — | — | -0.02 | -0.04 | -0.01 | -0.01 | -0.02 | -0.02 | 0.01 | 0.04 | 0.85* | 0.82* | 0.70 | 0.70 |
| $\omega$ | 0.92 | 0.92 | 0.88 | 0.81 | 0.85 | 0.86 | 0.86 | 0.85 | 0.91 | 0.90 | 0.91 | 0.90 |  |  |

*$p<0.05$; median values reported for Bayesian model.

Table 8.5  Standardized parameter estimates and score reliabilities ($\omega$) for Bayesian structural equation modeling (Models 2 and 3a) analyses of Gucciardi et al.'s (2015) model.

| | Mentally tough behavior | | Obsessive passion | | Harmonious passion | | Fear of failure | | Inspiration frequency | | Inspiration intensity | | $R^2$ | |
|---|---|---|---|---|---|---|---|---|---|---|---|---|---|---|
| | M2 | M3a | M2 | M3a | M2 | M3a | M2 | M3a | M2 | M3a | M2 | M3a | M2 | M3a |
| mt1 | 0.66* | 0.67* | — | — | — | — | — | — | — | — | — | — | 0.44 | 0.44 |
| mt2 | 0.72* | 0.72* | — | — | — | — | — | — | — | — | — | — | 0.51 | 0.51 |
| mt3 | 0.78* | 0.78* | — | — | — | — | — | — | — | — | — | — | 0.61 | 0.61 |
| mt4 | 0.75* | 0.75* | — | — | — | — | — | — | — | — | — | — | 0.57 | 0.57 |
| mt5 | 0.74* | 0.75* | — | — | — | — | — | — | — | — | — | — | 0.56 | 0.56 |
| mt6 | 0.76* | 0.76* | — | — | — | — | — | — | — | — | — | — | 0.58 | 0.58 |
| mt7 | 0.75* | 0.74* | — | — | — | — | — | — | — | — | — | — | 0.55 | 0.55 |
| mt8 | 0.77* | 0.78* | — | — | — | — | — | — | — | — | — | — | 0.60 | 0.60 |
| mt9 | 0.67* | 0.67* | — | — | — | — | — | — | — | — | — | — | 0.45 | 0.45 |
| mt10 | 0.70* | 0.70* | — | — | — | — | — | — | — | — | — | — | 0.49 | 0.48 |
| pas2 | — | — | 0.69* | 0.69* | 0.00 | 0.00 | 0.02 | 0.02 | -0.02 | -0.02 | -0.01 | -0.01 | 0.48 | 0.47 |
| pas4 | — | — | 0.63* | 0.63* | 0.08 | 0.09 | -0.05 | -0.05 | 0.06 | 0.06 | 0.08 | 0.08 | 0.57 | 0.57 |
| pas7 | — | — | 0.59* | 0.60* | 0.04 | 0.04 | 0.00 | 0.01 | -0.01 | -0.01 | 0.01 | 0.01 | 0.40 | 0.40 |
| pas9 | — | — | 0.57* | 0.56* | 0.02 | 0.02 | 0.06 | 0.06 | 0.03 | 0.03 | 0.02 | 0.02 | 0.39 | 0.40 |
| pas11 | — | — | 0.69* | 0.69* | 0.02 | 0.02 | -0.04 | -0.04 | 0.07 | 0.07 | 0.03 | 0.03 | 0.56 | 0.57 |
| pas12 | — | — | 0.59* | 0.58* | 0.01 | 0.01 | 0.06 | 0.06 | 0.00 | 0.00 | 0.00 | 0.00 | 0.38 | 0.38 |
| pas1 | — | — | -0.02 | -0.03 | 0.67* | 0.66* | -0.04 | -0.04 | 0.00 | -0.01 | -0.04 | -0.04 | 0.41 | 0.41 |
| pas3 | — | — | 0.01 | 0.01 | 0.63* | 0.63* | -0.03 | -0.04 | 0.08 | 0.08 | 0.05 | 0.05 | 0.54 | 0.54 |
| pas5 | — | — | 0.04 | 0.03 | 0.71* | 0.70* | -0.01 | -0.01 | -0.02 | -0.02 | -0.01 | -0.02 | 0.50 | 0.50 |
| pas6 | — | — | -0.19 | -0.19* | 0.79* | 0.79* | -0.03 | -0.04 | 0.01 | 0.00 | 0.00 | 0.00 | 0.52 | 0.52 |

| | | | | | | | | | | | | | | |
|---|---|---|---|---|---|---|---|---|---|---|---|---|---|---|
| pas8 | — | — | −0.01 | −0.01 | 0.70* | 0.71* | 0.02 | 0.02 | −0.02 | −0.02 | −0.01 | −0.01 | 0.48 | 0.48 |
| pas10 | — | — | −0.03 | −0.04 | 0.78* | 0.78* | 0.03 | 0.03 | −0.05 | −0.05 | 0.00 | −0.01 | 0.54 | 0.54 |
| fof1 | — | — | −0.09 | −0.08 | 0.01 | 0.01 | 0.74* | 0.74* | 0.00 | 0.00 | −0.02 | −0.01 | 0.54 | 0.54 |
| fof2 | — | — | 0.09 | 0.11 | −0.10 | −0.09 | 0.75* | 0.76* | −0.01 | −0.01 | −0.07 | −0.07 | 0.62 | 0.62 |
| fof3 | — | — | −0.02 | −0.01 | 0.04 | 0.04 | 0.80* | 0.80* | −0.05 | −0.05 | 0.01 | 0.01 | 0.63 | 0.63 |
| fof4 | — | — | −0.01 | −0.01 | −0.03 | −0.03 | 0.69* | 0.69* | 0.01 | 0.01 | 0.02 | 0.02 | 0.47 | 0.47 |
| fof5 | — | — | −0.08 | −0.08 | −0.01 | −0.01 | 0.64* | 0.64* | −0.01 | −0.01 | 0.00 | 0.00 | 0.41 | 0.41 |
| ins1 | — | — | −0.04 | −0.05 | 0.01 | 0.01 | −0.05 | −0.05 | 0.78* | 0.77* | 0.06 | 0.06 | 0.66 | 0.66 |
| ins3 | — | — | −0.01 | −0.02 | 0.02 | 0.01 | 0.04 | 0.04 | 0.85* | 0.84* | −0.03 | −0.03 | 0.68 | 0.68 |
| ins5 | — | — | −0.05 | −0.07 | 0.01 | 0.01 | 0.02 | 0.01 | 0.87* | 0.87* | −0.01 | −0.02 | 0.70 | 0.71 |
| ins7 | — | — | −0.01 | −0.01 | 0.00 | 0.00 | −0.03 | −0.03 | 0.79* | 0.79* | 0.07 | 0.07 | 0.71 | 0.71 |
| ins2 | — | — | 0.03 | 0.02 | 0.03 | 0.03 | −0.01 | −0.01 | 0.01 | 0.01 | 0.80* | 0.80* | 0.70 | 0.70 |
| ins4 | — | — | −0.02 | −0.03 | 0.01 | 0.01 | 0.03 | 0.02 | 0.00 | 0.00 | 0.84* | 0.84* | 0.71 | 0.71 |
| ins6 | — | — | −0.03 | −0.05 | 0.01 | 0.01 | 0.01 | 0.00 | 0.03 | 0.03 | 0.84* | 0.83* | 0.72 | 0.72 |
| ins8 | — | — | −0.04 | −0.04 | −0.01 | −0.01 | −0.02 | −0.02 | 0.04 | 0.04 | 0.83* | 0.82* | 0.70 | 0.70 |
| ω | 0.92 | 0.92 | 0.81 | 0.81 | 0.86 | 0.86 | 0.85 | 0.85 | 0.90 | 0.90 | 0.90 | 0.90 | 0.90 | 0.90 |

*p<0.05; median values reported for Bayesian model.

Table 8.6 Standardized parameter estimates and score reliabilities (ω) for Bayesian structural equation modeling (Models 2 and 3b) analyses of Gucciardi et al.'s (2015) model.

| | Mentally tough behavior | | Obsessive passion | | Harmonious passion | | Fear of failure | | Inspiration frequency | | Inspiration intensity | | $R^2$ | |
|---|---|---|---|---|---|---|---|---|---|---|---|---|---|---|
| | M2 | M3b | M2 | M3b | M2 | M3b | M2 | M3b | M2 | M3b | M2 | M3b | M2 | M3b |
| mt1 | 0.66* | 0.67* | — | — | — | — | — | — | — | — | — | — | 0.44 | 0.45 |
| mt2 | 0.72* | 0.71* | — | — | — | — | — | — | — | — | — | — | 0.51 | 0.51 |
| mt3 | 0.78* | 0.78* | — | — | — | — | — | — | — | — | — | — | 0.61 | 0.61 |
| mt4 | 0.75* | 0.75* | — | — | — | — | — | — | — | — | — | — | 0.57 | 0.57 |
| mt5 | 0.74* | 0.75* | — | — | — | — | — | — | — | — | — | — | 0.56 | 0.56 |
| mt6 | 0.76* | 0.76* | — | — | — | — | — | — | — | — | — | — | 0.58 | 0.58 |
| mt7 | 0.75* | 0.74* | — | — | — | — | — | — | — | — | — | — | 0.55 | 0.55 |
| mt8 | 0.77* | 0.78* | — | — | — | — | — | — | — | — | — | — | 0.60 | 0.60 |
| mt9 | 0.67* | 0.67* | — | — | — | — | — | — | — | — | — | — | 0.45 | 0.45 |
| mt10 | 0.70* | 0.70* | — | — | — | — | — | — | — | — | — | — | 0.49 | 0.49 |
| pas2 | — | — | 0.69* | 0.69* | 0.00 | 0.00 | 0.02 | 0.02 | -0.02 | -0.02 | -0.01 | -0.01 | 0.48 | 0.48 |
| pas4 | — | — | 0.63* | 0.63* | 0.09 | 0.09 | -0.05 | -0.05 | 0.06 | 0.06 | 0.08 | 0.08 | 0.57 | 0.57 |
| pas7 | — | — | 0.59* | 0.59* | 0.04 | 0.04 | 0.00 | 0.01 | -0.01 | -0.01 | 0.01 | 0.01 | 0.40 | 0.40 |
| pas9 | — | — | 0.57* | 0.57* | 0.02 | 0.02 | 0.06 | 0.06 | 0.03 | 0.03 | 0.02 | 0.02 | 0.39 | 0.39 |
| pas11 | — | — | 0.69* | 0.69* | 0.02 | 0.02 | -0.04 | -0.04 | 0.07 | 0.07 | 0.03 | 0.03 | 0.56 | 0.56 |
| pas12 | — | — | 0.59* | 0.59* | 0.01 | 0.01 | 0.05 | 0.06 | 0.00 | 0.00 | 0.00 | 0.00 | 0.38 | 0.38 |
| pas1 | — | — | -0.02 | -0.02 | 0.66* | 0.66* | -0.04 | -0.04 | -0.01 | 0.00 | -0.04 | -0.04 | 0.41 | 0.41 |
| pas3 | — | — | 0.01 | 0.02 | 0.63* | 0.63* | -0.03 | -0.03 | 0.08 | 0.08 | 0.05 | 0.05 | 0.54 | 0.53 |
| pas5 | — | — | 0.04 | 0.04 | 0.70* | 0.70* | -0.01 | -0.01 | -0.02 | -0.02 | -0.02 | -0.02 | 0.50 | 0.50 |
| pas6 | — | — | -0.19 | -0.19 | 0.79* | 0.79* | -0.03 | -0.04 | 0.00 | 0.01 | 0.00 | 0.00 | 0.52 | 0.52 |
| pas8 | — | — | -0.01 | -0.01 | 0.71* | 0.71* | 0.02 | 0.02 | -0.02 | -0.02 | -0.01 | -0.01 | 0.48 | 0.48 |

| | | | | | | | | | | | | | | |
|---|---|---|---|---|---|---|---|---|---|---|---|---|---|---|
| pas10 | — | — | −0.03 | −0.03 | 0.78* | 0.78* | 0.03 | 0.03 | −0.05 | −0.05 | 0.00 | 0.00 | 0.54 | 0.54 |
| fof1 | — | — | −0.09 | −0.09 | 0.01 | 0.01 | 0.74* | 0.74* | 0.00 | 0.00 | −0.01 | −0.01 | 0.54 | 0.54 |
| fof2 | — | — | 0.09 | 0.09 | −0.09 | −0.09 | 0.75* | 0.76* | −0.01 | −0.01 | −0.07 | −0.07 | 0.62 | 0.63 |
| fof3 | — | — | −0.02 | −0.02 | 0.04 | 0.04 | 0.80* | 0.80* | −0.05 | −0.05 | 0.01 | 0.01 | 0.63 | 0.63 |
| fof4 | — | — | −0.01 | −0.01 | −0.03 | −0.03 | 0.69* | 0.69* | 0.02 | 0.01 | 0.02 | 0.02 | 0.47 | 0.47 |
| fof5 | — | — | −0.08 | −0.08 | −0.01 | −0.01 | 0.64* | 0.64* | −0.01 | −0.01 | 0.00 | 0.00 | 0.41 | 0.41 |
| ins1 | — | — | −0.04 | −0.04 | 0.01 | 0.01 | −0.05 | −0.05 | 0.78* | 0.77* | 0.05 | 0.06 | 0.66 | 0.66 |
| ins3 | — | — | −0.02 | −0.01 | 0.01 | 0.01 | 0.04 | 0.04 | 0.84* | 0.84* | −0.03 | −0.03 | 0.68 | 0.68 |
| ins5 | — | — | −0.05 | −0.05 | 0.01 | 0.01 | 0.02 | 0.01 | 0.87* | 0.87* | −0.02 | −0.01 | 0.70 | 0.71 |
| ins7 | — | — | 0.00 | −0.01 | 0.00 | 0.00 | −0.03 | −0.03 | 0.79* | 0.78* | 0.07 | 0.07 | 0.71 | 0.71 |
| ins2 | — | — | 0.03 | 0.03 | 0.03 | 0.03 | −0.01 | −0.01 | 0.01 | 0.01 | 0.80* | 0.80* | 0.70 | 0.70 |
| ins4 | — | — | −0.02 | −0.02 | 0.01 | 0.01 | 0.03 | 0.03 | 0.00 | 0.00 | 0.84* | 0.84* | 0.71 | 0.71 |
| ins6 | — | — | −0.03 | −0.03 | 0.01 | 0.01 | 0.01 | 0.00 | 0.02 | 0.03 | 0.84* | 0.83* | 0.72 | 0.72 |
| ins8 | — | — | −0.04 | −0.04 | −0.01 | −0.01 | −0.02 | −0.02 | 0.04 | 0.04 | 0.82* | 0.82* | 0.70 | 0.70 |
| ω | 0.92 | 0.92 | 0.81 | 0.81 | 0.86 | 0.86 | 0.85 | 0.85 | 0.90 | 0.90 | 0.90 | 0.90 | | |

*$p < 0.05$; median values reported for Bayesian model.

Table 8.7 Standardized latent variable correlations and structural paths for Bayesian structural equation modeling (BSEM) analyses of Gucciardi et al. (2015) (Models 1–3).

| | Latent variable correlations | | | | | Structural paths |
| | 1 | 2 | 3 | 4 | 5 | Mentally tough behavior |
|---|---|---|---|---|---|---|
| **Model 1** | | | | | | |
| 1 Obsessive passion | — | 0.43 [0.26, 0.59] | 0.43 [0.25, 0.60] | 0.44 [0.26, 0.60] | 0.11 [−0.10, 0.33] | −0.09 [−0.22, 0.03] |
| 2 Harmonious passion | | — | 0.57 [0.38, 0.73] | 0.59 [0.40, 0.75] | −0.13 [−0.36, 0.11] | 0.18 [0.05, 0.32] |
| 3 Inspiration frequency | | | — | 0.82 [0.70, 0.90] | −0.11 [−0.36, 0.15] | 0.26 [0.08, 0.44] |
| 4 Inspiration intensity | | | | — | −0.13 [−0.37, 0.13] | 0.20 [0.01, 0.38] |
| 5 Fear of failure | | | | | — | −0.29 [−0.40, −0.18] |
| **Model 2** | | | | | | |
| 1 Obsessive passion | — | 0.51 [0.31, 0.68] | 0.45 [0.22, 0.65] | 0.44 [0.21, 0.63] | 0.18 [−0.07, 0.41] | −0.12 [−0.24, −0.01] |
| 2 Harmonious passion | | — | 0.62 [0.45, 0.77] | 0.65 [0.48, 0.79] | −0.05 [−0.31, 0.21] | 0.21 [0.09, 0.34] |
| 3 Inspiration frequency | | | — | 0.81 [0.70, 0.90] | −0.03 [−0.30, 0.24] | 0.24 [0.10, 0.38] |
| 4 Inspiration intensity | | | | — | −0.05 [−0.31, 0.22] | 0.21 [0.07, 0.35] |
| 5 Fear of failure | | | | | — | −0.27 [−0.37, −0.16] |
| **Model 3a** | | | | | | |
| 1 Obsessive passion | — | 0.51 [0.32, 0.69] | 0.46 [0.24, 0.66] | 0.45 [0.23, 0.64] | 0.17 [−0.08, 0.41] | −0.17 [−0.26, −0.07] |
| 2 Harmonious passion | | — | 0.62 [0.45, 0.77] | 0.65 [0.48, 0.79] | −0.05 [−0.31, 0.21] | 0.23 [0.13, 0.33] |
| 3 Inspiration frequency | | | — | 0.81 [0.70, 0.90] | −0.02 [−0.29, 0.25] | 0.24 [0.14, 0.35] |
| 4 Inspiration intensity | | | | — | −0.04 [−0.30, 0.22] | 0.22 [0.12, 0.33] |
| 5 Fear of failure | | | | | — | −0.26 [−0.35, −0.17] |
| **Model 3b** | | | | | | |
| 1 Obsessive passion | — | 0.51 [0.31, 0.68] | 0.45 [0.22, 0.65] | 0.44 [0.21, 0.63] | 0.19 [−0.07, 0.42] | −0.11 [−0.24, 0.01] |
| 2 Harmonious passion | | — | 0.62 [0.44, 0.77] | 0.65 [0.47, 0.79] | −0.04 [−0.30, 0.22] | 0.21 [0.07, 0.35] |
| 3 Inspiration frequency | | | — | 0.81 [0.69, 0.90] | −0.02 [−0.29, 0.25] | 0.25 [0.09, 0.42] |
| 4 Inspiration intensity | | | | — | −0.04 [−0.31, 0.23] | 0.20 [0.03, 0.36] |
| 5 Fear of failure | | | | | — | −0.28 [−0.39, −0.17] |

Nevertheless, there are two notable differences worth mentioning. First, the credibility intervals around the structural paths in Model 3a were smaller than those of Model 2, suggesting greater certainty in the posterior distribution. Second, the structural path from obsessive passion to mentally tough behavior was of a magnitude that is important in Model 2 ($\beta = -0.12$, 95% CI $= -24$, $-0.01$) but not for Model 3b ($\beta = -0.11$, 95% CI $= -24$, $0.01$), although the strength of the association was similar.

# Summary

Our goals in this chapter were to provide a nontechnical introduction to key concepts associated with ESEM and Bayesian estimation, illustrating their application in M*plus*. Through a reanalysis of a published paper on the motivational correlates of mentally tough behavior among adolescent tennis players (Gucciardi et al., 2015), we introduced readers to the notion that both statistical techniques provide researchers with a flexible analytical framework in which they can enhance the synergy between substance and method (Marsh & Hau, 2007). Both ESEM and Bayesian estimation accommodate cross-loadings in measurement models that are normally forced to be zero, allowing less inflated parameter estimation of residual covariance and structural paths (Marsh et al., 2014; Muthén & Asparouhov, 2012). Unlike frequentist statistics, which repeatedly test the same null hypothesis, Bayesian estimation permits the explicit integration of prior knowledge or beliefs with new data, thereby providing results that represent a revised or updated state of affairs (Zyphur & Oswald, 2015).

Given the flexibility of ESEM and Bayesian estimation, it is difficult to demonstrate the full potential of each statistical approach in a single chapter. Indeed, many of the techniques outlined in this book can accommodate ESEM and Bayesian estimation. For example, Bayesian estimation can be used to examine experimental designs using ANOVA (Zyphur & Oswald, 2015) and mediation effects in randomized clinical trials (Pirlott, Kisbu-Sakarya, DeFrancesco, Elliot, & MacKinnon, 2012). ESEM can be used to analyze bifactor measurement models (Morin et al., in press; Myers, Martin, Ntoumanis, Celimli, & Bartholomew, 2014), invariance tests across samples and time (see Marsh et al., 2014), and autoregressive cross-lagged models (see Morin et al., 2013). Interested readers are encouraged to consult examples from sport and exercise science (see Appendices 8.1 and 8.2) and beyond (e.g., Muthén, & Asparouhov, 2012; van de Schoot et al., 2014; Zyphur & Oswald, 2015) in order to enable an understanding of the full potential of ESEM and Bayesian estimation.

As with any statistical technique, it is important to consider the strengths of an approach against its potential shortcomings. Perhaps most pertinent to ESEM and Bayesian estimation, the flexibility of these techniques (e.g., accommodating item cross-loadings) should not come at the cost of sound instrument development or parsimonious models. It is important that researchers devote careful consideration to the quality of item indicators and theoretical or methodological issues as alternative explanations for the existence of small cross-loadings in measurement models. In terms of model selection, a comparison of ICM-CFA and ESEM measurement models appears warranted as a first step; when model-data fit and parameter estimates are similar, researchers should retain the more parsimonious ICM-CFA model for subsequent analyses (Marsh et al., 2014). The justification of noninformative and informative priors is a key issue with Bayesian analysis. As the specification priors are not straightforward, detailed descriptions of the source of priors are required to enable readers to judge the veracity of the prior beliefs and their influence on updated knowledge (i.e., posterior distribution) and to replicate and/or extend any particular study (van de Schoot & Depaoli, 2014; Zyphur & Oswald, 2015).

The introduction of user-friendly statistical software such as M*plus* has enhanced the accessibility of advanced statistical techniques to new generations of researchers. In this chapter, we have provided a foundational introduction to two such techniques, namely, ESEM (Asparouhov & Muthén, 2009; for a review, see Marsh et al., 2014) and Bayesian estimation (for reviews, see Kaplan & Depaoli, 2012; Levy & Choi, 2013; van de Schoot & Depaoli, 2014; van de Schoot et al., 2014; Zyphur & Oswald, 2015) within an SEM framework. We have shown readers how to implement these analyses, interpret their corresponding outputs, and present the results in a format suitable for publication in a peer-reviewed manuscript. It is our hope that this chapter will instill confidence in applied researchers with limited statistical training to enhance their knowledge of ESEM and Bayesian estimation and utilize these analytical methods in their future work.

# References

Asparouhov, T., & Muthén, B. (2009). Exploratory structural equation modeling. *Structural Equation Modeling, 16*, 397–438.

Bandalos, D. L. (2014). Relative performance of categorical diagonally weighted least squares and robust maximum likelihood estimation. *Structural Equation Modeling, 21*, 102–116.

Browne, M. W. (2001). An overview of analytic rotation in exploratory factor analysis. *Multivariate Behavioral Research, 36*, 111–150.

Chen, F. F. (2007). Sensitivity of goodness of fit indexes to lack of measurement invariance. *Structural Equation Modeling, 14*, 464–504.

Cole, D. A., Ciesla, J. A., & Steiger, J. H. (2007). The insidious effects of failing to include design-driven correlated residuals in latent-variable covariance structure analysis. *Psychological Methods, 12*, 381–398.

Gelman, A., Carlin, J. B., Stern, H. S., Dunson, D. B., Vehtari, A., & Rubin, D. B. (2013). *Bayesian data analysis* (3rd ed.). Boca Raton, FL: CRC Press.

Guay, F., Morin, A. J. S., Litalien, D., Valois, P., & Vallerand, R. J. (2015). Application of exploratory structural equation modeling to evaluate the Academic Motivation Scale. *Journal of Experimental Education, 83*, 51–82.

Gucciardi, D. F., & Hanton, S. (in press). Mental toughness: Critical reflections and future considerations. In R. J. Schinke, K. R. McGannon, & B. Smith (Eds.), *The Routledge international handbook of sport psychology*. Routledge.

Gucciardi, D. F., Jackson, B., Hanton, S., & Reid, M. (2015). Motivational correlates of mentally tough behaviors in tennis. *Journal of Science and Medicine and Sport, 18*, 67–71.

Kaplan, D., & Depaoli, S. (2012). Bayesian structural equation modeling. In R. H. Hoyle (Ed.), *Handbook of structural equation modeling* (pp. 650–673). New York, NY: Guilford.

Levy, R., & Choi, J. (2013). Bayesian structural equation modeling. In G. R. Hancock & R. O. Mueller (Eds.), *Structural equation modeling: A second course* (2nd ed., pp. 563–623). Charlotte, NC: Information Age Publishing.

Link, W. A., & Eaton, M. J. (2012). On thinning of chains in MCMC. *Methods in Ecology and Evolution, 3*, 112–115.

Marsh, H. W., & Hau, K.-T. (2007). Application of latent variable models in educational psychology: The need for methodological-substantive synergies. *Contemporary Educational Psychology, 32*, 151–171.

Marsh, H. W., Hau, K.-T., & Grayson, D. (2005). Goodness of fit evaluation in structural equation modeling. In A. Maydeu-Olivares & J. McArdle (Eds.), *Psychometrics. A Festschrift for Roderick P. McDonald* (pp. 275–340). Hillsdale, NJ: Erlbaum.

Marsh, H. W., Morin, A. J. S., Parker, P. D., & Kaur, G. (2014). Exploratory structural equation modelling: An integration of the best features of exploratory and confirmatory factor analyses. *Annual Review of Clinical Psychology, 10*, 85–110.

McAdams, D. P., & Pals, J. L. (2006). A new big five: Fundamental principles for an integrative science of personality. *American Psychologist, 61*, 204–217.

McDonald, R. P. (1970). The theoretical foundations of principal factor analysis, canonical factor analysis and alpha factor analysis. *British Journal of Mathematical Psychology, 23*, 1–21.

Morin, A. J. S., Arens, A. K., & Marsh, H. W. (in press). A bifactor exploratory structural equation modeling framework for the identification of distinct sources of construct-relevant psychometric multidimensionality. *Structural Equation Modeling*. doi: 10.1080/10705511.2014.961800

Morin, A. J. S., Marsh, H. W., & Nagengast, B. (2013). Exploratory structural equation modeling. In G. R. Hancock, & R. O. Mueller (Eds.), *Structural equation modeling: A second course* (2nd ed., pp. 395–436). Charlotte, NC: Information Age Publishing.

Muthén, B. O., & Asparouhov, T. (2012). Bayesian structural equation modeling: A more flexible representation of substantive theory. *Psychological Methods, 17*, 313–335.

Muthén, L. K., & Muthén, B. (2012). *Mplus user's guide* (7th ed.). Los Angeles, CA: Muthén & Muthén.

Myers, N. D., Martin, J. J., Ntoumanis, N., Celimli, S., & Bartholomew, K. J. (2014). Exploratory bifactor analysis in sport, exercise and performance psychology: A substantive-methodological synergy. *Sport, Exercise and Performance Psychology, 3*, 258–272.

Pirlott, A. G., Kisbu-Sakarya, Y., DeFrancesco, C. A., Elliot, D. L., & MacKinnon, D. P. (2012). Mechanisms of motivational interviewing in health promotion: A Bayesian mediation analysis. *International Journal of Behavioral Nutrition and Physical Activity, 9*, 69.

Rhemtulla, M., Brosseau-Laird, P. E., & Savalei, V. (2012). When can categorical variables be treated as continuous? A comparison of robust continuous and categorical SEM estimation methods under suboptimal conditions. *Psychological Methods, 17*, 354–373.

Satorra, A., & Bentler, P. N. (1999). A scaled difference chi-square test statistic for moment structure analysis. UCLA Statistic Series, No. 260. Retrieved from http://statistics.ucla.edu/preprints/uclastat-preprint-1999:19

van de Schoot, R., & Depaoli, S. (2014). Bayesian analyses: Where to start and what to report. *The European Health Psychologist, 16*(2), 75–84.

van de Schoot, R., Kaplan, D., Denissen, J., Asendorpf, J. B., Neyer, F. J., & van Aken, M. A. G. (2014). A gentle introduction to Bayesian analysis: Applications to developmental research. *Child Development, 85*, 842–860.

Zyphur, M. J., & Oswald, F. L. (2015). Bayesian estimation and inference: A user's guide. *Journal of Management, 41*, 390–420.

# 9

# A gentle introduction to mixture modeling using physical fitness performance data

**Alexandre J. S. Morin[1] and John C. K. Wang[2]**

[1] *Institute for Positive Psychology and Education, Australian Catholic University, Strathfield, NSW, Australia*
[2] *Physical Education and Sports Science, National Institute of Education, Nanyang Technological University, Singapore*

## General Introduction

Writing a gentle nontechnical introduction to mixture models is a challenge given the scope and complexity of this method. Years ago, multiple regression was presented as a generic framework for the analysis of relations between continuous or categorical predictors, their interactions, and a continuous outcome (Cohen, 1968). Multiple regression was later shown to be a special case of canonical correlation analysis, where multiple outcomes could be considered simultaneously (Knapp, 1978). Structural equation modeling (SEM) was then presented as an even broader framework (Bagozzi, Fornell, & Larcker, 1981), allowing for the estimation of sequences of relations between continuous latent variables (i.e., factors) corrected for measurement error. The generalized SEM (GSEM) framework now integrates SEM and mixture models, allowing for the estimation of relations between any type of continuous and categorical observed and latent variables (Muthén, 2002; Skrondal &

*An Introduction to Intermediate and Advanced Statistical Analyses for Sport and Exercise Scientists*, First Edition.
Edited by Nikos Ntoumanis and Nicholas D. Myers.
© 2016 John Wiley & Sons, Ltd. Published 2016 by John Wiley & Sons, Ltd.
Companion website: www.wiley.com/go/ntoumanis/sport

Rabe-Hesketh, 2004). The key difference between SEM and GSEM is that SEM is *variable-centered*, yielding results reflecting a synthesis of relations observed in the total sample and assuming that all individuals are drawn from a single population. GSEM relaxes this assumption by considering the possibility that the relations differ across subgroups of participants.

GSEM thus combines SEM with a mixture modeling *person-centered* framework aiming to identify relatively homogeneous subgroups of participants, also called latent classes or profiles, differing qualitatively and quantitatively from one another in relation to (i) specific observed and/or latent variable(s) and/or (ii) relations among observed and/or latent variables (Borsboom, Mellenbergh, & Van Heerden, 2003; Morin & Marsh, 2015). Person-centered analyses are thus *typological* in nature, resulting in a classification system designed to help categorize individuals more accurately into qualitatively and quantitatively distinct subpopulations (e.g., Bergman, 2000). The resulting profiles are also *prototypical* in nature, with all participants having a probability of membership in all profiles based on their degree of similarity with the profiles' specific configurations (McLachlan & Peel, 2000). More precisely, profile membership is not known *a priori* but rather inferred from the data and represented by a latent categorical variable where each category represents an inferred subpopulation. Because these profiles are latent, participants are not "forced" into a single profile, but are rather assigned a probability of membership in all profiles.

Mixture models have been around for decades (Gibson, 1959; Lazarsfeld & Henry, 1968), but it is their integration within GSEM, coupled with the development user-friendly statistical packages (e.g., Latent GOLD: Vermunt & Magidson, 2005; Mplus: Muthén & Muthén, 1998–2014; GLLAMM: Rabe-Hesketh, Skrondal, & Pickles, 2004), that have given these models a very high level of flexibility and popularity. Indeed, GSEM makes possible the extraction of subgroups differing from one another on any part of any type of SEM model. For this reason, a complete coverage of all possibilities provided by mixture models and GSEM is clearly beyond the scope of an introductory chapter and some choices had to be made. Thus, we elected to focus on a series of models aiming to provide a broad overview of the possibilities offered by this framework, as implemented in the Mplus package. Although mixture models can be used indirectly (in a *variable-centered* manner) to obtain more exact estimates of nonlinearity, nonnormality, and interactions among variables (Bauer, 2005), we focus on direct (*person-centered*) applications of mixture models where the latent categorical variable is assumed to reflect substantively meaningful subpopulations (Borsboom et al., 2003), adopting the perspective that "the real added value of person-centered approaches is heuristic: human beings naturally conceptualize things and persons in terms of categories and a person-centered approach is better suited to these natural mindsets than a variable-centered approach, for an equivalent predictive value" (Morin, Morizot, Boudrias, & Madore, 2011, p. 76). We assume that readers have a good understanding of structural equation models (Chapter 5), tests of measurement invariance (Chapter 6), and latent growth modeling (Chapter 7) covered elsewhere in this book.

The models illustrated in this chapter are represented in Figure 9.1, where octagons represent categorical latent variables ($C1$ to $Ci$), squares represent manifest variables ($X1$ to $Xi$ for indicators, $P$ for predictors, $O$ for outcomes), and circles represent continuous latent factors (here, the intercepts $\alpha$ and slopes $\beta$ of latent growth models; see Chapter 7), We start our illustration with latent profile analyses (LPA; Model 1 in Figure 9.1), a model-based approach to the classification of participants based on their scores on a set of indicators (e.g., Morin, Morizot et al., 2011; Wang, Biddle, Liu, & Lim, 2012). We then illustrate how to test the invariance of LPA solutions across observed subgroups of participants (Eid, Langeheine, & Diener, 2003; Kankaraš, Moors, & Vermunt, 2011), how to integrate predictors and outcomes to a LPA solution (Model 2 in Figure 9.1; Asparouhov & Muthén, 2014; Wang, Liu, Chatzisarantis, &

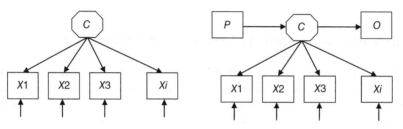

Model 1: Latent profile analysis                    Model 2: Latent profile analysis with covariates

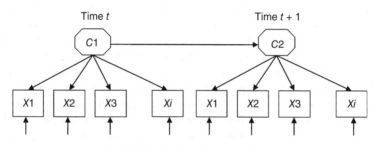

Model 3: Latent transition analysis

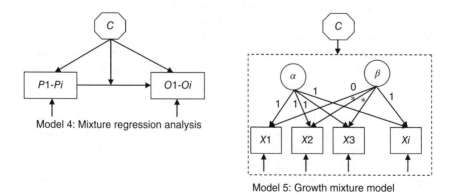

Model 4: Mixture regression analysis

Model 5: Growth mixture model

*Figure 9.1    Representation of key models illustrated in this chapter.*

Lim, 2010), and how to test for the longitudinal stability of LPA solutions using latent transition analyses (LTA; Model 3 in Figure 9.1; e.g., Collins & Lanza, 2009; Kam, Morin, Meyer, & Topolnytsky, 2014). Next, we illustrate the estimation of mixture regression models (MRM; Henson, Reise, & Kim, 2007; Morin, Scalas, & Marsh, 2015), allowing for the identification of subgroups differing from one another at the level of the relations among constructs, in addition to the levels of the constructs themselves (Model 4 in Figure 9.1). Finally, we illustrate growth mixture models (GMM), allowing for the identification of subgroups of participants following distinct longitudinal trajectories (Model 5 in Figure 9.1; e.g., Grimm, Ram, & Estabrook, 2010; Morin, Maïano, Nagengast, Marsh, Morizot & Janosz, 2011).

# Utility of the Method in Sport and Exercise Science

In sport and exercise science, most quantitative research uses *variable-centered* approaches as the main form of analysis. These *variable-centered* approaches describe relations among *variables* and address questions regarding the relative contributions that predictor variables can make to an outcome or the way variables can be grouped together. The use of (M)ANOVAs, regressions, factor analysis, and SEM are examples of *variable-centered* approaches.

*Person-centered* analyses focus on relations among *individuals* and more specifically investigate the way individuals can be grouped together based on their similarity on a set of indicators or the differential way variables relate to one another in these specific subgroups. Cluster analyses have often been used to achieve such classifications. However, cluster analyses (i) are highly reactive to the clustering algorithm, measurement scales, and distributions; (ii) do not provide clear guidelines to select the optimal number of profiles in the sample; (iii) rely on rigid assumptions; (iv) assume that participants correspond to a single profile (i.e., they are *typological* without being *prototypical*); and (v) have not been integrated to the GSEM framework. In contrast, mixture models provide a model-based approach to classification that is (i) integrated into the GSEM framework, (ii) extract *prototypical* profiles, (iii) rely on less stringent assumptions that can often be relaxed or empirically tested, (iv) can easily accommodate covariates, and (v) are associated with indices to help in the selection of the optimal model (Magidson & Vermunt, 2002, 2004; Vermunt & Magidson, 2002).

For these reasons, LPA appear to be gaining popularity in sport and exercise science as providing a more robust, less subjective, and more generalizable typological approach (Wang et al., 2012). The desire to classify objects, or persons, to better make sense of our environments has always been present across the social, psychological, and health disciplines that form the core of sport and exercise science and can be traced back to the Greek philosophers (e.g., Bergman, 2000; Bergman & Trost, 2006). The reasons why researchers would want to incorporate mixture models to their research are numerous: (i) to simply categorize individuals, (ii) to investigate whether a specific latent construct should be represented as a categorical entity rather than as a continuum (e.g., Borsboom et al., 2003; Masyn, Henderson, & Greenbaum, 2010), or (iii) to investigate the invariance of measurement models (see Chapter 6) across the full range of unobserved latent subpopulations present in a sample (Tay, Newman, & Vermunt, 2011).

There is a wide variety of applications of mixture models in sport and exercise science. At the most basic level, LPA aims to identity relatively homogenous subgroups of participants presenting similar patterns of scores on a set of categorical or continuous indicators. In this chapter, we illustrate LPA using fitness performance data, which are common in sport and exercise science. Wang et al. (2012) previously demonstrated the use of LPA in profiling physical and sedentary behavior patterns. However, LPA are not limited to physical data but can easily involve psychological (such as achievement goal profiles or personality types) or social (such as types of team motivational climates) data. For instance, Wang et al. (2010) estimated profiles of students based on their perceptions of the motivational climate of their physical education classes and then tested the association between these profiles and students achievement goals and affect. LPA can easily be extended to test the invariance of a profile solution across any meaningful subgroups of participants, such as different sports, levels of practice, or countries, or even across time points using LTA. Rather than classifying participants based on scores on a set of indicators, MRM can be used to extract subgroups of participants differing from one another in regard to the relations between sets of variables. For instance, Morin, Marsh, Nagengast, and Scalas (2014) used MRM to identify subgroups for which perceived actual and ideal levels of physical appearance were differentially related to more global self-conceptions. Finally, GMM is useful in studying dynamic patterns of change over time and in locating profiles presenting distinct longitudinal trajectories. For example, Morin, Maïano, Marsh, Nagengast, and Janosz (2013) used GMM to extract subgroups of adolescents presenting distinct longitudinal trajectories of global self-esteem (GSE). They identified four distinct trajectories showing (i) low and unstable levels of GSE, (ii) moderate levels of GSE, (iii) high and very stable levels of GSE, and (iv) a switching pattern characterized by low and unstable levels of GSE at the start of secondary school but high and stable levels a few years later.

# The Substantive Example(s)

This illustration relies on a sample of 10 000 students (5 000 boys; 5 000 girls) who annually completed physical fitness tests for 7 years, starting in grade four of primary school (aged 9–10) until the fourth year of secondary school (aged 15–16). These students come from 217 primary and 167 secondary Singaporean schools. In Singapore, all healthy students are required to participate annually in the National Physical Fitness Award (NAPFA) test, starting in Grade 4. The NAPFA is a high-stakes test conducted according to strict testing protocols: NAFPA testers must receive two days of training and be certified by the Singapore Sports Council, schools are required to inform the Ministry of Education (MOE) about test dates, and MOE performs random inspections of testing procedures.

The NAPFA involves six tests, recognized as reliable and valid indicators of physical fitness (Giam, 1981; Jackson, 2006): (i) Sit-ups: The maximum number of bent-knee sit-ups in one minute; (ii) Broad jumps: The better of two standing broad jumps distance; (iii) Sit and reach: The better of two sit-and-reach forward distances; (iv) Pull-ups: The maximum number of overhand-grasp regular pull-ups (males over 14) or overhand-grasp inclined pull-ups (females and males younger than 14) in half a minute; (v) Shuttle run: The faster of two attempts to complete a 4 times 10 m shuttle run; (vi) Run–walk: The minimum time taken for a 1.6 km (primary school) or 2.4 km (secondary school) run–walk. These tests are attempted on the same day, with 2–5 min rest between them, apart from the run–walk test which may be attempted on a different day within a 2-week period. As the norms for these tests differ as a function of grade and gender, scores were standardized within grade and gender. For details on time-related trends on these tests, see Wang, Pyun, Liu, Lim, and Li (2013).

Results on tests (i), (ii), and (iv) can be combined into single indicator of physical strength, results on tests (v) and (vi) can be combined into a single indicator of cardiovascular fitness, whereas test (iii) reflects flexibility. For some analyses (MRM, GMM), we relied on these global indicators (physical strength; cardiovascular fitness) computed as the factor scores from a fully invariant longitudinal confirmatory factor analytic model (see Appendix 9.1, also see Chapters 5 and 6).

This data set comes from an official government testing program and has a restricted access. We are thus unable to share it with readers. However, mixture models are computer- and time-intensive analyses for which users often struggle to get the models to converge properly on a well-replicated solution. Because of this, we strongly advocate users to use their own practice data sets.

In this illustration, we start by estimating LPA across separate samples of boys and girls in order to identify subgroups of participants with distinct profiles of physical fitness. To illustrate the inclusion of covariates, we use previous levels of body mass index (BMI; the only meaningful covariate available in this data set) to predict profile membership and use profile membership to predict later BMI. Then, we verify whether these LPA solutions are invariant across gender groups. Afterward, we rely on LTA to test whether these cross-sectional results remain the same across the combined pubertal and secondary school transition. To this end, we selected Grade 5 (primary) as the first measurement point (at which all participants are unlikely to have experienced the onset of puberty) and the third year of secondary school (at which all participants are likely to be through major pubertal changes). For consistency, all preliminary analyses leading to these LTA are thus based on Grade 5 students. To provide an alternative perspective of the estimation of relations between physical fitness and BMI, we also illustrate the use of MRM to extract profiles differing in the relations between predictors and later levels of BMI. Finally, we illustrate the use of GMM to extract profiles differing on their longitudinal trajectories of physical strength and cardiovascular fitness. Annotated input codes used to estimate the illustrated models are provided in Appendices 9.14–9.37. However, we first address two critical issues that are common to mixture models.

## Class Enumeration in Mixture Models

Conventional goodness-of-fit indices (e.g., CFI, RMSEA) are not available for mixture models. Mixture models require that solutions including differing number of latent profiles be contrasted in order to select the final solution in a mainly exploratory manner (but see Finch & Bronk, 2011, for confirmatory applications). Typically, solutions including one latent profile up to a number of latent profiles that is higher than expectations are estimated and contrasted. Here, we contrasted models including one to eight profiles. To help in the selection of the optimal number of profiles, multiple sources of information can be considered. Clearly, the most important criteria in this decision are the substantive meaning and theoretical conformity of the solution (Marsh, Lüdtke, Trautwein, & Morin, 2009) as well as its statistical adequacy (e.g., absence of negative variance estimates). This last verification is important as mixture models frequently converge on improper solutions. Such improper solutions suggest that the model may have been overparameterized in terms of requesting too many latent profiles or allowing too many parameters to differ across profiles (Bauer & Curran, 2003; Chen, Bollen, Paxton, Curran, & Kirby, 2001); more parsimonious models may thus be superior.

Several indicators also help in this decision: the Akaike information criterion (AIC), the consistent AIC (CAIC), the Bayesian information criterion (BIC), and the sample size-adjusted BIC (SABIC). A lower value on these indicators suggests a better-fitting model. Likelihood ratio tests (LRTs) are inappropriate for comparisons of models including different number of profiles but may be used to compare models based on the same variables and number of profiles.[1] However, for purposes of class enumeration, LRT approximations are available: the standard and adjusted Lo, Mendell, and Rubin's (2001) LRTs (LMR/aLMR, typically yielding the same conclusions—here, we only report the aLMR) and the bootstrap LRT (BLRT; McLachlan & Peel, 2000). These tests compare a $k$-profile model with a $k-1$-profile model, and nonsignificant $p$ values suggest that the $k-1$ profile model should be retained. Finally, the entropy indicates the precision with which the cases are classified into the profiles, with larger values (closer to 1) indicating fewer classification errors. The entropy should not be used to determine the optimal model, but nevertheless provides a useful summary of the classification accuracy of a model.

Simulation studies show that the BIC, SABIC, CAIC, and BLRT are particularly effective in choosing the model which best recovers the sample's true parameters (Henson et al., 2007; McLachlan & Peel, 2000; Nylund, Asparouhov, & Muthén, 2007; Peugh & Fan, 2013; Tein, Coxe, & Cham, 2013; Tofighi & Enders, 2008; Tolvanen, 2007; Yang, 2006). When these indicators fail to retain the optimal model, the AIC, ABIC, and BLRT tend to overestimate the number of profiles, whereas the BIC and CAIC tend to underestimate it. However, since these tests are all variations of tests of statistical significance, the class enumeration procedure can still be heavily influenced by sample size (Marsh et al., 2009). More precisely, with sufficiently large sample sizes, these indicators may keep on suggesting the addition of profiles without

---

[1] LRTs are computed as minus two times the difference in the log-likelihood of the nested models and interpreted as chi-squares with degrees of freedom equal to the difference in the number of free parameters between models. With MLR estimation, LRTs need to be divided by a scaling correction composite, cd, where (i) $cd = (p0 \times c0 - p1 \times c1)/(p0 - p1)$, (ii) $p0$ and $p1$ are the number of free parameters in the nested and comparison models, and (iii) $c0$ and $c1$ are the scaling correction factors for the nested and comparison models (Satorra & Bentler, 1999).

ever reaching a minimum. In these cases, information criteria should be graphically presented through "elbow plots" illustrating the gains associated with additional profiles (Morin, Maïano et al., 2011; Petras & Masyn, 2010). In these plots, the point after which the slope flattens out indicates the optimal number of profiles.

## The Estimation of Mixture Models

In this study, all models were estimated using the robust maximum likelihood estimator available in Mplus 7.2 (Muthén & Muthén, 1998–2014). Although we aim to provide a nontechnical introduction to mixture models, technically oriented readers may consult McLachlan and Peel (2000); Muthén and Shedden (1999), and Skrondal and Rabe-Hesketh (2004). An important challenge in mixture models is to avoid converging on a local solution (i.e., a false maximum likelihood). This problem often stems from inadequate start values. It is thus recommended to estimate the model with as many random sets of start values as possible (Hipp & Bauer, 2006; McLachlan & Peel, 2000), keeping in mind that more random starts requires more computational time. Here, due to the availability of powerful computers, we used 5 000 random sets of start values for LPA (10 000 for more complex LTA, MRM, and GMM), 100 iterations for each random start (1 000 for complex models), and retained the 200 best starts for final optimization (500 for complex models). In practice, we recommend using at least 3000 sets of random starts, 100 iterations, and to retain at least 100 for final stage optimization. These values can be increased when the final solution is not sufficiently replicated (Appendix 9.2). Finally, it is possible to control for the non-independence of the observations due to nesting within larger units (e.g., schools) using Mplus design-based correction (Appendix 9.3).

# The Synergy

## LPA of Grade 5 Students and Tests of Invariance across Gender Groups

The results of the class enumeration procedure used to determine the optimal number of latent profiles to describe NAPFA scores for boys and girls attending Grade 5 are reported in Table 9.1. In these models, the six NAPFA tests were used as profile indicators, and their means and variances were freely estimated in all profiles.[2] Although we relied on classical LPAs assuming conditional independence, we discuss

---

[2] Freely estimating the variances of the LPA indicators within profiles requires relaxing Mplus defaults which constrains them to be invariant across profiles. This more flexible parameterization does not involve reliance on the untested and unrealistic implicit assumption that all profile groups will present the same level of within-profile variability (see e.g., Morin, Maïano, et al., 2011), and has been shown to help recover the population true parameters (Peugh & Fan, 2013). However, this specification may not always be possible to implement (e.g., for more complex models or smaller sample sizes) and often tends to result in convergence problems—suggesting that more parsimonious models with invariant variances should be estimated. Our recommendation would be to always start with these more flexible models and reduce model complexity when necessary.

Table 9.1 Results from the latent profile analyses (Grade 5).

| Model | LL | #fp | Scaling | AIC | CAIC | BIC | ABIC | Entropy | aLMR | BLRT |
|---|---|---|---|---|---|---|---|---|---|---|
| *Class enumeration, boys* | | | | | | | | | | |
| 1 Profile | −39009.296 | 12 | 1.1352 | 78042.591 | 78131.795 | 78119.795 | 78081.663 | NA | NA | NA |
| 2 Profile | −35991.611 | 25 | 1.4041 | 72033.222 | 72219.061 | 72194.061 | 72114.621 | 0.768 | ≤0.001 | ≤0.001 |
| 3 Profile | −34941.597 | 38 | 1.4072 | 69959.194 | 70241.671 | 70203.671 | 70082.921 | 0.780 | ≤0.001 | ≤0.001 |
| 4 Profile | −34128.854 | 51 | 1.4119 | 68359.707 | 68738.820 | 68687.820 | 68525.762 | 0.819 | ≤0.001 | ≤0.001 |
| 5 Profile | −33659.337 | 64 | 1.4003 | 67446.674 | 67922.424 | 67858.424 | 67655.057 | 0.827 | ≤0.001 | ≤0.001 |
| 6 Profile | −33409.163 | 77 | 1.3617 | 66972.325 | 67544.712 | 67467.712 | 67223.035 | 0.805 | ≤0.001 | ≤0.001 |
| 7 Profile | −33218.378 | 90 | 1.3384 | 66616.755 | 67285.778 | 67195.778 | 66909.793 | 0.796 | ≤0.001 | ≤0.001 |
| 8 Profile | −33054.893 | 103 | 1.3359 | 66315.787 | 67081.447 | 66978.447 | 66651.152 | 0.790 | 0.004 | ≤0.001 |
| *Class enumeration, girls* | | | | | | | | | | |
| 1 Profile | −39137.000 | 12 | 1.1317 | 78298.000 | 78387.230 | 78375.230 | 78337.098 | NA | NA | NA |
| 2 Profile | −37026.139 | 25 | 1.3237 | 74102.279 | 74288.173 | 74263.173 | 74183.732 | 0.698 | ≤0.001 | ≤0.001 |
| 3 Profile | −36132.889 | 38 | 1.3303 | 72341.779 | 72624.338 | 72586.338 | 72465.588 | 0.789 | ≤0.001 | ≤0.001 |
| 4 Profile | −35608.657 | 51 | 1.4121 | 71319.315 | 71698.539 | 71647.539 | 71485.480 | 0.774 | ≤0.001 | ≤0.001 |
| 5 Profile | −35237.664 | 64 | 1.3754 | 70603.329 | 71079.218 | 71015.218 | 70811.850 | 0.791 | ≤0.001 | ≤0.001 |
| 6 Profile | −35055.796 | 77 | 1.3995 | 70265.591 | 70838.145 | 70761.145 | 70516.469 | 0.771 | 0.031 | ≤0.001 |
| 7 Profile | −34924.944 | 90 | 1.4579 | 70029.888 | 70699.107 | 70609.107 | 70323.121 | 0.760 | 0.329 | ≤0.001 |
| 8 Profile | −34806.684 | 103 | 1.5504 | 69819.369 | 70585.253 | 70482.253 | 70154.958 | 0.739 | 0.652 | ≤0.001 |

| Model | LL | #fp | Scaling | AIC | CAIC | BIC | ABIC | Entropy | LRT | df |
|---|---|---|---|---|---|---|---|---|---|---|
| *Final 5-profile model, including correction for nesting* | | | | | | | | | | |
| Boys | −33659.337 | 64 | 2.9958 | 67446.674 | 67922.424 | 67858.424 | 67655.057 | 0.827 | NA | NA |
| Girls | −35237.664 | 64 | 3.0487 | 70603.329 | 71079.218 | 71015.218 | 70811.850 | 0.791 | NA | NA |
| *Invariance of the LPA solution* | | | | | | | | | | |
| Configural | −75279.495 | 129 | 3.2672 | 150816.991 | 151865.480 | 151736.480 | 151326.539 | 0.866 | NA | NA |

(*Continued*)

Table 9.1  (*Continued*)

| Model | LL | #fp | Scaling | AIC | CAIC | BIC | ABIC | Entropy | LRT | df |
|---|---|---|---|---|---|---|---|---|---|---|
| Structural (M) | −75 305.956 | 99 | 3.6807 | 150 809.912 | 151 614.567 | 151 515.567 | 151 200.961 | 0.866 | 27.815 | 30 |
| Dispersion (M, V) | −75 460.796 | 69 | 4.6163 | 151 059.592 | 151 620.412 | 151 551.412 | 151 332.142 | 0.864 | 202.561* | 30 |
| Distributional (M, P) | −75 326.302 | 95 | 3.7025 | 150 842.603 | 151 614.747 | 151 519.747 | 151 217.853 | 0.865 | 12.865 | 4 |
| *Deterministic invariance* | | | | | | | | | | |
| Free | −72 635.877 | 103 | 3.5199 | 145 477.754 | 146 312.624 | 146 209.624 | 145 882.307 | 0.867 | NA | NA |
| Invariant | −72 662.917 | 99 | 3.5986 | 145 523.835 | 146 326.283 | 146 227.283 | 145 912.678 | 0.867 | 34.400* | 4 |
| *Predictive invariance* | | | | | | | | | | |
| Free | −87 691.334 | 106 | 3.6233 | 175 594.667 | 176 459.838 | 176 353.838 | 176 016.987 | 0.856 | NA | NA |
| Invariant | −87 720.652 | 101 | 3.7506 | 175 643.305 | 176 467.666 | 176 366.666 | 176 045.704 | 0.855 | 55.746* | 5 |

LL, model log-likelihood; #fp, number of free parameters; scaling, scaling factor associated with MLR log-likelihood estimates; AIC, Akaike information criteria; CAIC, constant AIC; BIC, Bayesian information criteria; ABIC, sample size-adjusted BIC; aLMR, adjusted Lo–Mendell–Rubin likelihood ratio test; BLRT, bootstrap likelihood ratio test; LRT, likelihood ratio test; df, degrees of freedom associated with the LRT; M, means; V, variances; P, class probabilities.
*$p \leq 0.01$.

alternative specifications in Appendix 9.4. As mentioned previously, it is typical for the indicators used in the class enumeration process, due to their sensitivity to sample size, to keep on suggesting the addition of profiles without ever reaching a minimum. This is what happened here, potentially due to the large sample size. We thus graphed, in Figure 9.2 for boys and Appendix 9.5 for girls, elbow plots representing the gains associated with additional profiles. These figures suggest that the improvement in fit reaches a plateau at 5 profiles and becomes negligible thereafter. Based on a detailed examination of the 5-profile solution, together with neighboring 4- and 6-profile solutions, the decision was made to retain 5 profiles for both genders based on clear qualitative differences between profiles, theoretical conformity, lack of small profiles (≤1–5% of cases), nonredundancies between profiles, and convergence across gender.

Once the 5-profile solution has been retained for both gender groups (see Appendices 9.14 and 9.15 for basic input files), it becomes possible to conduct more formal tests of invariance of this solution across genders. The sequence of invariance tests proposed here can easily be extended to the comparison of any subgroups of participants. This sequence is based on, and extends, a similar sequence previously proposed for latent class solutions (where the profile indicators are categorical rather than continuous, as in LPA; Eid et al., 2003; Kankaraš et al., 2011). This sequence starts with the verification of whether the same number of profiles can be identified in all subgroups. Once this has been ascertained, a multiple-group model of configural invariance where the same model, with the same number of profiles, is simultaneously estimated in all groups without added constraints (Appendix 9.17). Then, it becomes possible to test whether the profiles themselves are similar across samples in terms of being characterized by similar levels on the profile indicators (i.e., structural invariance; Appendix 9.18)—in this example, the NAPFA tests. Evidence of configural and structural invariance (see Chapter 6) is a prerequisite to subsequent tests. When the

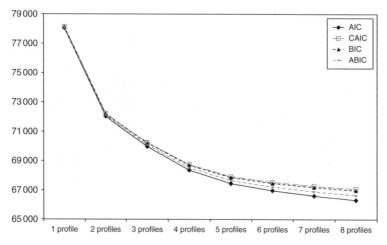

*Figure 9.2    Elbow plot of the information criteria for the LPA, boys, Grade 5.*

number and structure of the profiles differ across samples, all analyses must be conducted separately, and further tests of invariance are neither possible nor relevant.

The third step tests whether the within-profile variability on the indicators is similar across samples (i.e., dispersion invariance; Appendix 9.19). LPAs do not assume that all individuals share the exact same configuration of indicators within each profile, but rather allow for within-profile variability. Testing for dispersion invariance involves testing whether the profiles are more or less internally consistent across samples. Regardless of whether dispersion invariance is supported, the fourth step assesses whether the size of the profiles is similar across samples (i.e., distributional invariance; Appendix 9.20). Predictors and outcomes can then be added to the most invariant model, starting minimally with a model of structural invariance. The fifth step tests whether the relations between predictors (i.e., Grade 4 BMI) and profile membership are invariant or moderated across samples (i.e., deterministic invariance; Appendices 9.21 and 9.22). Finally, the sixth step assesses whether the relations between profiles and outcomes (i.e., Grade 6 BMI) replicate across samples (i.e., predictive invariance; Appendices 9.23 and 9.24).

The results from these tests of invariance are reported in the lower section of Table 9.1 and support the structural and distributional invariance of the profiles (i.e., lower or equivalent values on the information criteria, nonsignificant LRTs), but not their dispersion invariance (i.e., higher values on the information criteria, significant LRT). We thus retained a model in which the within-profile means and relative sizes were invariant across gender. The results from this model are reported in Appendix 9.6 and depicted in Figure 9.3. The first profile describes 10.05% of the sample presenting well below average scores on physical strength indicators (sit-ups, pull-ups, broad jumps), slightly below average scores on the indicator of flexibility (sit and reach), and well above average scores on cardiovascular fitness indicators (shuttle run, run–walk). We chose the label "Fit-Cardio" to describe this profile. The second profile describes 35.60% of the

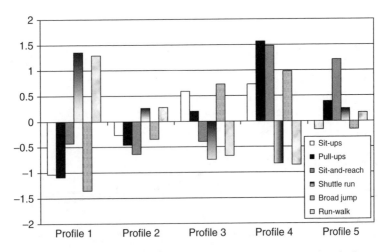

*Figure 9.3    Within-profile means for the LPA solution, Grade 5.*

sample presenting slightly below average scores on indicators of physical strength and flexibility and slightly above average scores on cardiovascular fitness indicators. We chose the label "Average Fitness with Low Flexibility" to describe this profile.

The third profile (26.25%) is characterized by below average scores on indicators of cardiovascular fitness and flexibility and above average scores on indicators of physical strength. We chose the label "Moderately Strong" to describe this profile. The fourth profile (10.34%) presents below average scores on indicators of cardio-vascular fitness but well above average scores on indicators of physical strength and flexibility. We chose the label "Strong and Flexible" to describe this profile. Finally, the fifth profile (17.77%) presents scores that are close to average on indicators of physical strength and cardiovascular fitness but well above average scores of flexibility. We chose the label "Flexible" to describe this profile. As discussed previously, the profiles means and sizes were found to be invariant across gender, but not the variance estimates. Gender-specific estimates of variability, which can easily be compared using the confidence intervals (CI) routinely provided with Mplus outputs, are reported in Appendix 9.6. The estimates in bold are those that differ across gender. Here, these results mainly show higher levels of variability for girls (relative to boys) in Profile 2 (Average Fitness with Low Flexibility) on most indicators and in Profile 4 (Strong and Flexible) on the run–walk test.

## Inclusion of Covariates in LPA Solutions

A critical advantage of mixture models over alternative procedures (e.g., cluster analyses) is the ability to include covariates (predictors and outcomes) directly in the model rather than to rely on two-step procedures where profile membership information is saved to an external file and used in a new series of analyses. Although covariates should not qualitatively change the profiles per se (Marsh et al., 2009), this helps to limit type 1 errors by combining analyses and have been shown to systematically reduce biases in the estimation of the model parameters, especially those describing the relations between the covariates and the profiles (which otherwise tend to be underestimated; Bolck, Croon, & Hagenaars, 2004; Clark & Muthén, 2009; Lubke & Muthén, 2007).

Before including covariates to the model, a critical question that needs to be answered is whether these covariates are logically and theoretically conceptualized as having an impact on profile membership (predictors) or as being impacted by pro-file membership (outcomes). In both cases, we recommend that covariates be included to the model after the class enumeration procedure has been completed. This method allows for the verification of the stability of the model following covariates inclusion (Marsh et al., 2009; Tofighi & Enders, 2008). But, more importantly, the inclusion or exclusion of covariates should not change the substantive interpretation of the pro-files. Observing such a change would indicate a violation of the assumption that covariates predict membership into profiles or are predicted by it and would rather show that the nature of the profiles is dependent on the choice of the predictors (Marsh et al., 2009; Morin, Morizot et al., 2011). Using the procedure described in Appendix 9.2, involving the use of the start values from the final unconditional solution, typically prevents running into such interpretation problems, especially when there are few covariates. However, should such problems be encountered in the estimation process, Mplus has recently implemented a series of AUXILIARY procedures to include covariates without allowing them to influence the nature of the profiles. We refer the reader to Asparouhov and Muthén (2014) for advice on the implementation of these alternative procedures.

The predictor (Grade 4 BMI) was directly incorporated to the model by way of a multinomial logistic regression,[3] whereas the outcome (Grade 6 BMI) was directly incorporated as a distal outcome. At the bottom of Table 9.1, we contrast the results of the models in which the relations between these covariates and the profiles were freely estimated across gender, with models in which these relations where constrained to invariance. These results suggest that neither the deterministic nor the predictive invariance of the LPA solution was supported, showing that all of these relations are moderated by gender. The results from these analyses (using the fifth profile "Flexible" as comparison profile; see Appendix 9.7) globally show that higher levels of BMI in Grade 4 increase the likelihood of membership into Profile 1 (Fit-Cardio), particularly among girls, but decrease the likelihood of membership into the third (Moderately Strong) and fourth (Strong and Flexible) profiles, particularly among boys. Regarding the outcomes, BMI levels in Grade 6 appeared to be higher in Profile 1 (Fit-Cardio) than in Profiles 2 (Average Fitness with Low Flexibility) and 5 (Flexible) and higher in these profiles than in Profiles 3 (Moderately Strong) and 4 (Strong and Flexible). Furthermore, BMI levels in Grade 6 are higher for girls corresponding to Profile 5 (Flexible) than to Profile 2 (Average Fitness with Low Flexibility), whereas no such difference could be observed for boys.

## LTA

Although LTA (e.g., Collins & Lanza, 2009; Kam, Morin, Meyer, & Topolnytsky, 2015, in press) may appear complex at first sight, they mainly involve the estimation of LPA solutions at two separate time points and provide a way to estimate the connections between these two solutions (i.e., the transitions between profile membership over time). In their most simple expression, LTA involve the estimation of LPA solutions based on the same set of indicators including the same number of profiles at both time points and provide a way to test the longitudinal invariance of LPA

---

[3] In multinomial logistic regressions, each predictor has $k-1$ (with $k$ being the number of profiles) effects for each possible pairwise comparison of profiles. Each regression coefficient reflects the expected increase, for each one unit increase in the predictor, in the log odds of the outcome (i.e., the probability of membership in one profile vs. another). For greater simplicity, odds ratios (ORs) are typically reported and reflect the change in the likelihood of membership in a target profile versus a comparison profile associated for each unit of increase in the predictor. For example, an OR of 3 suggests that each unit of increase in the value of the predictor is associated with participants being three times more likely to be member of the target profile (vs. the comparison profile). ORs under 1 correspond to negative logistic regression coefficients and suggest that the likelihood of membership in the target profile is reduced (e.g., an OR of 0.5 shows that a one unit increase in the predictor reduces by 50% the likelihood of being a member of the target, vs. comparison, profile).

solutions. However, LTA can be extended to tests of the longitudinal connections between any type of mixture models, whether or not they are based on the same set of indicators (see, e.g., Nylund-Gibson, Grimm, Quirk, & Furlong, 2014). To illustrate these models, we started with the estimation of separate LPA solutions, using all six NAPFA tests, in Grade 5 and the third year of secondary school. The results from these analyses are reported in Appendix 9.8 and support the superiority of a 5-profile model at both time points. From this evidence of configural invariance, these two LPA models were combined into a single LTA model (Appendix 9.25) through which it is possible to test the structural (Appendix 9.26), dispersion (Appendix 9.27), and distributional (Appendix 9.28) invariance of the model across time. These results show that the structural invariance of the model was not supported, precluding further tests of invariance.

Grade 5 profiles are already illustrated in Figure 9.3, whereas Secondary 3 profiles are illustrated in Figure 9.4. The relative sizes of all profiles and transition probabilities are presented in Table 9.2. These results show that Profile 1 (Fit-Cardio) remains unchanged across time points and that most members of Profile 1 in Grade 5 remain within the same profile in Secondary 3 (63%) or switch to profiles showing an average level of fitness on most indicators (14.5% switch to Profile 2, 21.1% switch to Profile 5). Profile 2, which was globally average in Grade 5, remains similarly average in Secondary 3 while presenting lower levels of upper body strength (pull-ups) and higher levels of flexibility. Over time, the relative size of this profile decreased from 36.51% to 19.94%. Most members of Profile 2 in Grade 5 transitioned either to Profile 2 (23.8%) or to the new average Profile 5 (53.9%) in Secondary 3. Profile 3 remains of the same relative size and moderately strong across time, but presents higher levels of flexibility in Secondary 3. Most members of this profile in Grade 5 remain in the same profile in Secondary 3 (70%). Conversely, Profile 4 presents lower levels of flexibility, as well as of middle and lower body strength (sit-ups

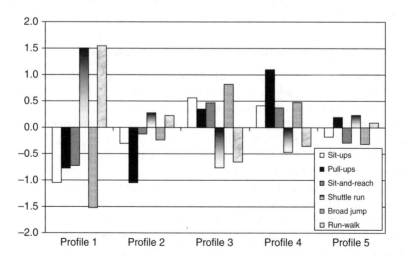

*Figure 9.4    Within-profile means for the LPA solution, Secondary 3.*

Table 9.2    Profile proportions and transitions probabilities for the latent transition analyses.

| | Transition probabilities to Secondary 3 profiles | | | | | Relative size (%) |
|---|---|---|---|---|---|---|
| | Pr.1 (fit-cardio) | Pr.2 (average, low upper body) | Pr.3 (moderately strong) | Pr.4 (strong upper body) | Pr.5 (average) | |
| Grade 5 profiles | | | | | | |
| Pr.1 (Fit-Cardio) | 0.630 | 0.145 | 0.003 | 0.011 | 0.211 | 11.06 |
| Pr.2 (Average Fitness, Low Flexibility) | 0.074 | 0.238 | 0.102 | 0.047 | 0.539 | 36.51 |
| Pr.3 (Moderately Strong) | 0.007 | 0.061 | 0.700 | 0.105 | 0.127 | 25.26 |
| Pr.4 (Strong and Flexible) | 0.005 | 0.072 | 0.769 | 0.064 | 0.090 | 10.34 |
| Pr.5 (Flexible) | 0.069 | 0.360 | 0.150 | 0.038 | 0.383 | 16.81 |
| Relative size (%) | 10.93 | 19.94 | 31.80 | 6.11 | 31.21 | |

and broad jumps) and was relabeled "Strong (Upper Body)" rather than "Strong and Flexible". This profile remains relatively small in size across time points and relatively stable in terms of membership (76.9%). Finally, Profile 5 is the most changed over time, substantially increases in size (from 16.81% to 31.21%), and now mainly presents an average level on all indicators. Globally members of Profile 5 in Grade 5 tend to remain members of "average" profiles in Secondary 3 (36% in Profile 2; 38.3% in Profile 5).

## Mixture Regression Analyses of Grade 5 Students

There are relatively few examples of MRM in the literature (e.g., Morin et al., 2015; Van Horn et al., 2009), which is surprising given the potential of MRM to identify subgroups of participants differing at the levels of estimated relations between constructs. Here, we use MRM to estimate subgroups of participants differing from one another on the relations between Grade 5 BMI, physical strength, cardiovascular fitness and flexibility, and Grade 6 BMI. Controlling for previous levels of BMI provides a direct test of the relations between the physical fitness indicators and later increases or decreases in BMI levels (for a discussion of the similarity between this operationalization and models involving change scores, see Morin et al., 2015). In addition, the mean and variance of all predictors and outcomes were freely estimated in all profiles. The free estimation of the outcomes' means and variance is typical in MRM. These means and variances, respectively, reflect the intercepts and residuals of the regressions of the outcomes on the predictors, making them essential to the estimation of profile-specific regression equations (Henson et al., 2007; Wedel, 2002). The free estimation of the predictors' means and variances provides additional flexibility and practical utility for the classification of current and later cases with incomplete information (Ingrassia, Minotti, & Vittadini, 2012; Wedel, 2002). Such models also reveal potential interactions among predictors, resulting in profiles in which the relations among constructs may differ as a function of predictors' levels (Bauer, 2005; Bauer & Shanahan, 2007). As for LPA (see footnote 2), we recommend to start with a model where all of these parameters are freely estimated across profiles and, failing to obtain converging or proper solutions, to fall back on simpler models where the variances are specified as equal between profiles. If this is not sufficient, then it is possible to move on to models where the predictors' means are also constrained to equality across profiles.

The results from MRM conducted separately for Grade 5 boys and girls are reported in Appendix 9.9. For boys and girls, the information criteria kept on decreasing up to a 6-profile solution, but this decrease reached a plateau around 3-profile and became negligible afterward. Similarly, the aLMR supported the 3-profile solution in both groups (see Appendix 9.29 for input). An examination of alternative solutions further supported the decision to retain three profiles based on the observation of greater theoretical meaningfulness and convergence between boys and girls, whereas solutions with more profiles tended to include very small ($\leq$1–5% of cases), redundant, or meaningless profiles. We then tested the invariance of this MRM solution across genders (Appendix 9.30) using a sequence of invariance tests similar to the one presented for LPA but starting by an additional test of invariance of the regression coefficients (Appendix 9.31), followed by tests of structural (Appendix 9.32), dispersion (Appendix 9.33), and distributional (Appendix 9.34) invariance. Although some LRT proved significant, information criteria kept on decreasing—or presenting only negligible levels of increases—across the full sequence, supporting the complete invariance of the model. This conclusion is also supported by the examination of the parameter estimates from the various models in the sequence. The detailed results from this invariant 3-profile solution are reported in Table 9.3.

Looking at the mean differences across profiles provides valuable information. Profile 2 (20.74% of the sample) presents the highest BMI of all profiles in Grade 5, the lowest level of physical strength, a midrange level of flexibility, but the highest level of cardiovascular fitness. In contrast, Profile 3 (37.90%) presents average levels on all indicators. Finally, Profile 1 already presents moderately low levels of BMI in Grade 5, the highest levels of physical strength and flexibility of all profiles, but the lowest levels of cardiovascular fitness. Comparing the regression coefficients across profiles is even more informative. For instance, BMI appears to be most stable in Profile 1, showing that low levels of BMI in Grade 5 tend to persist over time, and least stable in Profile 2, showing that kids with high levels of BMI can expect improvements over time. Even more interesting is the observation that higher levels of physical strength and cardiovascular fitness both predict decreases in BMI over time in Profile 2, whereas none of the NAPFA indicators predicts changes in BMI level in Profile 1. In Profile 3, only a small negative relation between physical strength and later decreases in BMI can be observed. These results clearly support

Table 9.3 Results from the final 3 class MRM solution.

| Means | Profile 1 | | Profile 2 | | Profile 3 | | |
|---|---|---|---|---|---|---|---|
| | Mean | Confidence interval (CI) | Mean | Confidence interval (CI) | Mean | Confidence interval (CI) | Comparisons |
| BMI (Gr.5) | −0.415 | [−0.491; −0.340] | 0.972 | [0.820; 1.124] | −0.350 | [−0.444; −0.256] | 2 > 1 = 3 |
| Strength (Gr.5) | 0.429 | [0.353; 0.506] | −0.770 | [−0.901; −0.638] | 0.231 | [0.132; 0.331] | 1 > 3 > 2 |
| Cardio (Gr.5) | −0.436 | [−0.515; −0.356] | 0.751 | [0.622; 0.880] | −0.222 | [−0.323; −0.122] | 2 > 3 > 1 |
| Flexibility (Gr.5) | 1.301 | [1.241; 1.361] | −0.115 | [−0.266; 0.037] | −0.222 | [−0.627; −0.532] | 1 > 2 > 3 |

| Variances | Variance | CI | Variance | CI | Variance | CI | Comparisons |
|---|---|---|---|---|---|---|---|
| BMI (Gr.5) | 0.427 | [0.361; 0.493] | 1.067 | [0.924; 1.210] | 0.456 | [0.386; 0.526] | 2 > 1 = 3 |
| Strength (Gr.5) | 0.667 | [0.631; 0.702] | 0.711 | [0.671; 0.751] | 0.676 | [0.641; 0.711] | 1 = 2 = 3 |
| Cardio (Gr.5) | 0.699 | [0.662; 0.737] | 0.660 | [0.625; 0.695] | 0.691 | [0.654; 0.728] | 1 = 2 = 3 |
| Flexibility (Gr.5) | 0.298 | [0.264; 0.332] | 0.919 | [0.774; 1.064] | 0.211 | [0.188; 0.233] | 2 > 1 = 3 |

| Regressions | b (s.e.) | CI | β | b (s.e.) | CI | β | b (s.e.) | CI | β | |
|---|---|---|---|---|---|---|---|---|---|---|
| Intercept | -0.042 (0.021)* | [-0.084; 0.000] | | 0.069 (0.037) | [-0.003; 0.142] | | -0.042 (0.022) | [-0.085; 0.001] | | |
| BMI (Gr.5) | 0.906 (0.011)** | [0.885; 0.928] | 0.918 | 0.831 (0.019)** | [0.793; 0.869] | 0.826 | 0.887 (0.012)** | [0.864; 0.911] | 0.900 | 1 > 2; 1 = 3; 2 = 3 |
| Strength (Gr.5) | -0.063 (0.046) | [-0.153; 0.026] | -0.080 | -0.367 (0.107)** | [-0.576; -0.158] | -0.298 | -0.103 (0.044)* | [-0.190; -0.016] | -0.127 | 2 > 1; 1 = 3; 2 = 3 |
| Cardio (Gr.5) | -0.058 (0.048) | [-0.152; 0.036] | -0.075 | -0.257 (0.115)* | [-0.481; -0.032] | -0.201 | -0.080 (0.044) | [-0.167; 0.006] | -0.100 | 1 = 2 = 3 |
| Flexibility (Gr.5) | 0.011 (0.013) | [-0.014; 0.036] | 0.010 | 0.007 (0.018) | [-0.028; 0.042] | 0.006 | -0.006 (0.014) | [-0.033; 0.022] | -0.004 | 1 = 2 = 3 |
| $R^2$ (boys) | 0.847 (0.014)** | | | 0.717 (0.015)** | | | 0.824 (0.016)** | | | |
| $R^2$ (girls) | 0.831 (0.016)** | | | 0.667 (0.031)** | | | 0.824 (0.014)** | | | |

Note: $b$, unstandardized regression coefficient; s.e., standard error of the estimate; $\beta$, standardized regression coefficient.

*$p \leq 0.05$.

**$p \leq 0.01$.

the efficacy of improvements in cardiovascular fitness as a way to help kids with high BMI to regain more normative BMI levels.

## Latent Basis Growth Mixture Analyses: Cardiovascular Fitness

No introduction to mixture modeling would be complete without a presentation of GMM, which allows for the estimation of subgroups of participants presenting distinct longitudinal trajectories on one—or many—outcome(s) of interest over time. However, GMMs are complex and can easily deserve a complete chapter in their own right. For this reason, we present a longer description of these models in Appendix 9.10 (also see Grimm et al., 2010; Morin, Maïano et al., 2011; Ram & Grimm, 2009), but here we present two short illustrations based on nonlinear specifications that we find to be particularly useful. Using the global indicator of cardiovascular fitness across the seven time waves, we estimated a latent basis GMM (Model 5 in figure 9.1; for details, see Appendices 9.10 and 9.35; for an illustration, see Morin et al., 2013), which provides a flexible way to estimate longitudinal trajectories differing in shape across multiple profiles of participants. In this illustration, all parameters from the model were freely estimated across profiles.

The results of the class enumeration procedure for models including 1–5 classes (models with more than 5 classes systematically converged on improper solutions and nonreplicated local maximum, suggesting that these models were inappropriate due to overparameterization) are reported in Appendix 9.11. These results generally support the 3-profile solution, which is illustrated in Figure 9.5. Detailed parameter estimates from this model are presented in Appendix 9.12. The first profile corresponds to 26.5% of the sample presenting levels of cardiovascular fitness that remain high over the course of the follow-up while showing a U-shaped trajectory characterized by an initial decrease (i.e., negative loadings on the slope factor) followed by an increase (positive loadings on the slope factor). The overall level of change over time (the mean of the slope factor, reflecting the level of change between the first and last

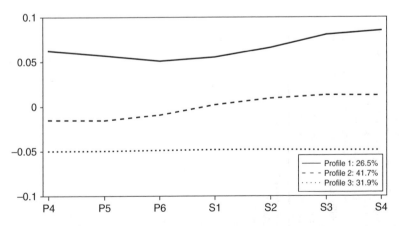

*Figure 9.5    Graph of the final latent basis GMM of cardiovascular fitness trajectories.*

time point, respectively, fixed to be 0 and 1) is significant, and the loadings on this slope factor reflect the proportion of the total change occurring at each time point (e.g., the decrease between Time 1 and 2 corresponds to 23.9% of the total change, as represented by a significant loading of −0.239 on the slope factor). The second profile (41.7%) presents moderate levels of cardiovascular fitness that tend to increase over the course of the study, particularly around the time of the transition to secondary school (as shown by an important increase in the factor loadings on the slope factor at this time point). Finally, the third profile (31.9%) presents low and stable (as shown by a nonsignificant slope factor mean) levels of cardiovascular fitness. Although differences in the average levels of the trajectories may appear minimal, we note that there is a substantial level of between-person variability within each of the profiles showing that within-profile differences may be even more pronounced than between-profile differences around trajectories showing on the average either a U-shaped (Profile 1), increasing (Profile 2), or stable (profile 3) longitudinal profile. We finally note that the time-specific residuals remain globally similar across profiles and of a typical magnitude. It is important to carefully examine these residuals as they may sometimes considerably enrich the interpretation of the profiles (e.g., see Morin, Rodriguez, Fallu, Maïano, & Janosz, 2012; Morin et al., 2013), although not in this specific application.

## Piecewise Growth Mixture Analyses: Physical Strength

As a final illustration, we estimated piecewise GMM using the global indicator of physical strength (see Appendices 9.10 and 9.36). Piecewise models allow for the estimation of a change in the direction of longitudinal trajectories before and after a transition point here represented by the entry into secondary school. To keep this model as simple as possible, we estimated models involving linear trajectories before and after the transition point, although more complex nonlinear models can also be estimated. Here, all parameters from the model were freely estimated across profiles. However, most models converged on improper solutions, mainly due to the presence of negative estimates of the time-specific residuals—something that frequently occur in GMM when the time-specific residuals are allowed to be freely estimated across time waves and profiles. However, before moving to more parsimonious representations involving the inclusion of unrealistic invariance constraints on the time-specific residuals or other model parameters, it is possible to constrain the time-specific residuals to take a value ≥ 0 as part of the estimation process in order to help the model to converge on a proper solution (see Appendix 9.37; for examples of this procedure in the estimation of similarly complex models, see Marsh et al., 2012, 2013, 2014). A limitation of this procedure is that the LMR/aLMR is not available with constrained estimation.

In Appendix 9.11, we report the results of the class enumeration process for the unconstrained (noting that the solutions are improper but provide access to the aLMR) and constrained models including 1–5 classes. These results generally support the 4-profile solution, which is illustrated in Figure 9.6. Parameter estimates from this model are presented in Appendix 9.13. Profile 1 corresponds to 24% of the population

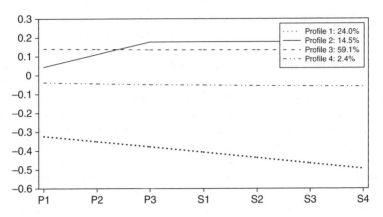

*Figure 9.6    Graph of the final piecewise GMM of physical strength trajectories.*

presenting low and decreasing levels of physical strength, a decrease that is unaffected by the transition to secondary school as illustrated by almost identical average values on the first (describing growth in primary school) and second (describing growth in secondary school) slope factors. The second profile is encouraging and describes 14.5% of the population who start the study with an average level of physical strength which increases over time over the course of primary school and stabilizes at high levels afterward, as illustrated by a significant and positive first slope followed by a nonsignificant second slope. The third profile describes the majority of the sample (59.1%) for whom levels of physical strength remain high and stable (as illustrated by nonsignificant slope factors) over the course of the study. Finally, the fourth latent profile describes a small number of participants (2.4%) who present moderate levels of physical strength that remain stable over the course of the study. The latent correlations estimated between the growth factors also reveal another interesting difference between the profiles. In Profiles 1, 2, and 3, the correlation between the intercept and both slope factors is significant and negative, suggesting that students with lower initial levels of physical strength present more pronounced levels of growth over time across both the primary and secondary school years. In contrast, these correlations are significant and positive in Profile 4, showing that for individuals with midrange levels of psychical strength, higher initial levels that are associated with more pronounced increase over time. Finally, although the two slope factors appear to be uncorrelated in Profiles 1 and 3, they are negatively related in Profile 2 (showing that greater increases in primary school are associated with lower increases in secondary school) and positively related in Profile 4. Again, we note that the time-specific residuals remain globally similar across profiles and of a typical magnitude.

# Summary

Mixture modeling is a person-centered approach to data analysis that is both typological and prototypical in nature, seeking to classify individuals according to the unique characteristics they possess. This introductory chapter presented an illustration of the use of LPA using a set of fitness performance data. In this illustration, LPA was used to identify subgroups of participants with distinct profiles of physical fitness performance. Prior and subsequent BMI levels were used as predictors and outcomes to illustrate the inclusion of covariates into the LPA model. We showed that the covariates can be used to verify the stability of the LPA model. In addition, we demonstrated how to test the invariance of LPA solutions across genders and across time points using LTA. We then illustrated the use of MRM to test how the relations between a set of predictors (Grade 5 BMI, physical strength, cardiovascular fitness, and flexibility) on a single outcome (Grade 6 BMI) differed across subgroups of participants. Finally, we demonstrated the GMM to extract profiles in terms of the longitudinal trajectories of physical strength and cardiovascular fitness. In doing so, we provided guidance stemming from both the statistical literature and extensive practical experience in the implementation of these models in order to help potential users to get the most out of these models.

While it is neither possible nor realistic to present all the possibilities provided by mixture modeling within a single introductory chapter targeting applied researchers, we aimed to provide interested readers with a nontechnical introduction to mixture models that was as broad a possible and highlighted the possible usage of these models in sport and exercise science. As we have noted all along, the methods presented here only remain the tip of the iceberg of the possibilities provided by mixture models. We hope our presentation may have motivated readers to pursue their own exploration.

One important point to highlight is that the methods of analysis need to match with the scientific problem under investigation. Although mixture models are by nature exploratory, a theory-based approach is typically required to guide the selection of the optimal solution and to converge on a meaningful interpretation of the results. In addition, because LPA, MRM, and GMM focus on individual-level variables, it is possible that contextual factors (such as class, teachers, schools, etc.) need to be taken into account. In the current application, clustering of students into schools was taken into account whenever possible. However, an interesting extension of the models presented here is the estimation of multilevel mixture models allowing for the estimation of profiles at multiple levels of analyses (e.g., Asparouhov & Muthén, 2008).

Finally, it is also important to reinforce the point that person- and variable-centered approaches should be viewed as complementary rather than opposite. When combined, these approaches have the potential to provide incredibly rich mutually reinforcing yet complementary views of the same reality (Bergman & Trost, 2006). Combining a focus on variables and average relations with a focus on persons and similarities can be seen as opening different windows on the same world.

# Acknowledgments

This chapter was made possible in part by a grant from the Australian Research Council awarded to the first author (DP140101559).

# References

*Key references are marked by an asterisk\**

Asparouhov, T., & Muthén, B.O. (2008). Multilevel mixture models. In G.R. Hancock, & K.M. Samuelsen (Eds.), *Advances in latent variable mixture models* (27–51). Charlotte, NC: Information Age.

*Asparouhov, T., & Muthén, B.O. (2014). Auxiliary variables in mixture modeling: Three-step approaches using Mplus. *Structural Equation Modeling, 21*, 1–13.

Bagozzi, R.P., Fornell, C., & Larcker, D. (1981). Canonical correlation analysis as a special case of a structural relations model. *Multivariate Behavioral Research, 16*, 437–454.

Bauer, D.J. (2005). A semiparametric approach to modeling nonlinear relations among latent variables. *Structural Equation Modeling, 12*, 513–535.

Bauer, D.J., & Curran, P.J. (2003). Distributional assumptions of growth mixture models over-extraction of latent trajectory classes. *Psychological Methods, 8*, 338–363.

Bauer, D.J., & Shanahan, M.J. (2007). Modeling complex interactions: Person-centered and variable-centered approaches. In T. Little, J. Bovaird & N. Card (Eds.), *Modeling ecological and contextual effects in longitudinal studies of human development* (pp. 255–283). Mahwah, NJ: Lawrence Erlbaum.

Bergman, L.R. (2000). The application of a person-oriented approach: Types and clusters. In L.S. Bergman, R.B. Cairns, L.-G. Nilsson, & L. Nystedt (Eds.), *Developmental science and the holistic approach* (pp. 137–154). Mahwah, NJ: Erlbaum.

Bergman, L.R., & Trost, K. (2006). The person-oriented versus the variable-oriented approach: Are they complementary, opposites, or exploring different worlds? *Merrill-Palmer Quarterly, 52*(3), 601–632.

Bolck, A., Croon, M., & Hagenaars, J. (2004). Estimating latent structure models with categorical variables: One-step versus three-step estimators. *Political Analysis, 12*, 3–27.

*Borsboom, D., Mellenbergh, G.J., & van Heerden, J. (2003). The theoretical status of latent variables. *Psychological Review, 110*, 203–218.

Chen, F., Bollen, K.A., Paxton, P., Curran, P.J., & Kirby, J. (2001). Improper solutions in structural models: Causes, consequences, strategies. *Sociological Methods & Research, 29*, 468–508.

*Clark, S.L., & Muthén, B.O. (2009). *Relating latent class analysis results to variables not included in the analysis. Technical Report.* Los Angeles, CA: Muthén & Muthén.

Cohen, J. (1968). Multiple regression as a general data-analytic system. *Psychological Bulletin, 70*, 426–443.

Collins, L.M., & Lanza, S.T. 2009. *Latent class and latent transition analysis: With applications in the social, behavioral, and health sciences.* New York: John Wiley & Sons.

*Eid, M., Langeheine, R., & Diener, E. (2003). Comparing typological structures across cultures by multigroup latent class analysis. A primer. *Journal of Cross-Cultural Psychology, 34*, 195–210.

*Finch, W.H., & Bronk, K.C. (2011). Conducting confirmatory latent class analysis using Mplus. *Structural Equation Modeling, 18*, 132–151.

Giam, C. (1981). Physical fitness: Definition & assessment. *Singapore Medical Journal, 22*, 176–181.

Gibson, W.A. (1959). Three multivariate models: Factor analysis, latent structure analysis, and latent profile analysis. *Psychometrika, 24*, 229–252.

*Grimm, K.J., Ram, N. & Estabrook, R. (2010). Nonlinear structured growth mixture models in Mplus and OpenMx. *Multivariate Behavioral Research, 45*, 887–909.

Henson, J.M., Reise, S.P., & Kim, K.H. (2007). Detecting mixtures from structural model differences using latent variable mixture modeling: A comparison of relative model fit statistics. *Structural Equation Modeling, 14*, 202–226.

*Hipp, J.R., & Bauer, D.J. (2006). Local solutions in the estimation of growth mixture models. *Psychological Methods, 11*, 36–53.

Ingrassia, S., Minotti, S.C., & Vittadini, G. (2012). Local statistical modeling via cluster-weighted approach with elliptical distributions. *Journal of Classification, 29*, 363–401.

Jackson, A.S. (2006). The evolution and validity of health-related fitness. *Quest, 58*, 160–175.

*Kam, C., Morin, A.J.S., Meyer, J.P., & Topolnytsky, L. (2015, in press). Are commitment profiles stable and predictable? A latent transition analysis. *Journal of Management.* doi:10.1177/0149206313503010

*Kankaraš, M., Moors, G., & Vermunt, J.K. (2011). Testing for measurement invariance with latent class analysis. In E. Davidov, P. Schmidt, & J. Billiet (Eds.), *Cross-cultural analysis: Methods and applications* (pp. 359–384). New York, NY: Routledge.

Knapp, T.R. (1978). Canonical correlation analysis: A general parametric significance testing system. *Psychological Bulletin, 85*, 410–416.

Lazarsfeld, P.F., & Henry, N.W. (1968). *Latent structure analysis.* Boston, MA: Houghton Mifflin.

Lo, Y., Mendell, N., & Rubin, D. (2001). Testing the number of components in a normal mixture. *Biometrika, 88*, 767–778.

Lubke, G. & Muthén, B. (2007). Performance of factor mixture models as a function of model size, criterion measure effects, and class-specific parameters. *Structural Equation Modeling, 14*, 26–47.

Magidson, J., & Vermunt, J.K. (2002). Latent class models for clustering: A comparison with K-Means. *Canadian Journal of Marketing Research, 20*, 37–44.

*Magidson, J., & Vermunt, J.K. (2004). Latent class models. In D. Kaplan (ed.), *Handbook of quantitative methodology for the social sciences* (pp. 175–198). Newbury Park, CA: Sage.

Marsh, H.W., Lüdtke, O., Nagengast, B., Trautwein, U., Morin, A.J.S., Abduljabbar, A.S., & Köller, O. (2012). Classroom climate and contextual effects: Methodological issues in the evaluation of group-level effects. *Educational Psychologist, 47*(2), 106–124.

*Marsh, H.W., Lüdtke, O., Trautwein, U., & Morin, A.J.S. (2009). Latent profile analysis of academic self-concept dimensions: Synergy of person- and variable-centered approaches to the internal/external frame of reference model. *Structural Equation Modeling, 16*, 1–35.

*Masyn, K., Henderson, C., & Greenbaum, P. (2010). Exploring the latent structures of psychological constructs in social development using the Dimensional-Categorical Spectrum. *Social Development, 19*, 470–493.

*McLachlan, G., & Peel, D. (2000). *Finite mixture models.* New York: Wiley.

*Morin, A.J.S., Maïano, C., Marsh, H.W., Nagengast, B., & Janosz, M. (2013). School life and adolescents' self-esteem trajectories. *Child Development, 84*, 1967–1988.

*Morin, A.J.S., Maïano, C., Nagengast, B., Marsh, H.W., Morizot, J., & Janosz, M. (2011). Growth mixture modeling of adolescents trajectories of anxiety: The impact of untested invariance assumptions on substantive interpretations. *Structural Equation Modeling, 18*(4), 613–648.

*Morin, A.J.S., & Marsh, H.W. (2015). Disentangling shape from levels effects in person-centered analyses: An illustration based university teacher multidimensional profiles of effectiveness. *Structural Equation Modeling, 22*(1), 39–59.

Morin, A.J.S., Marsh, H.W., Nagengast, B., & Scalas, L.F. (2014). Doubly latent multilevel analyses of classroom climate: An illustration. *The Journal of Experimental Education, 82*, 143–167.

*Morin, A.J.S., Morizot, J., Boudrias, J.-S., & Madore, I., (2011). A multifoci person-centered perspective on workplace affective commitment: A latent profile/factor mixture Analysis. *Organizational Research Methods, 14*, 58–90.

*Morin, A.J.S., Rodriguez, D., Fallu, J.-S., Maïano, C., & Janosz, M. (2012). Academic achievement and adolescent smoking: A general growth mixture model. *Addiction, 107*, 819–828.

*Morin, A.J.S., Scalas, L.F., & Marsh, H.W. (2015). Tracking the elusive actual-ideal discrepancy model within latent subpopulations. *Journal of Individual Differences, 36* (2), 65–72.

*Muthén, B. O. (2002). Beyond SEM: General latent variable modeling. *Behaviormetrika, 29*, 81–117.

Muthén, L. K., & Muthén, B. O. (1998–2014). *Mplus user's guide*. Los Angeles, CA: Muthén & Muthén.

Muthén, B., & Shedden, K. (1999). Finite mixture modeling with mixture outcomes using the EM algorithm. *Biometrics, 55*, 463–469.

Nylund, K.L., Asparouhov, T., & Muthén, B. (2007). Deciding on the number of classes in latent class analysis and growth mixture modeling: A Monte Carlo simulation study. *Structural Equation Modeling, 14*, 535–569.

Nylund-Gibson, K.L., Grimm, R., Quirk, M., & Furlong, M. (2014). A latent transition mixture model using the three-step specification. *Structural Equation Modeling, 21*, 439–454.

*Petras, H., & Masyn, K. (2010). General growth mixture analysis with antecedents and consequences of change. In A.R. Piquero, & D. Weisburd (Eds.), *Handbook of quantitative criminology* (pp. 69–100). New York, NY: Springer.

Peugh, J., & Fan, X. (2013). Modeling unobserved heterogeneity using latent profile analysis: A Monte Carlo simulation. *Structural Equation Modeling, 20*, 616–639.

Rabe-Hesketh, S., Skrondal, A., & Pickles, A. (2004). *GLLAMM Manual*. U.C. Berkeley Division of Biostatistics Working Paper Series (Working Paper 160).

*Ram, N., & Grimm, K.J. (2009). Growth mixture modeling: A method for identifying differences in longitudinal change among unobserved groups. *International Journal of Behavioral Development, 33*, 565–576.

Satorra, A., & Bentler, P. (1999). *A scaled difference chi-square test statistic for moment structure analysis*. Technical Report, University of California, Los Angeles, CA.

*Skrondal, A., & Rabe-Hesketh, S. (2004). *Generalized latent variable modeling: Multilevel, longitudinal, and structural equation models*. New York, NY: Chapman & Hall/CRC.

Tay, L., Newman, D.A., & Vermunt, J.K. (2011). Using mixed-measurement item response theory with covariates (MM-IRT-C) to ascertain observed and unobserved measurement equivalence. *Organizational Research Methods, 14*, 147–176.

Tein, J.-Y., Coxe, S., & Cham, H. (2013). Statistical power to detect the correct number of classes in latent profile analysis. *Structural Equation Modeling, 20*, 640–657.

Tofighi, D., & Enders, C. (2008). Identifying the correct number of classes in growth mixture models. In G.R. Hancock & K.M. Samuelsen (Eds.), *Advances in latent variable mixture models* (pp. 317–341). Charlotte, NC: Information Age.

Tolvanen, A. (2007). *Latent growth mixture modeling: A simulation study*. Ph.D. dissertation, Department of Mathematics, University of Jyväskylä, Jyväskylä, Finland.

Van Horn, M.L., Jaki, T., Masyn, K., Ramey, S.L., Smith, J., & Antaramian, S. (2009). Assessing differential effects: Applying regression mixture models to identify variations in the influence of family resources on academic achievement. *Developmental Psychology, 45*, 1298–1313.

Vermunt, J.K., & Magidson, J. (2002). Latent class cluster analysis. In J. Hagenaars & A. McCutcheon (Eds.), *Applied latent class models* (pp. 89–106). New York: Cambridge.

Vermunt, J.K., & Magidson, J. (2005). *Latent Gold 4.0*. Belmont, MA: Statistical Innovations.

Wang, J.C.K., Biddle, S.J.H., Liu, W.C., & Lim, B.S.C. (2012). A latent profile analysis of sedentary and physical activity patterns. *Journal of Public Health, 20*, 367–373.

Wang, J.C.K., Liu, W.C., Chatzisarantis, N.L.D., & Lim, B.S.C. (2010). Influence of perceived motivational climate on achievement goals in physical education: A structural equation mixture modeling analysis. *Journal of Sport & Exercise Psychology, 32*, 324–338.

Wang, J.C.K., Pyun, D.Y., Liu, W.C., Lim, B.S.C., & Li, F. (2013). Longitudinal changes in physical fitness performance in youth: A multilevel latent growth curve modeling approach. *European Physical Education Review, 19*, 329–346.

Wedel, M. (2002). Concomitant variables in finite mixtures. *Statistica Neerlandica, 56*, 362–375.

Yang, C. (2006). Evaluating latent class analyses in qualitative phenotype identification. *Computational Statistics & Data Analysis, 50*, 1090–1104.

# 10

# Multilevel (structural equation) modeling

## Nicholas D. Myers[1], David E. Conroy[2], and Marietta Suarez[1]

[1] School of Education and Human Development, University of Miami, Coral Gables, FL, USA
[2] College of Health & Human Development, The Pennsylvania State University, University Park, PA USA

## General Introduction

Applications of multilevel modeling (MLM) can be found within many influential journals in sport and exercise science. For example, in *Exercise and Sport Sciences Reviews* (*ESSR*), Lee and Cubbin (2009) argued for the use of multilevel ecological frameworks to better understand disparities in physical activity. In *Medicine and Science in Sports and Exercise* (*MSSE*), King, Satariano, Marti, and Zhu (2008) discussed the need to consider multiple levels of influence (e.g., people, place, and time) when trying to understand walking behavior. In the *British Journal of Sports Medicine* (*BJSM*), Elferink-Gemser, Visscher, van Duijn, and Lemmink (2006) used a multilevel model to explore the development of interval endurance capacity in youth field hockey athletes. In the *Scandinavian Journal of Medicine and Science in Sports* (*SJMSS*), Barkoukis, Taylor, Chanal, and Ntoumanis (2014) fitted a multilevel model to examine the relation of student motivation and student grades across time. We believe that applications of MLM will continue to play an important role in sport and exercise science.

*An Introduction to Intermediate and Advanced Statistical Analyses for Sport and Exercise Scientists*, First Edition.
Edited by Nikos Ntoumanis and Nicholas D. Myers.
© 2016 John Wiley & Sons, Ltd. Published 2016 by John Wiley & Sons, Ltd.
Companion website: www.wiley.com/go/ntoumanis/sport

As evidenced in several chapters within the current text, applications of structural equation modeling (SEM) can also be found within many influential journals in sport and exercise science. For example, in *ESSR*, Duncan, Duncan, Strycker, and Chaumeton (2004) provided preliminary findings from a longitudinal study of youth physical activity. In *MSSE*, Motl, Dishman, Felton, and Pate (2003) investigated self-motivation and physical activity among black and white adolescent girls. In the *BJSM*, Smith and Hale (2004) examined the factor structure of a bodybuilding dependence scale. In the *SJMSS*, Felton and Jowett (2013) explored links between coach interpersonal behaviors, coach–athlete relationships, and athletes' psychological need satisfaction and well-being. As with MLM, we believe that applications of SEM will continue to play an important role in sport and exercise science.

## Multilevel Structural Equation Modeling

The idea of forming a more general model to flexibly combine the strengths of both MLM and SEM has been of interest in the methodological community for several decades (e.g., Goldstein & McDonald, 1988; Muthén, 1989; Schmidt, 1969). A flexible and user-friendly implementation of multilevel structural equation modeling (MSEM) exists in Mplus software (Muthén & Muthén, 1998–2012). We believe that applications of MSEM soon will begin to play an important role in sport and exercise science because (i) both MLM and SEM have already proven to be frequently used and (ii) the combination of MLM and SEM into MSEM provides the opportunity to investigate a wide array of research questions of interest in sport and exercise science. The current chapter will focus on single-population, two-level MSEM for continuous endogenous variables.

This chapter provides a somewhat detailed accounting of the fuller statistical model as parameterized in Mplus (Muthén & Asparouhov, 2008) within which MSEM exists and that can include, as special cases, many of the models focused on in other chapters of the current book. Providing a detailed accounting within the current chapter may prove useful for researchers in sport and exercise science when particular methodological issues are encountered (e.g., sample size determination and/or power estimation) that require the researcher to provide related information. Subsequent sections in this chapter will provide specific worked examples from sport and exercise science wherein the somewhat abstract statistical model presented in this section may be viewed in a more concrete way.

The single-population, two-level MSEM can be expressed in three equations.[1] While the examples in this chapter will focus on reduced versions of these equations, the fuller statistical model is presented as a broader methodological framework within which some of the next generation of sport and exercise research may occur. The range of parameter estimates typically available in both MLM and SEM is available in MSEM. To make explicit the structure of the nonindependence of the data, let the subscript $i$ denote Level-1 (or "within") units and the subscript $j$ denote Level-2

---

[1] The notation system used in the current chapter generally is consistent with that used by Preacher, Zyphur, and Zhang (2010).

(or "between") units (or parameters that are free to vary across clusters if the subscript $j$ is attached to them), respectively.[2]

The first equation can be described as the measurement model:

$$\mathbf{y}_{ij} = \mathbf{v}_j + \mathbf{\Lambda}_j \mathbf{\eta}_{ij} + \mathbf{K}_j \mathbf{x}_{ij} + \mathbf{\varepsilon}_{ij} \tag{10.1}$$

where

$p$ is the number of observed dependent variables

$m$ is the number of latent variables across Level-1 ($m_w$) and Level-2 ($m_B$)

$q$ is the number of observed exogenous variables

$\mathbf{y}_{ij} = p x 1$ vector containing observed endogenous variables

$\mathbf{v}_j = p x 1$ vector of intercepts

$\mathbf{\Lambda}_j = p x m$ partitioned matrix of ($\mathbf{y}$ on $\mathbf{\eta}$) regression coefficients, $\left[ \mathbf{\Lambda}_W \mid \mathbf{\Lambda}_B \right]$

$\mathbf{\eta}_{ij} = m x 1$ partitioned vector of latent variables, $\begin{bmatrix} \mathbf{\eta}_W \\ \hline \mathbf{\eta}_B \end{bmatrix}$

$\mathbf{K}_j = p x q$ matrix of ($\mathbf{y}$ on $\mathbf{x}$) regression coefficients

$\mathbf{x}_{ij} = q x 1$ vector of observed exogenous variables

$\mathbf{\varepsilon}_{ij} = p x 1$ vector of residuals for $\mathbf{y}$

$\Theta = p x p$ covariance matrix for $\mathbf{\varepsilon}$

The second equation can be described as a latent variable model (e.g., specifying structural relationships at Level-1):

$$\mathbf{\eta}_{ij} = \mathbf{\alpha}_j + \mathbf{B}_j \mathbf{\eta}_{ij} + \mathbf{\Gamma}_j \mathbf{x}_{ij} + \mathbf{\zeta}_{ij} \tag{10.2}$$

where

$\mathbf{\eta}_{ij} = m x 1$ partitioned vector of latent variables, $\begin{bmatrix} \mathbf{\eta}_W \\ \hline \mathbf{\eta}_B \end{bmatrix}$

$\mathbf{\alpha}_j = m x 1$ partitioned vector of intercepts for $\mathbf{\eta}$, $\begin{bmatrix} \mathbf{0}_W \\ \hline \mathbf{\alpha}_B \end{bmatrix}$

$\mathbf{B}_j = m x m$ partitioned matrix of ($\mathbf{\eta}$ on $\mathbf{\eta}$) regression coefficients, $\begin{bmatrix} \mathbf{B}_W & \mid & \mathbf{0}_{W \times B} \\ \hline \mathbf{0}_{B \times W} & \mid & \mathbf{0}_B \end{bmatrix}$

$\mathbf{\Gamma}_j = m x q$ partitioned matrix of ($\mathbf{\eta}$ on $\mathbf{x}$) regression coefficients, $\left[ \mathbf{\Gamma}_W \mid \mathbf{0}_B \right]$

$\mathbf{x}_{ij} = q x 1$ partitioned vector of observed exogenous variables, $\begin{bmatrix} \mathbf{x}_W \\ \hline \mathbf{0}_B \end{bmatrix}$

---

[2] This type of a "level" description (e.g., Level-1, Level-2, etc.) probably is more consistent with an MLRM approach than it is with an MSEM approach (e.g., within, between, etc.). While this type of a "level" description is relatively common in sport and exercise science, it is noted that focusing on the type of variability being modeled (e.g., within, between, etc.) and less on the level at which a variable is measured (e.g., Level-1, Level-2, etc.) may be useful in some cases.

$\zeta_{ij} = px1$ partitioned vector of residuals for $\eta$, $\begin{bmatrix} \zeta_W \\ 0_B \end{bmatrix}$

$\Psi = mxm$ covariance matrix for $\zeta$

The third equation can be described as the latent variable model at Level-2:

$$\eta_j = \mu + B\eta_j + \Gamma x_j + \zeta_j \tag{10.3}$$

where

$r$ is the number of random effects allowed for within the previous two equations

$s$ is the number of observed cluster-level exogenous variables

$\eta_j = rx1$ stacked vector of random effects.

$\mu = rx1$ vector of fixed intercepts for $\eta_j$

$B = rxr$ matrix of ($\eta_j$ on $\eta_j$) fixed regression coefficients

$\Gamma = rxs$ matrix of ($\eta_j$ on $x_j$) fixed regression coefficients

$x_j = sx1$ vector of observed cluster-level exogenous variables

$\zeta_j = rx1$ vector of residuals for $\eta_j$

$\Psi = rxr$ covariance matrix for $\zeta_j$

# Utility of the Methodology in Sport and Exercise Science

Multilevel data, sometimes referred to as hierarchical (or nested) data, are common in sport and exercise science research. A commonly observed hierarchical structure has repeated observations nested within participants (e.g., Elferink-Gemser et al., 2006). Time-varying data collected at repeated measurement occasions can be viewed as Level-1 variables, while time-invariant data from the individual participants can be viewed as Level-2 variables.[3] MLM accommodates nested data and can be defined as a statistical model that has two or more distinct hierarchical levels, with variables at each of these levels, and a theoretical interest in relationships at one or more of, or across, these levels (Hox & Roberts, 2010).

Cross-sectional data can also be viewed as multilevel. For example, walking behavior data may be collected from people who reside in neighborhoods that differ dramatically in walkability (e.g., King et al., 2008). Suppose that within a particular study, the relevant population of neighborhoods was viewed as large and that some of the randomly sampled neighborhoods were assigned to an experimental treatment condition (e.g., an intervention designed to increase walking), while other

---

[3] This two-level description is consistent with a univariate approach to change modeling (often implemented by users of dedicated MLRM software). A multivariate approach to change modeling (often implemented by users of Mplus) considers this to be a one-level model.

neighborhoods were assigned to the control condition (e.g., treatment as usual). From a conceptual perspective, variability in individual walking behaviors may be attributable to both person-level characteristics (e.g., self-regulation, health status, etc.) and neighborhood-level characteristics (e.g., experimental treatment vs. control condition, crime rates, etc.). This design is often referred to as a cluster randomized trial. MLM enables researchers to partition variability in the outcome(s) by level (e.g., person and neighborhood level) and allows for modeling within and across these levels simultaneously.

Researchers in sport and exercise science may recognize MLM from multiple labels including mixed (non)linear models, random coefficient models, covariance components models, and hierarchical linear and nonlinear models (or merely as HLM). We adopt the nomenclature of Hox and Roberts (2010) and classify MLM into two (useful but nonexhaustive) groups: multilevel regression modeling (MLRM) and MSEM. In general, MLRMs have an observed outcome or outcomes at Level-1, regression coefficients as outcomes at Level-2 and above, and generally observed independent variables. In general, MSEM have latent or observed outcomes at each level, latent or observed independent variables, and typically at least as much flexibility as MLRM with regard to the measurement and latent variable models that may be imposed (e.g., see Equations 10.1–10.3).

To date, MLM in sport and exercise science generally has been conceptualized within MLRM (e.g., Silverman & Solmon, 1998; Zhu, 1997) although applications of MSEM have begun to emerge (e.g., Myers, Beauchamp, & Chase, 2011). Recent didactic reviews of MLRM as applied in sport and exercise science (e.g., Gaudreau, Fecteau, & Perreault, 2010) and biobehavioral medicine (e.g., Myers et al., 2012) are available. Gaudreau et al. focused on modeling dyadic data in HLM software. Myers et al. focused on 2-level and 3-level MLRM examples and provided supplemental digital content for related diagrams, equations, interpretations of terms (http://links. lww.com/PSYMED/A53), and input and output from both Mplus software and SAS software (http://links.lww.com/PSYMED/A54). The examples detailed in the next section of this chapter were selected to demonstrate some applications available in MSEM that take advantage, at least to some extent, of the flexible latent variable and measurement equations available in SEM.

# The Substantive Examples

This section conceptualizes two specific examples in sport and exercise science within the MSEM framework. The first example is consistent with theoretical models of sport coaching and self-efficacy theory and has a cross-sectional data structure wherein athletes (i.e., Level-1) are nested within teams (i.e., Level-2). The second example is consistent with a social-cognitive approach to physical activity promotion and has a longitudinal data structure wherein repeated measures of motivation and physical activity (i.e., Level-1) are nested within people who are randomly assigned to different intervention groups (i.e., Level-2). These conceptualizations will provide relevant examples for subsequent demonstration in the synergy section.

Multilevel mediation is present in both examples and is reflective of many theories and data structures in sport and exercise science wherein indirect, as well as direct and total, effects are theorized (at least implicitly) and the data are nested. A general MSEM framework for assessing multilevel mediation has been proposed as a flexible alternative to other MLM-based approaches (Preacher et al., 2010). There is evidence for the utility of using the MSEM framework for assessing mediation in multilevel data (Preacher, Zhang, & Zyphur, 2011). A numeric notation system proposed by Krull and Mackinnon (2001), and slightly modified by Preacher et al. (2010), for describing two-level mediation will be adopted in this chapter. Let $X$–$M$–$Y$ be replaced with numbers to reflect the level at which a variable (or a set of related variables, such as indicators of a latent variable) is measured.

## Coaching Competency–Collective Efficacy–Team Performance: 1–1–2

Scholars of coaching leadership have long noted that "the ultimate effects that coaching behavior exerts are mediated by the meaning that players attribute to them" (Smoll & Smith, 1989, p. 1527). Accordingly, athletes' perceptions of a coach's behavior play a central role in several theoretical models of sport coaching (e.g., Côté & Gilbert, 2009; Jowett & Ntoumanis, 2004). More specifically, within Horn's (2002) working model of coaching effectiveness, athletes' perceptions and evaluations of a coach's behavior (e.g., coaching competency) mediate the influence that a coach's behavior has on athletes' self-perceptions, beliefs (e.g., collective efficacy), and attitudes, which in turn directly affects athletes' motivation and performance. Specifying that coaching competency exerts a direct effect on collective efficacy and that collective efficacy exerts a direct effect on team performance is consistent with Horn's model.

*Coaching Competency* (*X*). Myers and colleagues (Myers, Feltz, Maier, Wolfe, & Reckase, 2006) operationally defined coaching competency as athletes' perceptions of their head coach's ability to affect athletes' learning and performance. Coaching competency has been conceptualized as multidimensional (e.g., motivation, game strategy, technique, character building, and physical conditioning) at the athlete level and unidimensional at the team level (Myers, Chase, Beauchamp, & Jackson, 2010). Indicators of coaching competency will be measured at Level-1 (i.e., $X = 1$) in this example.

*Collective Efficacy* (*M*). Bandura (1997) defined collective efficacy as a group's shared belief in its conjoint capabilities to organize and execute the courses of action required to produce given levels of attainments. Collective efficacy has played a prominent role in sport and exercise research (Feltz, Short, & Sullivan, 2008). Collective efficacy has typically been conceptualized as unidimensional and multilevel and measured by multiple indicators (Myers & Feltz, 2007). A commonly used method to assess collective efficacy involves measuring each athlete's beliefs in relation to a particular team performance. Indicators of collective efficacy will be measured at Level-1 (i.e., $M = 1$) in this example.

*Team Performance* (*Y*). The effect of collective efficacy on team performance has been studied extensively in sport and exercise (Feltz & Lirgg, 1998). Team performance has typically been conceptualized as unidimensional and measures at Level-2 and sometimes measured by multiple indicators (Myers, Payment, & Feltz, 2004). Indicators of team performance will be measured at Level-2 (i.e., $Y = 2$) in this example.

## Action Planning Intervention–Physical Activity Action Plans–Physical Activity: 2–1–1

Physical activity plays an important role in preserving health as evidenced by inverse correlations between usual physical activity levels and the prevalence of chronic diseases such as cardiovascular disease, diabetes, and some forms of cancer (US Department of Health and Human Services, 2008). Although emerging adults are among the most active segments of the adult population and many perceive themselves as invulnerable to health threats, over 45% fail to attain the recommended level of aerobic physical activity (Carlson, Fulton, Schoenborn, & Loustalot, 2010). Normative trends indicate that physical activity levels decrease as adulthood progresses (Carlson et al., 2010), so interventions to promote physical activity and habit formation in the emerging adulthood stage may be valuable for long-term health preservation/promotion.

Implementation planning, a social-cognitive behavior change technique, is a known pathway to habit formation (Aarts & Dijksterhuis, 2000). It involves forming detailed "if…then…" plans for engaging in a desired behavior in a particular context (e.g., *if* it is 5 p.m. and I am at my dorm, *then* I will go to the fitness center to run on the treadmill for 30 min) and consistently improves goal achievement including increasing physical activity levels (Carraro & Gaudreau, 2013). Interventions that prompt and support people in forming implementation plans for physical activity should contribute to people forming more well-defined plans and subsequently engaging in greater physical activity than if they had not formed those plans. Of course, physical activity motivation and behavior vary from day to day (Conroy, Elavsky, Doerksen, & Maher, 2013), so there is an inherent multilevel structure involved when evaluating the effects of an implementation planning intervention on motivation and behavior.

*Action Planning Intervention (X).* For illustration, consider a study in which participants are randomly assigned in equal numbers to either a no-treatment control group or to receive an eHealth physical activity intervention. The intervention consists of an e-mail prompt with links to a branching web questionnaire that facilitates implementation planning for physical activity (cf. Maher & Conroy, 2015). Upon clicking on the link, the website prompts the individual to identify *when* they plan to engage in physical activity that day, *where* they will engage in physical activity, and *how* they will engage in moderate-to-vigorous-intensity physical activity. Responses to the *when* questions form the *if…* part of the plan, and responses to the *where* and *how* questions form the *then…* part of the plan (e.g., *if* it's 5 p.m., *then* I will run for 30 min on the treadmill in the fitness center of my dorm). Suppose that these prompts take 1 min to complete and will be delivered daily at 8:00 a.m. for six consecutive days (i.e., Day 1–Day 6) for the purpose of indirectly increasing physical activity by increasing physical activity action plans. Assignment to the action planning intervention condition (i.e., 0 = intervention not delivered, 1 = intervention delivered) will be measured at Level-2 (i.e., $X = 2$) in this example.

*Physical Activity Action Plans* (*M*). Daily physical activity action plans can be assessed by considering the strength of an individual's plan in regard to when, where, and how physical activity is intended to occur (e.g., Maher & Conroy, 2015). A commonly used method to create a physical activity action plan score is to create an average across the indicators at each time point. Suppose that physical activity action plan is measured at 8:15 a.m. for seven consecutive days (i.e., Day 0, Day 1–Day 6) using a prospective prompt (e.g., an e-mail reminder to form a physical activity action plan for the day). The physical activity action plans score will be measured at Level-1 (i.e., $M = 1$) in this example.

*Physical Activity* (*Y*). Daily physical activity often is assessed by measuring the duration of time an individual engages in different intensities of physical activity (e.g., Booth, 2000). It is relatively common to create a single daily physical activity score representing energy expended in physical activity. Suppose that physical activity is measured at the end of the day (i.e., just prior to going to sleep) for seven consecutive days (i.e., Day 0, Day 1–Day 6). The physical activity score will be measured at Level-1 (i.e., $Y = 1$) in this example.

# The Synergy

This section demonstrates, via the two examples from the previous section, how to visually depict, determine degrees of freedom (df), parameterize, perform related analyses, and interpret related results. For each example, the reader can reproduce the results by accessing the relevant dataset (available at the publisher supported website) and the annotated Mplus input file. Some key output will be summarized in the tables, but the reader can generate the fuller output by saving the input file and the dataset in the same folder and then running the input file in Mplus.[4]

Data were simulated (i.e., artificial) for both examples. The simulated datasets incorporated some parameterizations based on existing real datasets (e.g., estimates of the parameter values) when such data were available to the authors. When existing data were not available, parameter values were selected by the authors. The population data-generating model for both examples is available from the first author upon request. In both examples, the data were drawn from a multivariate normal distribution.

Total sample size (*N*) for the first example was $N = 20\,000$ because the number of Level-2 units (i.e., teams or "*J*") was $J = 1000$ and the number of Level-1 units within each *j* (i.e., athletes or "$n_j$") was $n_j = 20$. For the second example, $N = 1400$ because the number of Level-2 units (i.e., participants) was $J = 200$ and the number of Level-1 units within each *j* (i.e., repeated measures) was $n_j = 7$. These sample size values were selected because they represented values within a range for which related simulation evidence exists (e.g., Preacher et al., 2011).

---

[4] In several cases, input statements provided were not necessary, but such input was retained for peda-gogical purposes. A complete treatment of syntax writing in Mplus is available in Muthén and Muthén (1998–2012).

# Coaching Competency–Collective Efficacy–Team Performance: 1–1–2

Figure 10.1 visually depicts a simplified version of an MSEM for this example. Some model parameters (e.g., variances) and identification constraints were omitted from the figure to reduce clutter, but both of these types of simplifications will be fully accounted for in subsequent sections. The structure of each measurement model generally was consistent with Myers et al. (2010) in regard to coaching competency and Myers et al. (2004) in regard to collective efficacy and team performance. At the athlete level, direct effects were not specified from the five dimensions of coaching competency to collective efficacy because we are unaware of any existing research (or theory) to inform decisions regarding the relative magnitude of each direct effect. At the team level, specifying the two direct effects (from coaching competency to collective efficacy and from collective efficacy to team performance) and the indirect effect (from coaching competency to team performance through collective efficacy) was consistent with Horn's (2002) model. A direct effect from coaching competency to team performance was not specified because we are unaware of any a priori theory that explicitly supports such a specification.

*Determine df.* The df can be determined a priori for the model by subtracting the total number of parameters to be estimated ($q$) from the total number of observations available for the analysis ($u$). Level, however, may need to be considered when determining both $q$ (i.e., $q_{\text{Level-1}}$ and $q_{\text{Level-2}}$) and $u$ (i.e., $u_{\text{Level-1}}$ and $u_{\text{Level-2}}$). Figure 10.1 depicts the observations available for analysis.

The level at which an observed variable is measured and modeled can impact $u$. Most (i.e., 24 of 29) of the observed variables (i.e., $x1, \dots, m7$) were measured at the athlete level and were modeled at both levels. The observed variables associated with team performance, however, were measured and modeled at the team level only. At the athlete level, $u_{\text{Level-1}}$ can be determined by finding the value of $p(p+1)/2$, where $p$ is the number of observed variables. The value of $u_{\text{Level-1}}$ is 300 (i.e., 24(24+1)/2). At the team level, $u_{\text{Level-2}}$ can be determined by finding the value of $p(p+3)/2$. The value of $u_{\text{Level-2}}$ is 464 (i.e., 29(29+3)/2). The value of $u$ is 764 (i.e., $u_{\text{Level-1}} + u_{\text{Level-2}}$) for this example.

The total number of parameters to be estimated in the full version of this model is 153 (i.e., $q_{\text{Level-1}} + q_{\text{Level-2}}$). The number of parameters to be estimated at the athlete level (i.e., $q_{\text{Level-1}}$) is 64. The number of parameters to be estimated at the team level (i.e., $q_{\text{Level-2}}$) is 89. The df for this example are 611 because df $= u - q$ (i.e., 764 – 153).

*Parameters to Be Estimated.* We return to the three equations introduced in the MSEM section of the General Introduction to provide a detailed accounting of the specific parameters to be estimated in this example. The Mplus input file will be written in a way to emphasize consistency with the notation used in this section. Tables will be formatted in a way to emphasize consistency with the notation used in this section.

*Equation 10.1.* This equation (i.e., the measurement model) reduces to $\mathbf{y}_{ij} = \mathbf{v} + \Lambda\eta_{ij} + \varepsilon_{ij}$, and an expansion of it with respect to the current example is

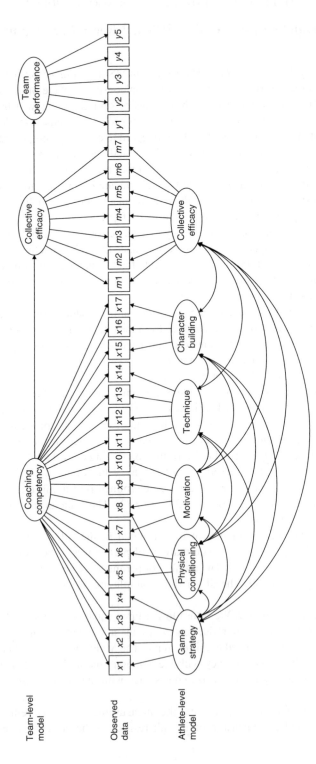

*Figure 10.1 A simplified version of an MSEM for the coaching competency–collective efficacy–team performance (i.e., 1–1–2) example. Some model parameters (e.g., variances) and identification constraints were omitted to reduce clutter. The full version of this model, where all model parameters and identification constraints are represented, is available in Tables 10.1 and 10.2.*

available in Appendix 10.1.[5] At the athlete level, 43 parameters are estimated (i.e., 19 pattern coefficients or "loadings," $\lambda$, and 24 residual variances, $\theta$). At the team level, 84 parameters are estimated (i.e., 29 intercepts, $\nu$, 26 loadings, and 29 residual variances). The magnitude of parameter values within matrices that are likely to be of special interest in practice (e.g., $\Lambda$) was consistent with key findings from Myers et al. (2010) in regard to coaching competency and Myers et al. (2004) in regard to collective efficacy and team performance.

*Equation 10.2.* This equation (e.g., a latent variable model specifying structural relationships at Level-1) reduces to $\eta_{ij} = \zeta_{ij}$, and an expansion of it with respect to the current example is available in Appendix 10.2. At the athlete level, 21 parameters are estimated (i.e., a saturated covariance matrix, $\Psi$, for the six latent variables at the athlete level: game strategy, physical conditioning, motivation, technique, character building, and collective efficacy). The magnitude of parameter values within $\Psi$ in regard to coaching competency was consistent with key findings from Myers et al. (2010). The magnitude of parameter values within $\Psi$ in regard to coaching competency and collective efficacy was set equal to an arbitrary correlation value of 0.25 because we are unaware of existing research that has estimated these parameters.

*Equation 10.3.* This equation (e.g., a latent variable model at Level-2) reduces to $\eta_j = B\eta_j + \zeta_j$, and an expansion of it with respect to the current example is available in Appendix 10.3. At the team level, 5 parameters are estimated (i.e., 2 direct effects, $\beta$; 1 variance; and 2 residual variances, $\psi$). The two direct effects (from coaching competency to collective efficacy and from collective efficacy to team performance) and the indirect effect (from coaching competency to team performance through collective efficacy) likely would be of considerable interest in practice. Parameter values were arbitrarily selected such that the variance accounted for in collective efficacy and team performance was equal to 9 and 16%, respectively.

*Analyses.* The input file provided in Appendix 10.4 demonstrates a way of implementing this example in Mplus. Some brief annotations within the input file are provided, denoted by the presence of a "!" and followed by italicized text. The input file was written in a way to emphasize consistency with the notation used in Equations 10.1–10.3. The default estimator in Mplus for this type of model was used (i.e., maximum likelihood robust ("MLR")) to fit the data.

An assumption was that athletes' responses to the coaching competency and collective efficacy items were nonindependent of the team within which each athlete was nested. Item-level intraclass correlation (ICC) values were reported to provide a summary of the degree of nonindependence. An ICC value $\geq 0.05$ was viewed as potentially meaningful (e.g., Julian, 2001). Team was the cluster variable from this point forward. The indexes of model-data fit reported were the exact fit test ($\chi_R^2$), root mean square error of approximation (RMSEA), standardized root mean square residual (SRMR), comparative fit index (CFI), and nonnormed fit index (NNFI).

The standard error for the indirect effect of coaching competency on team performance provided by Mplus was obtained using the delta method, which assumed

---

[5] The term expansion is meant to communicate that the elements within the arrays will be made explicit.

that the effect was drawn from a normal distribution. To relax this assumption, a 95% CI was obtained for the indirect effect using Monte Carlo methods for assessing mediation (MacKinnon, Lockwood, & Williams, 2004) by using an online utility (Selig & Preacher, 2008). R code generated by the online utility (http://quantpsy.org/medmc/medmc.htm) is provided in Appendix 10.5.

*Results.* The model fits the data $\chi_R^2(611) = 629.37$, $p = 0.295$, RMSEA $= 0.001$, SRMR$_{within} = 0.005$, SRMR$_{between} = 0.023$, CFI $= 1.00$, and TLI $= 1.00$. Item-level ICC values ranged from 0.16 to 0.35 (see Table 10.1). These values provided evidence for the assumption that athlete responses to the coaching competency and collective efficacy items were nonindependent of the team within which each athlete was nested.

Table 10.1 provided all of the parameter estimates at the athlete level, but only facets of the model typically of primary interest in applied research will be discussed. Standardized loadings ($\lambda^0$) ranged from 0.18 to 0.73 for the coaching competency indicators and from 0.62 to 0.72 for the collective efficacy indicators. Variance accounted for ranged from 0.34 to 0.53 for the coaching competency indicators and from 0.38 to 0.52 for the collective efficacy indicators. Correlations between pairs of latent variables ($\psi$) ranged from 0.57 to 0.83 within the dimensions of coaching competency and from 0.26 to 0.27 between the dimensions of coaching competency and collective efficacy.

Table 10.2 provided all of the parameter estimates at the team level, but only facets of the model typically of primary interest in applied research will be discussed. Standardized loadings ($\lambda^0$) ranged from 0.73 to 0.97 for the coaching competency indicators, from 0.88 to 0.98 for the collective efficacy indicators, and from 0.65 to 0.85 for team performance indicators. Variance accounted for ranged from 0.53 to 0.95 for the coaching competency indicators, from 0.77 to 0.95 for the collective efficacy indicators, and from 0.43 to 0.72 for team performance indicators. The direct effect ($\beta$) from coaching competency, 0.28, was statistically significant, $p < 0.001$, and accounted for 8% of the variance in collective efficacy. The direct effect ($\beta$) from collective efficacy, 0.78, was statistically significant, $p < 0.001$, and accounted for 19% of the variance in team performance. The indirect effect of coaching competency on team performance through collective efficacy, 0.22, was statistically significant, $p < 0.001$, with a 95% CI of [0.16, 0.29].

## Action Planning Intervention–Physical Activity Action Plans–Physical Activity: 2–1–1

The two-level description provided for this example up to this point is consistent with a univariate approach to change modeling as often implemented by users of dedicated MLRM software. A multivariate approach to change modeling, as often implemented by users of Mplus, considers this to be a one-level model (see Bauer, 2003, for a thorough description). From this point forward, a one-level description of this model generally will be adopted.

Figure 10.2 visually depicts a simplified version of this example (see Cheong, MacKinnon, & Khoo, 2003, for a fuller treatment of parallel process latent growth curve modeling). Some model parameters (e.g., variances) and identification constraints were omitted from the figure to reduce clutter, but both of these types of

Table 10.1    Intraclass correlation values, parameter estimates, and $R^2$ at the athlete level from the coaching competency–collective efficacy–team performance example: 1–1–2.

| Variable | ICC | $\lambda$(SE) | $\lambda^0$ | $\theta$(SE) | $R^2$ |
|---|---|---|---|---|---|
| $x1$ | 0.28 | 1.00 | 0.64 | 0.27(0.01) | 0.41 |
| $x2$ | 0.25 | 1.16(0.02) | 0.66 | 0.33(0.01) | 0.43 |
| $x3$ | 0.18 | 1.29(0.02) | 0.64 | 0.45(0.01) | 0.41 |
| $x4$ | 0.25 | 1.21(0.02) | 0.68 | 0.31(0.01) | 0.47 |
| $x8$ | — | 0.34(0.03) | 0.18 | — | — |
| $x5$ | 0.32 | 1.00 | 0.73 | 0.30(0.01) | 0.53 |
| $x6$ | 0.30 | 0.99(0.01) | 0.71 | 0.33(0.01) | 0.50 |
| $x7$ | 0.28 | 1.00 | 0.62 | 0.38(0.01) | 0.39 |
| $x8$ | 0.16 | 0.77(0.03) | 0.46 | 0.43(0.01) | 0.37 |
| $x9$ | 0.28 | 1.22(0.02) | 0.69 | 0.39(0.01) | 0.48 |
| $x10$ | 0.25 | 1.05(0.02) | 0.63 | 0.40(0.01) | 0.40 |
| $x11$ | 0.26 | 1.00 | 0.71 | 0.28(0.01) | 0.50 |
| $x12$ | 0.22 | 0.88(0.01) | 0.62 | 0.34(0.01) | 0.39 |
| $x13$ | 0.30 | 0.93(0.01) | 0.69 | 0.27(0.01) | 0.48 |
| $x14$ | 0.23 | 0.97(0.01) | 0.67 | 0.33(0.01) | 0.45 |
| $x15$ | 0.25 | 1.00 | 0.68 | 0.36(0.01) | 0.46 |
| $x16$ | 0.22 | 1.05(0.01) | 0.70 | 0.34(0.01) | 0.49 |
| $x17$ | 0.26 | 0.79(0.01) | 0.58 | 0.36(0.01) | 0.34 |
| $m1$ | 0.29 | 1.00 | 0.64 | 0.27(0.01) | 0.41 |
| $m2$ | 0.25 | 1.20(0.02) | 0.67 | 0.32(0.01) | 0.45 |
| $m3$ | 0.18 | 1.32(0.02) | 0.64 | 0.46(0.01) | 0.41 |
| $m4$ | 0.25 | 1.22(0.02) | 0.68 | 0.32(0.01) | 0.46 |
| $m5$ | 0.16 | 1.36(0.02) | 0.72 | 0.31(0.01) | 0.52 |
| $m6$ | 0.31 | 1.35(0.02) | 0.71 | 0.34(0.01) | 0.50 |
| $m7$ | 0.35 | 1.13(0.02) | 0.62 | 0.38(0.01) | 0.38 |

$\Psi$ (with standardized estimates above the diagonal)

| | $\eta_G$ | $\eta_P$ | $\eta_M$ | $\eta_T$ | $\eta_C$ | $\eta_{CE}$ |
|---|---|---|---|---|---|---|
| $\eta_G$ | 0.18(0.01) | 0.74 | 0.80 | 0.83 | 0.73 | 0.26 |
| $\eta_P$ | 0.19(0.01) | 0.34(0.01) | 0.61 | 0.65 | 0.57 | 0.26 |
| $\eta_M$ | 0.17(0.01) | 0.18(0.01) | 0.24(0.01) | 0.76 | 0.83 | 0.26 |
| $\eta_T$ | 0.19(0.01) | 0.20(0.01) | 0.20(0.01) | 0.29(0.01) | 0.72 | 0.27 |
| $\eta_C$ | 0.17(0.01) | 0.18(0.01) | 0.22(0.01) | 0.21(0.01) | 0.30(0.01) | 0.27 |
| $\eta_{CE}$ | 0.05(0.01) | 0.07(0.01) | 0.06(0.01) | 0.06(0.01) | 0.06(0.01) | 0.18(0.01) |

ICC = intraclass correlation; $\lambda$ = pattern coefficient; $\lambda^0$ = standardized pattern coefficient; $\theta$ = residual variance; $\psi$ = (co)variance; $\eta_G$ = game strategy; $\eta_P$ = physical conditioning; $\eta_M$ = motivation; $\eta_T$ = technique; $\eta_C$ = character building; $\eta_{CE}$ = collective efficacy.

simplifications will be fully accounted for in subsequent sections. The structure of each measurement model was consistent with estimating continuous latent variables for (i) initial status for both action plan and physical activity (e.g., baseline at Day

Table 10.2  Parameter estimates and variance accounted for at the team level from the coaching competency–collective efficacy–team performance example: 1–1–2.

| Variable | $\nu$(SE) | $\lambda$(SE) | $\lambda^0$ | $\theta$(SE) | $\beta$(SE) | $\psi$ | Indirect effect (SE) | $R^2$ |
|---|---|---|---|---|---|---|---|---|
| y1 | −0.01(0.03) | 1.00 | 0.67 | 0.59(0.029) | — | — | — | 0.45 |
| y2 | 0.00(0.03) | 1.10(0.05) | 0.76 | 0.42(0.023) | — | — | — | 0.58 |
| y3 | 0.03(0.03) | 1.27(0.06) | 0.85 | 0.31(0.021) | — | — | — | 0.72 |
| y4 | 0.02(0.03) | 1.07(0.05) | 0.75 | 0.43(0.024) | — | — | — | 0.56 |
| y5 | 0.00(0.03) | 0.95(0.05) | 0.65 | 0.57(0.029) | — | — | — | 0.43 |
| x1 | 0.00(0.01) | 1.00 | 0.91 | 0.03(0.002) | — | — | — | 0.84 |
| x2 | 0.00(0.02) | 1.07(0.03) | 0.93 | 0.03(0.002) | — | — | — | 0.87 |
| x3 | 0.01(0.01) | 0.93(0.03) | 0.88 | 0.04(0.003) | — | — | — | 0.77 |
| x4 | 0.01(0.02) | 1.12(0.03) | 0.97 | 0.01(0.001) | — | — | — | 0.95 |
| x5 | 0.00(0.02) | 1.37(0.03) | 0.96 | 0.02(0.002) | — | — | — | 0.93 |
| x6 | 0.00(0.02) | 1.34(0.03) | 0.96 | 0.02(0.002) | — | — | — | 0.92 |
| x7 | 0.00(0.02) | 1.09(0.03) | 0.86 | 0.06(0.004) | — | — | — | 0.73 |
| x8 | 0.00(0.01) | 0.86(0.03) | 0.90 | 0.02(0.002) | — | — | — | 0.82 |
| x9 | 0.00(0.02) | 1.02(0.04) | 0.73 | 0.14(0.007) | — | — | — | 0.53 |
| x10 | 0.02(0.02) | 0.99(0.03) | 0.81 | 0.07(0.005) | — | — | — | 0.66 |
| x11 | 0.00(0.02) | 1.10(0.03) | 0.93 | 0.03(0.002) | — | — | — | 0.87 |
| x12 | −0.01(0.01) | 0.98(0.02) | 0.93 | 0.02(0.002) | — | — | — | 0.87 |
| x13 | 0.01(0.02) | 1.16(0.03) | 0.95 | 0.02(0.002) | — | — | — | 0.91 |
| x14 | 0.00(0.02) | 1.08(0.03) | 0.97 | 0.01(0.002) | — | — | — | 0.93 |
| x15 | 0.01(0.02) | 1.03(0.03) | 0.85 | 0.06(0.004) | — | — | — | 0.72 |
| x16 | 0.00(0.02) | 1.07(0.03) | 0.96 | 0.01(0.002) | — | — | — | 0.92 |
| x17 | 0.00(0.02) | 0.91(0.03) | 0.79 | 0.07(0.004) | — | — | — | 0.62 |
| m1 | 0.01(0.01) | 1.00 | 0.89 | 0.04(0.003) | — | — | — | 0.80 |

| | | | | | | | |
|---|---|---|---|---|---|---|---|
| $m2$ | 0.03(0.02) | 1.06(0.03) | 0.94 | 0.02(0.002) | — | — | — | 0.87 |
| $m3$ | 0.00(0.02) | 0.95(0.03) | 0.88 | 0.04(0.003) | — | — | — | 0.77 |
| $m4$ | 0.01(0.02) | 1.12(0.03) | 0.98 | 0.01(0.001) | — | — | — | 0.95 |
| $m5$ | 0.00(0.01) | 0.83(0.02) | 0.91 | 0.02(0.002) | — | — | — | 0.82 |
| $m6$ | 0.03(0.02) | 1.37(0.03) | 0.96 | 0.02(0.002) | — | — | — | 0.93 |
| $m7$ | 0.02(0.02) | 1.32(0.04) | 0.90 | 0.06(0.004) | — | — | — | 0.81 |
| $\eta_{CC}$ | — | — | — | — | — | 0.15(0.01) | 0.22(0.03)[a] | — |
| $\eta_{TCE}$ | — | — | — | — | 0.28(0.03) | 0.14(0.01) | — | 0.08 |
| $\eta_{TP}$ | — | — | — | — | 0.78(0.07) | 0.38(0.03) | — | 0.19 |

$\nu$ = intercept coefficient; $\lambda$ = pattern coefficient; $\lambda^0$ = standardized pattern coefficient; $\theta$ = residual variance; $\beta$ = regression coefficient (estimate appears in the row of the outcome variable); $\psi$ = variance (residual variance in the case of $\eta_{CE}$ and $\eta_{TP}$); $\eta_{CC}$ = coaching competency; $\eta_{CE}$ = team collective efficacy; $\eta_{TP}$ = team performance. Estimate of the indirect effect appears in the row of the initial independent variable (i.e., $\eta_{CC}$ in this example).
[a]The standard error was obtained using the delta method. The 95% CI obtained using the Monte Carlo method for assessing mediation was [0.16, 0.29].

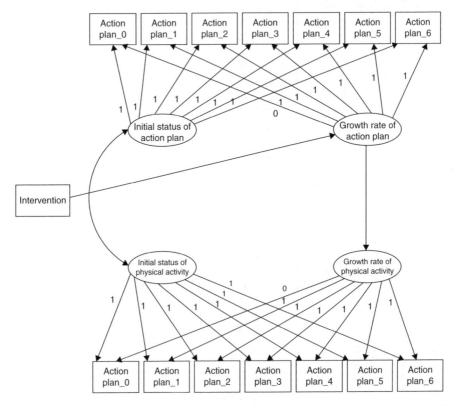

*Figure 10.2   A simplified version of the action planning intervention–physical activity action plans–physical activity example. Some model parameters (e.g., variances) and identification constraints were omitted to reduce clutter. The full version of this model, where all model parameters and identification constraints are represented, is available in Table 10.3.*

0—prior to the intervention) and (ii) growth rate for both action plan and physical activity, where a change from Day 0 to Day 1 was expected to be observed and then stabilized throughout the remainder of the study. Initial status of both action plan and physical activity was specified to covary. Direct effects were specified from the dummy-coded intervention variable to growth rate of action plan and from growth rate of action plan to growth rate of physical activity. Thus, consistent with the intention of the intervention, an indirect effect of the intervention on growth rate of physical activity through growth rate of action plan was specified.

*Determine df.* The df can be determined a priori for the model by subtracting the total number of parameters to be estimated ($q$) from the total number of observations available for the analysis ($u$). Figure 10.2 depicts the observations available for analysis. The value of $u$ can be determined by finding the value of $(p(p+3)/2)+i$, where $p$ is the number of observed dependent variables and $i$ is the additional information provided by the exogenous covariate (i.e., a covariance with each of the observed dependent variables). The value of $u$ is 133 (i.e., $119+14$) for this example. The total number of parameters to be estimated in the full version of this model is 25. The df for this example are 108 because $df = u - q$ (i.e., $133 - 25$).

*Parameters to Be Estimated.* We now transition to a reduced version of the three equations introduced in the MSEM section of the General Introduction to provide a detailed accounting of the parameters to be estimated in this single-level SEM. The $j$ subscript can be omitted from Equations 10.1 and 10.2. Equation 10.3 can be omitted entirely consistent with a one-level description of this model.

*Equation 10.1.* This equation (i.e., the measurement model) reduces to $\mathbf{y}_i = \mathbf{v} + \Lambda \boldsymbol{\eta}_i + \boldsymbol{\varepsilon}_i$, and an expansion of it with respect to the current example is available in Appendix 10.6.[5] Note that although no parameters are estimated in $\Lambda \boldsymbol{\eta}_i$, the growth factors and the shape of the trajectory are defined here. Sixteen parameters are estimated (i.e., 2 intercepts, $\mathbf{v}$, and 14 residual variances, $\theta$). A common intercept is estimated across the repeated measures of action planning, and another common intercept is estimated across the repeated measures of physical activity (see Khoo, 2001, for a rationale). Parameter values were arbitrarily selected such that the variance accounted for in the repeated measures of action planning and physical activity ranged from 50 to 58%.

*Equation 10.2.* This equation (e.g., a latent variable model specifying structural relationships) reduces to $\boldsymbol{\eta}_i = \boldsymbol{\alpha} + \mathbf{B}\boldsymbol{\eta}_i + \boldsymbol{\zeta}_i$, and an expansion of it with respect to the current example is available in Appendix 10.7. Nine parameters are estimated (i.e., 2 intercepts, $\alpha$; 2 direct effects, $\beta$; 4 variances; and 1 covariance, $\psi$). The two direct effects (from the intervention to growth rate of action plan and from growth rate of action plan to growth rate of physical activity) and the indirect effect (from the intervention to growth rate of physical activity through growth rate of action plan) likely would be of considerable interest in practice. Parameter values were selected such that the variance accounted for in growth rate of action plan and growth rate of physical activity was equal to 50 and 16%, respectively (Carraro & Gaudreau, 2013).

*Analyses.* The input file provided in Appendix 10.8 demonstrates a way of implementing this example in Mplus. Again, some brief annotations within the input file are provided, denoted by the presence of a "!" and followed by italicized text. As before, the input file was written in a way to emphasize consistency with the notation used in Equation 10.1 (see Appendix 10.6) and Equation 10.2 (see Appendix 10.7). The default estimator in Mplus for this type of model was used (i.e., maximum likelihood ("ML")) to fit the data. The indexes of model-data fit reported were the same as for the first example. The standard error for the indirect effect was obtained as described in the first example (see Appendix 10.9 for R code).

*Results.* The model fits the data $\chi^2(108) = 87.88, p = 0.922$, RMSEA $= 0.000$, 90% CI [0.000, 0.013], SRMR $= 0.047$, CFI $= 1.00$, and TLI $= 1.01$. Table 10.3 provided all of the parameter estimates (and each variance accounted for), but only facets of the model typically of primary interest in applied research will be discussed. Variance accounted for ranged from 0.52 to 0.59 for the physical activity action plan score and from 0.52 to 0.62 for the physical activity score. The significant variability in both initial status of action plan, 0.44, $p < 0.001$, and initial status of physical activity, 0.58, $p < 0.001$, provided evidence that participants differed on both of these

Table 10.3 Parameter estimates and variance accounted from the action planning intervention–physical activity action plans–physical activity example: 2–1–1.

| Variable | $\nu$(SE) | $\theta$(SE) | $\alpha$(SE) | $\beta$(SE) | $\psi$(SE) | Indirect effect (SE) | $R^2$ |
|---|---|---|---|---|---|---|---|
| m0 | −0.01(0.07)[a] | 0.42(0.06) | — | — | — | — | 0.52 |
| m1 | −0.01(0.07)[a] | 0.50(0.06) | — | — | — | — | 0.58 |
| m2 | −0.01(0.07)[a] | 0.53(0.06) | — | — | — | — | 0.56 |
| m3 | −0.01(0.07)[a] | 0.48(0.06) | — | — | — | — | 0.59 |
| m4 | −0.01(0.07)[a] | 0.53(0.06) | — | — | — | — | 0.56 |
| m5 | −0.01(0.07)[a] | 0.48(0.06) | — | — | — | — | 0.59 |
| m6 | −0.01(0.07)[a] | 0.49(0.06) | — | — | — | — | 0.58 |
| y0 | 0.10(0.08)[b] | 0.54(0.07) | — | — | — | — | 0.52 |
| y1 | 0.10(0.08)[b] | 0.49(0.06) | — | — | — | — | 0.60 |
| y2 | 0.10(0.08)[b] | 0.44(0.05) | — | — | — | — | 0.62 |
| y3 | 0.10(0.08)[b] | 0.63(0.07) | — | — | — | — | 0.53 |
| y4 | 0.10(0.08)[b] | 0.59(0.07) | — | — | — | — | 0.55 |
| y5 | 0.10(0.08)[b] | 0.61(0.07) | — | — | — | — | 0.54 |
| y6 | 0.10(0.08)[b] | 0.55(0.06) | — | — | — | — | 0.57 |
| Intervention | — | — | | | | 0.22(0.09)[c] | — |
| $\eta_{IS\_AP}$ | — | — | 0.00 | — | 0.44(0.06) | — | — |
| $\eta_{IS\_PA}$ | — | — | 0.00 | — | 0.58(0.08) | — | — |
| $\eta_{GR\_AP}$ | — | — | 0.02(0.07) | 0.68(0.09) | 0.13(0.05) | — | 0.48 |
| $\eta_{GR\_PA}$ | — | — | 0.00(0.08) | 0.33(0.12) | 0.11(0.05) | — | 0.19 |
| $\eta_{IS\_AP}$ & $\eta_{IS\_PA}$ | — | — | — | — | 0.27(0.05) | — | — |

$\nu$ = intercept coefficient; $\theta$ = residual variance; $\alpha$ = intercept coefficient; $\beta$ = regression coefficient (estimate appears in the row of the outcome variable); $\psi$ = variance or covariance; $\eta_{IS\_AP}$ = initial status of action plan; $\eta_{IS\_PA}$ = initial status of physical activity; $\eta_{GR\_AP}$ = growth rate of action plan; $\eta_{GR\_AP}$ = growth rate of physical activity. Estimate of the indirect effect appears in the row of the initial independent variable.

[a] First equality constraint.

[b] Second equality constraint.

[c] The standard error was obtained using the delta method. The 95% CI obtained using the Monte Carlo method for assessing mediation was [0.06, 0.41].

variables prior to the intervention. The correlation ($\psi$) between initial status of action plan and initial status of physical activity was 0.53. The statistically nonsignificant intercept for both growth rate of action plan, 0.02, $p = 0.780$, and growth rate of physical activity, 0.00, $p = 0.958$, provided evidence that the average growth rates in the no-treatment control group were flat. The direct effect ($\beta$) from the intervention to growth rate of action plan, 0.68, was statistically significant, $p < 0.001$, and accounted for 48% of the variance in growth rate of action plan. The direct effect ($\beta$) from growth rate of action plan to growth rate of physical activity, 0.33, was statistically significant, $p < 0.001$, and accounted for 19% of the variance in growth rate of physical activity. The indirect effect of intervention on growth rate of physical activity through growth rate of action plan, 0.22, was statistically significant, $p < 0.001$, with a 95% CI of [0.06, 0.41]. This provides evidence for the assertion that exposure to the intervention led to positive change in physical activity action plans over time, which, in turn, led to positive change physical activity over time.

## Summary

Applications of MLM can be found within many influential journals in sport and exercise science. Applications of SEM can also be found within many influential journals in sport and exercise science. We believe that applications of MSEM soon will begin to play an important role in sport and exercise science because (i) both MLM and SEM have already proven to be frequently used and (ii) the combination of MLM and SEM into MSEM provides the opportunity to investigate a wide array of research questions of interest in sport and exercise science. We hope that this chapter through its use of substantive examples to demonstrate how to visually depict, determine df, parameterize, perform related analyses, and interpret related results will expedite the use of MSEM in sport and exercise science. Our emphasis on MSEM should not be interpreted as advocating that all applications of MLM in sport and exercise science need to occur within the MSEM as opposed to MLRM.

The current chapter was limited in at least three ways. First, the chapter focused on single-population, two-level MSEM for continuous endogenous variables because we believe that this will be the most common application of MSEM application in sport and exercise science. Readers are referred to Jedidi and Ansari (2001), Muthén and Asparouhov (2008), and Rabe-Hesketh, Skrondal, and Pickles (2004) for introductions to Bayesian MSEM for heterogeneous populations and/or noncontinuous endogenous variables. Second, because both datasets were simulated (and with no model error present), the results that follow should be viewed as only a means for providing a relevant context for demonstration purposes. Third, sample size values selected in this chapter (Example 1: $N = 20\,000$, $J = 1000$, $n_j = 20$; Example 2: $N = 1400$, $J = 200$, $n_j = 7$) may be larger than what is often observed in practice. While the sample size values selected in this chapter represented values within a range for which related simulation evidence exists (e.g., Preacher et al., 2011), it may be useful for future research to demonstrate how Monte Carlo methods can be used to determine sample size and to estimate power for MSEM applications under model-data conditions commonly encountered in exercise and sport science.

# References

Aarts, H., & Dijksterhuis, A. (2000). Habits as knowledge structures: Automaticity in goal-directed behavior. *Journal of Personality & Social Psychology, 78*, 53–63.

Bandura, A. (1997). *Self-efficacy: The exercise of control.* New York, NY: Freeman.

Barkoukis, V., Taylor, I., Chanal, J., & Ntoumanis, N. (2014). The relation between student motivation and student grades in physical education: A 3-year investigation. *Scandinavian Journal of Medicine & Science in Sports, 24*, e406–e414.

Bauer, D. J. (2003). Estimating multilevel linear models as structural equation models. *Journal of Educational and Behavioral Statistics, 28*, 135–167.

Booth, M. L. (2000). Assessment of physical activity: An international perspective. *Research Quarterly for Exercise and Sport, 71*(2), S114–S120.

Carlson, S. A., Fulton, J. E., Schoenborn, C. A., & Loustalot, F. (2010). Trend and prevalence estimates based on the 2008 physical activity guidelines for Americans. *American Journal of Preventive Medicine, 39*, 305–313.

Carraro, N., & Gaudreau, P. (2013). Spontaneous and experimentally-induced action planning and coping planning for physical activity: A meta-analysis. *Psychology of Sport & Exercise, 14*, 228–248.

Cheong, J. W., MacKinnon, D. P., & Khoo, S. T. (2003). Investigation of mediational processes using parallel process latent growth curve modeling. *Structural Equation Modeling: A Multidisciplinary Journal, 10*, 238–262.

Conroy, D. E., Elavsky, S., Doerksen, S. E., & Maher, J. P. (2013). A daily process analysis of intentions and physical activity in college students. *Journal of Sport & Exercise Psychology, 35*(5), 493–502.

Côté, J., & Gilbert, W. (2009). An integrative definition of coaching effectiveness and expertise. *International Journal of Sport Science and Coaching, 4*, 307–323.

Duncan, S. C., Duncan, T. E., Strycker, L. A., & Chaumeton, N. R. (2004). A multilevel approach to youth physical activity research. *Exercise and Sport Sciences Reviews, 32*(3), 95–99.

Elferink-Gemser, M. T., Visscher, C., Van Duijn, M. A. J., & Lemmink, K. A. P. M. (2006). Development of the interval endurance capacity in elite and sub-elite youth field hockey players. *British Journal of Sports Medicine, 40*, 340–345.

Felton, L., & Jowett, S. (2013). "What do coaches do" and "how do they relate": Their effects on athletes' psychological needs and functioning. *Scandinavian Journal of Medicine & Science in Sports, 23*, e130–e139.

Feltz, D. L., & Lirgg, C. D. (1998). Perceived team and player efficacy in hockey. *Journal of Applied Psychology, 83*, 557–564.

Feltz, D. L., Short, S. E., & Sullivan, P. J. (2008). *Self-efficacy in sport.* Champaign, IL: Human Kinetics.

Gaudreau, P., Fecteau, M. C., & Perreault, S. (2010). Multi-level modeling of dyadic data in sport sciences: Conceptual, statistical, and practical issues. *Measurement in Physical Education and Exercise Science, 14*, 29–51.

Goldstein, H., & McDonald, R. P. (1988). A general model for the analysis of multilevel data. *Psychometrika, 53*, 455–467.

Horn, T. S. (2002). Coaching effectiveness in the sports domain. In T. S. Horn (Ed.), *Advances in sport psychology* (2nd ed., pp. 309–354). Champaign, IL: Human Kinetics.

Hox, J. J., & Roberts, J. K. (2010). Multilevel analysis: Where we were and where we are. In: J. J. Hox & J. K. Roberts (Eds.). *Handbook of advanced multilevel analysis* (pp. 3–11). New York, NY: Routledge.

Jedidi, K., & Ansari, A. (2001). Bayesian structural equation models for multilevel data. In G. A. Marcoulides & R. E. Schumacker (Eds.), *New developments and techniques in structural equation modeling* (pp. 129–157). New York, NY: Erlbaum.

Jowett, S., & Ntoumanis, N. (2004). The coach–athlete relationship questionnaire (CART-Q): Development and initial validation. *Scandinavian Journal of Medicine & Science in Sports, 14*, 245–257.

Julian, M. W. (2001). The consequences of ignoring multilevel data structures in nonhierarchical covariance modeling. *Structural Equation Modeling: A Multidisciplinary Journal, 8*, 325–352.

Khoo, S. T. (2001). Assessing program effects in the presence of treatment-baseline interactions: A latent curve approach. *Psychological Methods, 6*, 234–257.

King, A. C., Satariano, W. A., Marti, J., & Zhu, W. (2008). Multilevel modeling of walking behavior: Advances in understanding the interactions of people, place, and time. *Medicine and Science in Sports and Exercise, 40*, S584–S593.

Krull, J. L., & MacKinnon, D. P. (2001). Multilevel modeling of individual and group level mediated effects. *Multivariate Behavioral Research, 36*, 249–277.

Lee, R. E., & Cubbin, C. (2009). Striding toward social justice: The ecologic milieu of physical activity. *Exercise and Sport Sciences Reviews, 37*(1), 10.

MacKinnon, D. P., Lockwood, C. M., & Williams, J. (2004). Confidence limits for the indirect effect: Distribution of the product and resampling methods. *Multivariate Behavioral Research, 39*, 99–128.

Maher, J. P., & Conroy, D. E. (2015). Habit strength moderates the effects of daily action planning prompts on physical activity but not sedentary behavior. *Journal of Sport & Exercise Psychology, 37*(1): 97–107.

Motl, R. W., Dishman, R. K., Felton, G., & Pate, R. R. (2003). Self-motivation and physical activity among black and white adolescent girls. *Medicine & Science in Sports & Exercise, 35*, 128–136.

Muthén, B. O. (1989). Latent variable modeling in heterogeneous populations. *Psychometrika, 54*, 557–585.

Muthén, B. O., & Asparouhov, T. (2008). Growth mixture modeling: Analysis with non-Gaussian random effects. In G. Fitzmaurice, M. Davidian, G. Verbeke, & G. Molenberghs (Eds.), *Longitudinal data analysis* (pp. 143–165). Boca Raton, FL: Chapman & Hall/CRC.

Muthén, L. K., & Muthén, B. O. (1998–2012). *Mplus user's guide.* 7th ed., Los Angeles, CA: Muthén & Muthén.

Myers, N. D., & Feltz, D. L. (2007). From self-efficacy to collective efficacy in sport: Transitional methodological issues. In G. Tenenbaum & R.C. Eklund (Eds.), *The handbook of sport psychology* (3rd ed., pp. 799–819). New York, NY: Wiley.

Myers, N. D., Payment, C. A., & Feltz, D. L. (2004). Reciprocal relationships between collective efficacy and team performance in women's ice hockey. *Group Dynamics: Theory, Research, and Practice, 8*, 182–195.

Myers, N. D., Feltz, D. L., Maier, K. S., Wolfe, E. W., & Reckase, M. D. (2006). Athletes' evaluations of their head coach's coaching competency. *Research Quarterly for Exercise and Sport, 77*, 111–121.

Myers, N. D., Chase, M. A., Beauchamp, M. R., & Jackson, B. (2010). The coaching competency scale II – high school teams. *Educational and Psychological Measurement, 70*, 477–494.

Myers, N. D., Beauchamp, M. R., & Chase, M. A. (2011). Coaching competency and satisfaction with the coach: A multilevel structural equation model. *Journal of Sports Sciences, 29*, 411–422.

Myers, N. D., Brincks, A. M., Ames, A. J., Prado, G., Penedo, F. J., & Benedict, C. (2012). Multilevel modeling in psychosomatic medicine research. *Psychosomatic Medicine: Journal of Biobehavioral Medicine, 74*, 925–936.

Preacher, K. J., Zyphur, M. J., & Zhang, Z. (2010). A general multilevel SEM framework for assessing multilevel mediation. *Psychological Methods, 15*, 209–233.

Preacher, K. J., Zhang, Z., & Zyphur, M. J. (2011). Alternative methods for assessing mediation in multilevel data: The advantages of multilevel SEM. *Structural Equation Modeling: A Multidisciplinary Journal, 18*, 161–182.

Rabe-Hesketh, S., Skrondal, A., & Pickles, A. (2004). Generalized multilevel structural equation modeling. *Psychometrika, 69*, 167–190.

Schmidt, W. H. (1969). Covariance structure analysis of the multivariate random effects model. (Unpublished doctoral dissertation). University of Chicago.

Selig, J. P., & Preacher, K. J. (2008). *Monte Carlo method for assessing Mediation: An interactive tool for creating confidence intervals for indirect effects [Computer software]*. Available from http://quantpsy.org/ (accessed July 24, 2015).

Silverman, S., & Solmon, M. (1998). The unit of analysis in field research: Issues and approaches to design and data analysis. *Journal of Teaching in Physical Education, 17*(3), 270–284.

Sjöström, M., Ainsworth, B., Bauman, A., Bull, F., Craig, C., & Sallis, J. (2005). *Guidelines for data processing and analysis of the Intentional Physical Activity Questionnaire (IPAQ)— short and long forms*. Stockholm, Sweden: Karolinska Institute.

Smith, D., & Hale, B. (2004). Validity and factor structure of the bodybuilding dependence scale. *British Journal of Sports Medicine, 38*, 177–181.

Smoll, F. L., & Smith, R. E. (1989). Leadership behaviors in sport: A theoretical model and research paradigm. *Journal of Applied Social Psychology, 19*, 1522–1551.

US Department of Health and Human Services. (2008). Physical activity guidelines advisory committee report. Retrieved from http://www.health.gov/paguidelines/ (accessed July 24, 2015).

Zhu, W. (1997). A multilevel analysis of school factors associated with health-related fitness. *Research Quarterly for Exercise and Sport, 68*, 125–135.

# 11

# Application of meta-analysis in sport and exercise science

## Soyeon Ahn[1], Min Lu[1], G. Tyler Lefevor[1], Alicia L. Fedewa[2], and Seniz Celimli[1]

[1] *School of Education and Human Development, University of Miami, Coral Gables, FL, USA*
[2] *Department of Educational, School, and Counseling Psychology, University of Kentucky, Lexington, KY, USA*

## General Introduction

Meta-analysis,[1] or "analysis of analyses," was coined by Gene V. Glass (1976) in his presidential talk at the annual meeting of the American Educational Research Association. Meta-analysis (see footnote 1) is a tool that provides a cohesive picture of a phenomenon of interest by statistically integrating study findings on the "same" or "similar" phenomenon across a large collection of studies. It boasts a number of strengths, such as an increase in statistical power by including more samples from selected studies, which have made meta-analysis popular in many disciplines, including sport and exercise science (Becker & Ahn, 2012).

### Stages of Meta-Analysis

The general procedure for conducting a meta-analysis is almost identical to that for primary research. Cooper (1984) conceptualized meta-analysis in five stages, which he

---

[1] Other terms that have been interchangeably used in the literature include *research synthesis* and *quantitative review*.

*An Introduction to Intermediate and Advanced Statistical Analyses for Sport and Exercise Scientists*, First Edition.
Edited by Nikos Ntoumanis and Nicholas D. Myers.
© 2016 John Wiley & Sons, Ltd. Published 2016 by John Wiley & Sons, Ltd.
Companion website: www.wiley.com/go/ntoumanis/sport

further expanded to seven stages in 2010 (Cooper, 2010). Stage 1, *problem formulation*, involves formulating research questions and hypotheses. Stage 2, *data collection*, involves searching the literature and coding information from relevant studies. Stage 3, *data evaluation*, involves evaluating the quality of study and dealing with differences in the quality of studies. Stage 4, *data analysis*, involves analyzing and integrating effect sizes across studies. Stage 5, *presentation*, involves interpreting the cumulative evidence obtained through the analysis.

In each of the five stages, Cooper outlined questions to be addressed that would "enhance or undermine the trustworthiness of the conclusion" (2010, p. 11). These questions allow a researcher to better ensure the validity of the subsequent meta-analysis. Though important, space prevents a detailed discussion of each stage in the present chapter. The interested reader is referred to several excellent sources that give a more detailed description of questions for consideration in each stage of meta-analysis (Borenstein, Hedges, Higgins, & Rothstein, 2009; Cooper, 1984, 2010; Hedges & Olkin, 1985; Wanous, Sullivan, & Malinak, 1989). In this chapter, our focus is primarily on Stage 4 as our main goal is to illustrate how to apply meta-analytic methods in sport and exercise science.

# Key Elements of Meta-Analysis

Figure 11.1 shows a forest plot for a meta-analysis of 18 studies on the treatment effect of physical activity in reducing children's depression, which were included in a published meta-analysis conducted by Ahn and Fedewa (2011). The forest plot in Figure 11.1 presents four key elements for conducting a meta-analysis: (i) *individual studies*, (ii) the *effect size* of each study, (iii) the *variance* (or *standard error*) of each effect size as a measure of *precision*, and (iv) *study weight* (Borenstein et al., 2009).

The first column of this plot shows the study ID that is assigned to each of the 18 *individual studies* that examine treatment effect with physical activity by comparing the level of children's depression between a treatment and control group. These 18 studies examine the "same" or a "similar" phenomenon—the treatment effect of physical activity on children's depression. Therefore, the findings from those studies are comparable and can be synthesized in a meta-analysis.

From each of the individual studies included in a meta-analysis, a standardized mean difference ($d$) between the treatment and control groups on the level of children's depression is computed and serves as the *effect size* of each study. The effect sizes are shown in the second column of this plot. The standardized mean difference ($d$) in children's depression score ($X$) between treatment group ($t$) with physical activity and control group ($c$) is computed via $d = \left( \overline{X}_t - \overline{X}_c \right) / S_{\text{pooled}}$, with $S_{\text{pooled}} = \sqrt{[(n_t - 1)SD_t^2 + (n_c - 1)SD_c^2]/(n_t + n_c - 2)}$, where $n$ is sample size and $SD$ is standard deviation.

This effect size represents the difference in children's depression between the treatment and control groups on the standard metric and thus enables us to compare the effects across studies. A couple of other commonly used effect sizes are the correlation coefficient ($r$) and the odds ratio, both of which represent the strength and direction of the relationship of interest. In this example, a standardized mean difference

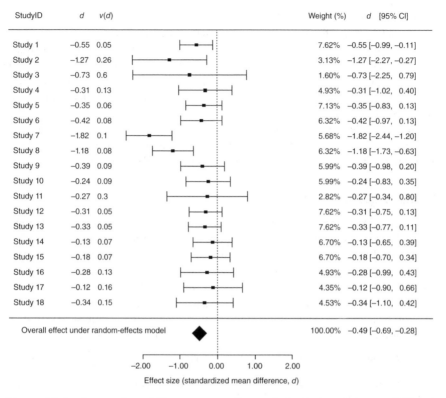

*Figure 11.1    Forest plot of 18 treatment effects of physical activity on children's depression included in Ahn and Fedewa (2011).*

of 0 (the center) represents no difference on children's depression between treatment and control groups: A negative value (falling left of the center) indicates a lower mean on children's depression in the treatment group and thus a beneficial effect of treatment, and a positive value (falling right of the center) indicates a higher mean on children's depression from treatment. As indicated in Figure 11.1, the strongest treatment effect (farthest from the center to the left) is found in study #7 with $d=-1.82$.

The next element of the meta-analysis is the *variance* of the effect size (or the *standard error*, the square root of the variance). Because the [within-study] variance of the effect size is known from the sampling distribution of the effect size, meta-analysis is also referred to as "level-1 variance-known or V-known application" (Raudenbush & Bryk, 2002, p. 207) in the multilevel modeling (hierarchical linear modeling) literature. In this plot, the variance of standardized mean difference (shown in the third column of this plot) is computed via $v(d) = [(n_t + n_c)/n_t n_c] + d^2 /[2(n_t + n_c)]$. The variance can be used to construct the confidence interval (CI) around the effect size (shown in the last column of this plot). The variance is a measure of *precision* of the estimated effect size. The bigger the variance of an effect size is, the wider the CI will be, which reflects a less precise effect size. In this example, study #3 has the widest CI around the effect size with the largest variance ($v(d)$=0.60), while study #1, study #12, and study #13 have the narrowest CI around the effect size with the smallest variances ($v(d)$=0.05).

The fourth element is *study weight* ($w$), which is displayed in the fifth column of this plot. Study weight varies in its size across the studies and is the inverse of the variance of the effect size. In meta-analysis, bigger weights are assigned to effect sizes that are estimated more precisely with smaller variance. In this example, the biggest study weights are assigned to study #1, study #12, and study #13 ($w$=7.62%), while the smallest study weight is assigned to study #3 ($w$=1.60%). Because the variance of the effect size is primarily dependent upon the sample size,[2] study effects are often known as being weighted by the sample size (Borenstein et al., 2009).

## Goals of Meta-Analysis

With the four key elements in mind, the researcher conducts a meta-analysis to reach two main goals. These include (i) to compute the overall effect size and (ii) to explore the potential variation in effect sizes. The first goal is to compute the overall effect size of study findings on the question of interest. This is referred as the *overall analysis*. On the forest plot shown in Figure 11.1, the overall effect of the 18 studies is shown on the bottom of the figure. The estimated overall effect is −0.49, with a 95% CI of −0.69 and −0.28, indicating a significant treatment effect of physical activity in lowering the level of children's depression. An overall effect is simply a weighted mean ($\bar{d}$) of the individual effects, computed via $\bar{d}_{..} = \sum_{i=1}^{k} w_i d_i / \sum_{i=1}^{k} w_i$, where $d_i$ is the effect size for the $i$th study for $i = 1, ..., k$, $k$ is the number of studies, and $w_i$ is the inverse-variance weight for the $i$th study.

Depending on whether the participants in the included studies were assumed to be sampled from a single population, a fixed- or random-effects model is chosen to estimate the overall effect (for a more extensive discussion, see Borenstein et al., 2009). Under the fixed-effects model, it is assumed that samples from selected studies come from the same population and they vary only due to the sampling error. Thus, the common effect is computed based solely on the effects inversely weighted by their sampling variance ($v_i$), $w_i = 1/v_i$. Under the random-effects model, it is assumed that samples from selected studies do not come from the same population and so the true effect varies across studies. Thus, an average effect is estimated based on the effect sizes inversely weighted by both the between-study difference[3] ($\sigma_\theta^2$) and their sampling variance ($v_i$), $w_i^* = 1/v_i^* = 1/(\sigma_\theta^2 + v_i)$.

The second goal of meta-analysis is to explore the potential sources of between-study variation in the effect sizes using exploratory variable(s), which is referred to as

---

[2] Other factors affecting the precision of the effect size are study design (Borenstein et al., 2009) and study quality (Cooper & Hedges, 1994).

[3] A number of methods are available for estimating the between-study variation ($\sigma_\theta^2$). These include an estimator proposed by Hunter and Schmidt (1990), an estimator by Hedges (1983), and estimator by Dersimonian and Laird (1986) and two estimators based on maximum likelihood (ML) estimation and restricted maximum likelihood (REML) estimation. Of these estimators, Viechtbauer (2005) showed that REML estimation provides the most unbiased and efficient estimator of between-study variance.

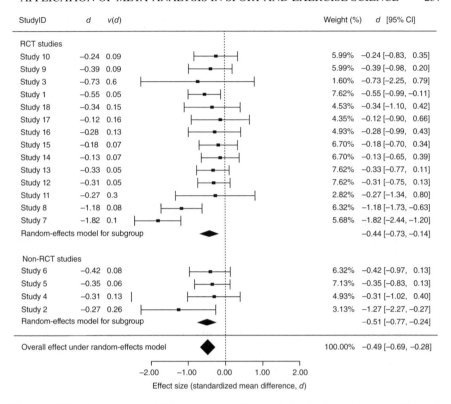

*Figure 11.2   Forest plot of 18 treatment effects of physical activity on children's depression by RCT versus non-RCT studies.*

*moderator analysis.* If the true effect size is consistent (and a fixed-effects model is adopted in estimating the overall analysis), the focus is solely on estimating an overall effect. However, when the true effect varies considerably across studies (and a random-effects model is adopted in estimating the overall analysis), the important task for the meta-analyst is to identify the source of variation. Figure 11.2 shows a forest plot with two subgroups, which differ by whether a randomized control trial (RCT) is used or not (non-RCT). In this example, the first fourteen studies were based on RCTs and yielded an overall effect of −0.44 with a 95% CI of −0.73 and −0.14, while the last four studies were based on non-RCTs and yielded the overall effect of −0.51 with a 95% CI of −0.77 and −0.24. This result indicates that no significant difference exists in the treatment effect between the RCT studies and the non-RCT studies as the CIs for two groups are overlapping.

For moderator analysis, either a fixed- or a mixed-effects model with a moderator is available. In particular, when an exploratory variable(s) is assumed to explain all the between-study difference in the effect sizes, a fixed-effects model with a moderator(s) is deemed appropriate. However, when an exploratory variable(s) is assumed to explain some but not all the between-study difference in the effect sizes, a mixed-effects model with a moderator analysis is more appropriate.

# Utility of the Methodology in Sport and Exercise Science

Based on the computerized searches of MEDLINE and PsycINFO in 2009, Becker and Ahn (2012) found that the change in the number of the published peer-reviewed meta-analyses in the area of sport and exercise science between 1975 and 2009 follows an exponential growth line, with an $R^2$ value of 0.99. This trend has continued in the last 5 years, with a total number of 108,227 peer-reviewed journal articles published between 2010 and 2015 in our informal searches of MEDLINE and PsycINFO conducted in February 2015 using the key terms "meta-analysis," "sports science," "kinesiology," and "exercise."

In his review of meta-analyses in sport and exercise research, Hagger (2006) pointed out that many researchers in the area employ the fixed-effects model, with only a few discussing differences between the fixed- and random-effects model. Hagger also noted that, when the effect (e.g., the effectiveness of physical activity) is examined on multiple outcomes/constructs (e.g., depression, self-concept, and externalizing problems), researchers in the area either summarize the effects by each outcome separately or conduct the moderator analysis comparing the effects by type of outcome. Likewise, when more than one effect size on several outcomes/constructs are extracted from the same study, yielding a multivariate data, the current practice in the area relies on the univariate meta-analysis. However, multivariate meta-analysis may be more appropriate for such data. Hagger recommended researchers adopt the best meta-analytic practice that is appropriate for the nature of the data and its underlying assumption.

Figure 11.3 presents a flowchart that can be used to guide meta-analytic researchers to choose the appropriate meta-analytic model. As shown in Figure 11.3, multivariate meta-analysis might be an appropriate option for multivariate data when (i) the number of effect sizes is sufficiently large and (ii) statistical information needed to compute the dependent effect sizes and their variance–covariance is available. Otherwise, univariate meta-analysis is likely more appropriate. Regardless of the meta-analytic approach used, the decision of whether to use a fixed- or a random-effects model for the overall analysis and whether to use a fixed- or a mixed-effects model for the moderator analysis should be made based on both theoretical and statistical assumptions about the nature of the data (one true effect size vs. multiple true effect sizes). More discussion on the choice of models can be found in Borenstein et al. (2009); Cooper and Hedges (1994); Cooper, Hedges, and Valentine (2009); and Hedges and Vevea (1998).

# The Substantive Example

Keeping the general guidelines on choosing either a univariate or a multivariate meta-analysis in mind, we illustrate a step-by-step example to demonstrate both methods using the free software R. Our illustration follows four steps: step 1,

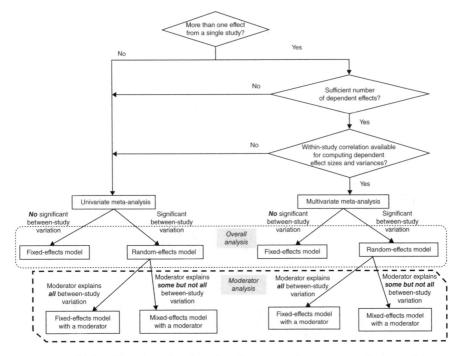

*Figure 11.3    Flowchart for choosing the appropriate meta-analytic model.*

*data management*; step 2, *test of the homogeneity assumption in effects*; step 3, *overall analysis*; and step 4, *moderator analysis*.

In this example, we use the data from a published meta-analysis (Craft, Magyar, Becker, & Feltz, 2003). Using correlation coefficients ($r$) as a primary effect-size measure, the main purposes of their meta-analysis were to examine the interrelationships between three subscales: cognitive anxiety, somatic anxiety, and self-concept measured by the Competitive State Anxiety Inventory (CSAI-2) and athletic performance. We further explore the potential moderators that might explain the variation observed across the effect sizes.

Craft et al. (2003) extracted 246 correlations from 29 independent studies (20 published and 9 unpublished studies) that report at least one correlation coefficient describing the relationship among cognitive anxiety, somatic anxiety, self-concept, and sport performance in athletes. Across the 29 included studies, the number of reported correlations from a single study varied from one to six, with a mean of 3.6 out of 6 possible correlations (i.e., $[4 \times 3]/2 = 6$). For the purpose of demonstration, we use a subset of the data that provides all six correlation coefficients among cognitive anxiety, somatic anxiety, self-concept, and sport performance in athletes.

Table 11.1 presents the 18 studies that provide all six correlations among the four variables of interest. These include (i) the correlation between cognitive anxiety and somatic anxiety (C1), (ii) the correlation between cognitive anxiety and self-confidence

Table 11.1  Relationships between three subscales of CSAI and athletic performance in 18 studies.

| ID | n | Gender | % Male | Correlation (r) | | | | | |
|---|---|---|---|---|---|---|---|---|---|
| | | | | C1 | C2 | C3 | C4 | C5 | C6 |
| Caruso 1990a | 24 | Male | 100 | 0.240 | -0.400 | -0.340 | -0.170 | 0.080 | 0.210 |
| Caruso 1990b | 27 | Male | 100 | 0.420 | -0.420 | -0.480 | -0.080 | 0.170 | -0.120 |
| Caruso 1990c | 30 | Male | 100 | 0.330 | -0.190 | -0.590 | -0.140 | -0.110 | 0.090 |
| Barnes 1986 | 14 | Male | 100 | 0.212 | -0.544 | -0.431 | -0.391 | -0.166 | 0.191 |
| Edwards 1996 | 45 | Female | 0 | 0.470 | -0.370 | -0.500 | 0.100 | 0.310 | -0.170 |
| Maynard 1995a | 24 | Male | 100 | 0.670 | -0.360 | -0.720 | -0.150 | -0.400 | 0.350 |
| Maynard 1995b | 24 | Male | 100 | 0.670 | -0.410 | -0.720 | -0.240 | -0.240 | 0.360 |
| Maynard 1995c | 24 | Male | 100 | 0.130 | -0.040 | -0.500 | -0.060 | -0.160 | 0.220 |
| Rodrigo 1990 | 51 | Male | 100 | 0.570 | -0.180 | -0.260 | -0.520 | -0.430 | 0.160 |
| McAuley | 7 | Female | 0 | 0.171 | -0.311 | -0.177 | 0.106 | -0.008 | -0.007 |
| Abouzekri 2010a | 61 | Male | 100 | 0.425 | -0.128 | -0.158 | 0.084 | 0.086 | -0.218 |
| Abouzekri 2010b | 61 | Male | 100 | 0.145 | -0.049 | -0.219 | 0.066 | 0.061 | -0.187 |
| Abouzekri 2010c | 61 | Male | 100 | 0.456 | -0.136 | -0.124 | 0.120 | -0.008 | -0.322 |
| Kais 2005a | 24 | Male | 100 | 0.500 | -0.520 | -0.500 | 0.290 | -0.150 | 0.000 |
| Kais 2005b | 24 | Male | 100 | 0.500 | -0.520 | -0.500 | 0.290 | -0.150 | 0.000 |
| Nicholls 2010 | 307 | Mixed | 82 | 0.490 | -0.200 | -0.380 | -0.080 | -0.030 | 0.130 |
| Otten 2009 | 243 | Mixed | 63 | 0.790 | -0.330 | -0.230 | -0.150 | -0.110 | 0.490 |
| Sanchez 2010 | 19 | Male | 100 | 0.109 | -0.668 | 0.690 | 0.130 | 0.542 | -0.158 |

*Note*: C1, correlation (r) between cognitive anxiety and somatic anxiety; C2, r between cognitive anxiety and self-confidence; C3, r between somatic anxiety and self-confidence; C4, r between cognitive anxiety and athletic performance; C5, r between somatic anxiety and athletic performance; C6, r between self-confidence and athletic performance.

(C2), (iii) the correlation between somatic anxiety and self- confidence (C3), (iv) the correlation between cognitive anxiety and athletic performance (C4), (v) the correlation between somatic anxiety and athletic performance (C5), and (vi) the correlation between self-confidence and athletic performance (C6). Sample size ($n$), gender (*gender*: male, female, and mixed-gender group), and % of male participants (*% male*) are also presented along with the six reported correlations.

# The Synergy

## Univariate Meta-Analysis

A univariate meta-analysis is first presented to investigate two distinct research questions: (i) what is the overall effect across studies? and (ii) is the variation in study effects explained by hypothesized moderating variables such as gender or race? In other words, overall and moderator analyses are conducted using the data provided. The overall relationships between each of the three subscales (i.e., cognitive anxiety, somatic anxiety, and self-concept) of the CSAI-2 and athletic performance (C4, C5, and C6 in Table 11.1) are first estimated. Then, the follow-up moderator analyses are conducted to examine the effect of gender as a potential moderator on the effect sizes. All analyses were conducted using the *metafor* package (Viechtbauer, 2010) written in the free statistical software R (R Development Core Team, 2014).

*Step 1: Data management.* The first step involves two main tasks for creating a dataset for univariate meta-analysis in the *R* statistical software. First, effect sizes extracted from the included studies should be stacked in a column. For instance, as shown in the dataset (*craft.txt*), the $r$ between somatic anxiety and performance are stacked and saved in a column called C5. For missing correlations, "NA" should be entered in the dataset. This can be done in Excel and should be saved as a "tab-delimited" file.

Once the "tab-delimited" dataset is imported to the *R* statistical software, the next step is to compute the effect size ($r$) and its variance. A transformation is recommended to stabilize the raw correlation, $r$ (Becker, 2000). Therefore, in this example the $r$ was transformed to Fisher's $z$ via $z_r = 0.5 \log(1 + r)/(1 - r)$ and then its associated variance ($v(z_r)$) was computed via $v(z_r) = 1/(n - 3)$. These transformations can all be easily done using the *escalc* function available in the *metafor* package written in the R statistical software (see Appendix 11.1 for R code).

*Step 2: Test of the homogeneity assumption in effects.* In step 2, we seek to determine whether to use a fixed- or random-effects model for an overall analysis. Theoretically, the relationship between each of the three subscales of the CSAI-2 and athletic performance would differ depending on a number of factors such as gender, ethnicity, muscle mass, and experience. Therefore, a random-effects model, which assumes that the true relationships between these variables vary from study to study, appears appropriate. In addition to our theoretical justification, we can test the assumption of homogeneity in effects regarding whether effects are from the same population.

The test of the homogeneity of variance of the effect sizes is based on the $Q_{\text{total}}$ statistic (Cooper et al., 2009), which quantifies a total observed variance in effect sizes across the $k$ studies computed via $Q_{\text{total}} = \sum_{i=1}^{k} w_i (r_i - r)^2$ where $w_i = 1/v_i$. Under the null hypothesis that all the studies come from the same population, the $Q_{total}$ follows a central chi-squared distribution with degrees of freedom equal to $k-1$. If the $Q_{total}$ is found to be statistically significant at a preset alpha level, it is assumed that study effects are not from the same population, suggesting that a random-effects model should be adopted for the overall analysis. Otherwise, a fixed-effects model should be adopted for the overall analysis.

In our example, $Q_{total}$ was computed using "rma" function available in the *metafor* package written in the R statistical software (see Appendix 11.1 for R code). The $Q_{total}$ statistics for C4, C5, and C6 are shown in the third column of Table 11.2. The tests of the homogeneity assumption in effect sizes indicate that statistically significant between-study variation exists in the relationship (C4) between cognitive anxiety and athlete performance ($Q_{total}(17)=28.57$, $p=0.04$), the relationship (C5) between somatic anxiety and athlete performance ($Q_{total}(17)=29.84$, $p=0.03$), and the relationship (C6) between self-confidence and athlete performance ($Q_{total}(17)=75.19$, $p<0.01$). These suggest that the overall relationships for C4, C5, and C6 should be estimated under the random-effects model, in which effects are assumed to come from different populations.

*Step 3: Overall analysis.* In step 3, the overall effect size is estimated under the chosen model using the *rma* function available in the *metafor* package written in the R statistical software (see Appendix 11.1 for R code). For our example, overall effects were estimated under the random-effects model, where study effects were weighted by the sum of the between-study variance $\left(\sigma_\theta^2\right)$ as well as the within-study variance ($v_i$). Under the random-effects model, the estimated overall correlations for C4, C5, and C6 were −0.06 (95% CI: −0.16, 0.05), −0.04 (95% CI: −0.14, 0.06), and 0.06 (95% CI: −0.07, 0.19), respectively, and they were all found to be not statistically

Table 11.2   Estimated correlations among each subscale of CSAI from the univariate meta-analysis.

| Interrelationship | $k$ | $Q_{total}$ | $df$ | $\bar{r}$ | 95% CI | |
|---|---|---|---|---|---|---|
| | | | | | LL | UL |
| Cognitive anxiety and athletic performance (C4) | 18 | 28.57* | 17 | −0.06 | −0.16 | 0.05 |
| Somatic anxiety and athletic performance (C5) | 18 | 29.84* | 17 | −0.04 | −0.14 | 0.06 |
| Self-confidence and athletic performance (C6) | 18 | 75.19** | 17 | 0.06 | −0.07 | 0.19 |

*Note*: $k$, number of effects.
*$p<0.05$.
**$p<0.01$.

significant. These results suggest that none of the three subscales (i.e., cognitive anxiety, somatic anxiety, and self-concept) of CSAI-2 is related to athletic performance. Figures 11.4, 11.5, 11.6, and Table 11.2 summarize the results based on a random-effects model on C4, C5, and C6.

*Step 4: Moderator analysis.* In step 4, when the significant amount of between-study variation in effect sizes exists (when the $Q_{total}$ is found to be significant in the preceding step), a series of moderator analysis can be performed to find the source of variation among the effects. For this example, we will use gender with three subgroups (female, male, and mixed-gender group) as a categorical moderator and the percentage of males in the sample (*p_male*) as a continuous moderator to see whether each of the relationships (C4, C5, and C6) significantly differs by gender (either *gender* or *p_male*).

The first step in a moderator analysis is to determine whether to use the fixed-versus mixed-effects model on theoretical and statistical bases. In particular, two pieces of the statistical evidence that helps researchers choose the model are the significance tests of (i) $Q_{model}$, which quantifies the amount of variation in effects explained by a moderator, and (ii) $Q_{error}$, which quantifies the amount of variation in effects unexplained by a moderator. When a moderator is assumed to explain all between-study variation in effects (i.e., $Q_{model}$ is significant, but $Q_{error}$ is not significant), a fixed-effects model with a moderator is deemed appropriate. When a moderator is

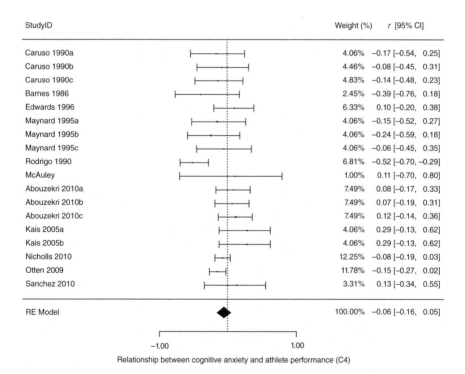

Figure 11.4    Forest plot of correlation between cognitive anxiety and athlete performance.

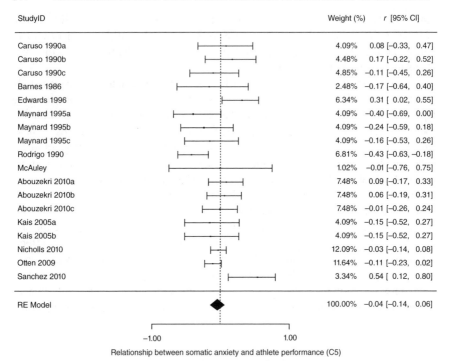

*Figure 11.5    Forest plot of correlation between somatic anxiety and athlete performance.*

assumed to explain some but not all between-study variation in effects (i.e., both $Q_{model}$ and $Q_{error}$ are significant), a mixed-effects model with a moderator is deemed appropriate. When $Q_{model}$ is not found to be statistically significant, another moderator should be sought out to explain the between-study variation in effects.

For our example, as shown in Table 11.3, none of moderators were found to significantly explain the between-study variation in the relationships (C4) between cognitive anxiety and athletic performance ($Q_{model}(1) = 0.02$, $p = 0.88$ for % of males in the sample; $Q_{model}(2) = 2.43$, $p = 0.30$ for gender) or the relationships (C5) between somatic anxiety and athletic performance ($Q_{model}(1) = 2.34$, $p = 0.13$ for % of males in the sample; $Q_{model}(1) = 5.58$, $p = 0.06$ for gender). Both moderators were found to significantly explain some but not all between-study variation in the relationship (C6) between self-confidence and athletic performance ($Q_{model}(1) = 7.21$, $p < 0.01$ and $Q_{error}(16) = 67.98$, $p < 0.01$ for % of males in the sample; $Q_{model}(2) = 31.55$, $p < 0.01$ and $Q_{error}(15) = 43.65$, $p < 0.01$ for gender). Therefore, a mixed-effects model was applied to perform a moderator analysis with percentage of males in the sample or gender.

Under the mixed-effects model with percentage of males in the sample as a continuous moderator, neither the intercept nor the slope was found to be statistically significant ($Q_{model}(2) = 0.0004$, $p = 0.98$). In particular, an insignificant intercept of 0.07 (95% CI: −0.36 and 0.47) suggests that the relationship between self-confidence

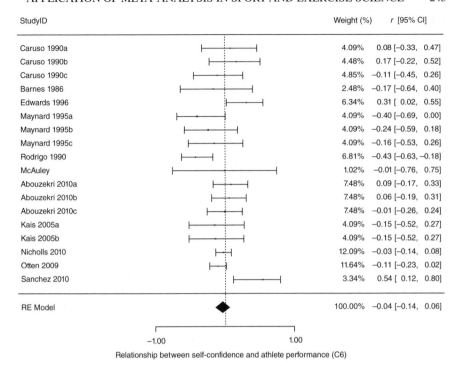

*Figure 11.6    Forest plot of correlation between self-confidence and athlete performance.*

and athletic performance was not significantly different from zero when females are included in the sample (% of males in the sample equals to zero). And an insignificant slope related to % of males of −0.0001 (95% CI: −0.005 and 0.005) suggests that the change in the relationship between self-confidence and athletic performance is not significant for an additional 1% increase in males in the sample.

Under the mixed-effects model with a gender as categorical moderator, the estimated relationship (C6) between self-confidence and athletic performance was not statistically significant for female-only ($\bar{r}$ = −0.14, 95% CI: −0.51 and 0.27) and male-only samples ($\bar{r}$ = 0.01, 95% CI: −0.13 and 0.15), while it was statistically significant for the mixed-gender sample ($\bar{r}$ = 0.32, 95% CI: 0.06 and 0.53). However, the estimated correlation between self-confidence and athletic performance was not significantly different among those three gender groups ($Q_{model}(2)$ = 6.44, $p$ = 0.09). Typically, when the $Q_{model}$ value is not significant for a moderator, separate group analyses are not conducted. However, they are conducted in this example for the purpose of illustration.

# Multivariate Meta-Analysis

A multivariate meta-analysis is performed on the same dataset to investigate research questions similar to those we examined in the univariate meta-analysis: (i) what is the overall effect across studies after accounting for interrelationships among multiple

Table 11.3    Results from univariate moderator analysis.

| Moderators | $k$ | $Q_{model}$ | $df_{model}$ | $Q_{error}$ | $df_{error}$ | $\bar{r}$ | 95% CI | |
|---|---|---|---|---|---|---|---|---|
| | | | | | | | LL | UL |
| *Cognitive anxiety and athletic performance (C4)* | | | | | | | | |
| % of males in the sample | 18 | 0.02 | 1 | 28.55* | 16 | – | – | – |
| Gender | 18 | 2.43 | 2 | 26.13* | 15 | – | – | – |
| *Somatic anxiety and athletic performance (C5)* | | | | | | | | |
| % of males in the sample | 18 | 2.34 | 1 | 27.50* | 16 | – | – | – |
| Gender | 18 | 5.58 | 2 | 24.25 | 15 | – | – | – |
| *Self-confidence and athletic performance (C6)* | | | | | | | | |
| % of males in the sample | 18 | 7.21**/0.0004† | 1 | 67.98** | 16 | | | |
| Intercept | | | | | | | 0.07 | –0.36 | 0.47 |
| Slope related to % of males in the sample | | | | | | | –0.0001 | –0.005 | 0.005 |
| Gender | 18 | 31.55**/6.44† | 2 | 43.64** | 15 | | | |
| Female | 14 | | | | | | –0.14 | –0.51 | 0.27 |
| Male | 2 | | | | | | 0.01 | –0.13 | 0.15 |
| Mixed-gender group | 2 | | | | | | 0.32* | 0.06 | 0.53 |

*Note*: $k$, number of effects; † $Q_{model}$ was estimated under the mixed-effects model.
*$p<0.05$.
**$p<0.01$.

effects? and (ii) is the variation in study effects explained by hypothesized moderating variables such as gender or race after accounting for interrelationships among multiple effects? In other words, overall and moderator analyses are conducted using the data, but the effects are estimated more precisely by incorporating nonzero correlations among dependent effect sizes (Becker, 2009; Kim & Becker, 2010; Nam, Mengersen, & Garthwaite, 2003).

Presently, the overall relationships between each of the three subscales (i.e., cognitive anxiety, somatic anxiety, and self-concept) of the CSAI-2 and athletic performance (C4, C5, and C6 in Table 11.1) after accounting for interrelationships among three subscales (i.e., cognitive anxiety, somatic anxiety, and self-concept: C1, C2, and C3 in Table 11.1) are first estimated. Then, follow-up moderator analyses are conducted to examine if each relationship varies by a potential moderator (i.e., gender) after accounting for interrelationships among three subscales (i.e., cognitive anxiety, somatic anxiety, and self-concept: C1, C2, and C3 in Table 11.1). A number of different data analytic techniques are available for multivariate meta-analysis; our presentation in this section is based on the generalized least squares (GLS) method (Becker, 1992, 2000). All analyses were conducted using the *mvmeta* package (Gasparrini, Armstrong, & Kenward, 2012) written in the free R statistical software (R Development Core Team, 2014).

*Step 1: Data management.* There are two main tasks for creating a dataset for multivariate meta-analysis. First, all the observed correlation values across the 18 studies are stacked in a column. As shown in the dataset (*craft.txt*), each of six correlations (C1–C6) among four measures extracted from the 18 studies is saved in each column and saved as a "tab-delimited" file.

Once the "tab-delimited" dataset is imported to the R software, the next step is to transform the six reported raw correlation values (C1–C6) to Fisher's $z$ values via $z_{st} = 0.5\log(1 + r_{st})/(1 - r_{st})$ where $r_{st}$ is observed correlation between $s$th and $t$th variables and four variable index labels $s$, $t$, $u$, and $v$ range from 1 to the number of variables in correlation matrix. Then, the associated within-study variance–covariance matrix for the transformed Fisher's $z$ values for each study should be computed using equations proposed by Olkin and Siotain (1976): $\text{var}(z_{st}) = 1/(n - 3)$ and $\text{cov}(z_{st}, z_{uv}) = SD_{st,uv} / \left[\left(1 - r_{st}^2\right)\left(1 - r_{uv}^2\right)\right]$. Appendix 11.2 provides R syntax code written by authors for computing within-study variance–covariance matrix for the transformed Fisher's $z$.

*Step 2: Test of the homogeneity assumption in effect-size vector.* In step 2, the test of the homogeneity assumption in an effect-size vector is performed in order to see whether the vector of effect-size measures is from the same population. For our example, a homogeneity test of the effect-size vector indicates that the set of six observed correlations do not come from the same (common) population ($Q_{\text{total}}(102) = 349.86$, $p < 0.01$), suggesting that a vector of overall correlations among four measures should be estimated under the random-effects model rather than the fixed-effects model. A multivariate homogeneity test was performed using "mvmeta" function available in the *mvmeta* package (see Appendix 11.2 for R code).

*Step 3: Overall analysis.* In step 3, a set of effect sizes on multiple measures is estimated using either a fixed- or random-effects model depending on the results of a multivariate homogeneity test described above. In our example, as suggested in step 2, overall relationships among four variables were estimated under the random-effects model.

Under the random-effects model, the estimated correlations among the four variables are shown in Tables 11.4 and 11.5. Of the six estimated correlations, three pairs of variables—cognitive anxiety and somatic anxiety ($\bar{r} = 0.47$, $z = 7.90$, $p < 0.01$, 95% CI: 0.36 and 0.56), cognitive anxiety and self-confidence ($\bar{r} = -0.26$, $z = -6.34$, $p < 0.01$, 95% CI: $-0.34$ and $-0.18$), and somatic anxiety and self-confidence ($\bar{r} = -0.34$, $z = -4.34$, $p < 0.01$, 95% CI: $-0.47$ and $-0.19$)—were found to be statistically significant. However, none of the three subscales of CSAI-2 (i.e., cognitive anxiety, somatic anxiety, and self-concept) were related to athletic performance: $-0.02$ (95% CI: $-0.13$, 0.08) for C4, $-0.004$ (95% CI: $-0.10$, 0.10) for C5, and 0.03 (95% CI: $-0.10$, 0.16) for C6. These were all estimated using *mvmeta* function available in the *mvmeta* package written in the R statistical software (see Appendix 11.2 for R code).

Table 11.4    Estimated correlations between three subscales of CSAI and athletic performance using multivariate meta-analysis.

| Interrelationship | k | $\bar{r}$ | 95% CI | |
| --- | --- | --- | --- | --- |
| | | | LL | UL |
| Cognitive anxiety and somatic anxiety (C1) | 18 | 0.47** | 0.36 | 0.56 |
| Cognitive anxiety and self-confidence (C2) | 18 | −0.26** | −0.34 | −0.18 |
| Somatic anxiety and self-confidence (C3) | 18 | −0.34** | −0.47 | −0.19 |
| Cognitive anxiety and athletic performance (C4) | 18 | −0.02 | −0.13 | 0.08 |
| Somatic anxiety and athletic performance (C5) | 18 | −0.004 | −0.10 | 0.10 |
| Self-confidence and athletic performance (C6) | 18 | 0.03 | −0.10 | 0.16 |

Note: k, number of effects.
**$p < 0.01$.

Table 11.5    Estimated correlation matrix among three subscales of CSAI and athletic performance using multivariate meta-analysis.

| | Cog | Som | SC | P |
| --- | --- | --- | --- | --- |
| Cognitive anxiety (Cog) | | | | |
| Somatic anxiety (Som) | 0.47** | | | |
| Self-confidence (Sc) | −0.26** | −0.34** | | |
| Performance (P) | −0.02 | −0.004 | 0.03 | |

Note: k, number of effects.
**$p < 0.01$.

Step 4: Moderator analysis. In step 4, a fixed-effects model with predictors or a mixed-effects model can be performed to explore the sources of between-study variations in a set of effect sizes on multiple measures. In our example, we used the percentage of male participants as a potential moderator and ran a mixed-effects model to see whether the effect sizes differed by the percentage of males in the sample (p_male). These were all estimated using "mvmeta" function available in the mvmeta package (see Appendix 11.2 for R code).

A significant $Q_{model}$ indicates that the percentage of male athletes significantly explained the between-study variation in a set of correlations among four variables ($Q_{model}(6) = 43.88$ [$Q_{total}$ of 349.86 estimated in step 2—$Q_{error}$ of 305.98 estimated in step 4], $p < 0.01$). As shown in Table 11.6, the relationship between cognitive anxiety and somatic anxiety was found to be statistically significant and positive for female athletes ($\bar{r} = 0.57$, $z = 3.11$, $p = 0.002$, 95% CI: 0.23 and 0.78). However, the relationship between cognitive anxiety and self-confidence was found to be negative and significant for female athletes ($\bar{r} = −0.31$, $z = −2.07$, $p = 0.03$, 95% CI: −0.55 and −0.02). Results suggest that cognitive anxiety is positively related to somatic anxiety but is negatively related to self-confidence among female athletes.

Table 11.6    Results from multivariate moderator analysis using percentage of males in the samples.

| Interrelationships | $\bar{r}$ | 95% CI | |
| --- | --- | --- | --- |
| | | LL | UL |
| *Cognitive anxiety and somatic anxiety (C1)* | | | |
| Intercept | 0.57** | 0.23 | 0.78 |
| % of males in the sample | −0.002 | −0.006 | 0.003 |
| *Cognitive anxiety and self-confidence (C2)* | | | |
| Intercept | −0.31* | −0.55 | −0.02 |
| % of males in the sample | 0.0005 | −0.003 | 0.004 |
| *Somatic anxiety and self-confidence (C3)* | | | |
| Intercept | −0.37 | −0.73 | 0.16 |
| % of males in the sample | 0.0002 | −0.006 | 0.006 |
| *Cognitive anxiety and athletic performance (C4)* | | | |
| Intercept | 0.08 | −0.28 | 0.41 |
| % of males in the sample | −0.001 | −0.005 | 0.003 |
| *Somatic anxiety and athletic performance (C5)* | | | |
| Intercept | 0.30 | −0.04 | 0.57 |
| % of males in the sample | −0.004 | −0.008 | 0.0002 |
| *Self-confidence and athletic performance (C6)* | | | |
| Intercept | 0.03 | −0.39 | 0.44 |
| % of males in the sample | 0.0001 | −0.005 | 0.005 |

*$p < 0.05$.
**$p < 0.01$.

# Summary

Since being introduced, meta-analysis has been widely used in sport and exercise science, and we believe that this will continue to be the case. The increased number of available computer programs for meta-analysis makes meta-analytic research more accessible than ever before. However, the ease of use of meta-analytic software might result in poorly conducted analyses unless researchers have a thorough understanding of the underlying principles of meta-analysis and its application appropriate for the nature of data as well as the underlying assumptions. Our hope is to guide researchers to adopt the best available meta-analytic practice. This chapter provided a brief overview of meta-analysis and discussed how to choose the most appropriate meta-analytic methods. We offered a step-by-step tutorial in R that illustrates the process of performing both univariate and multivariate meta-analysis using a real dataset in the area of sport and exercise science.

Univariate meta-analysis is an appropriate option for synthesizing the study effect of a single outcome/construct. However, researchers in practice are often interested in examining study effects on multiple outcomes/constructs rather than on a single one. In such cases, more than one effect size may be extracted from a study, and consequently, these effect sizes are dependent on one another, which leads to a multivariate scenario. Other circumstances that produce a multivariate data in meta-analysis are when multiple comparison groups are used within the study and their pairs are contrasted to address treatment effects (Gleser & Olkin, 1994, 2009; Ryan, Blakeslee, & Furst, 1986) and(or) when the same participants are measured on multiple outcomes over several time periods (Wei & Higgins, 2013a, 2013b).

Different univariate meta-analytic approaches are available for dealing with a multivariate data, including ignoring dependence of effect sizes, averaging dependent effect sizes, and separating effect sizes into independent subgroups and analyzing them separately by subgroup (Borenstein et al., 2009). However, when multivariate meta-analysis, with nonzero within-study correlations among dependent effect sizes (Becker, 2009; Kim & Becker, 2010; Nam et al., 2003) is used for data analysis, it provides more precise estimates and control for type I error rate. Although multivariate meta-analysis is known to hold many advantages (Becker, 1992, 2009; Becker & Schram, 1994; Gleser & Olkin, 2009; Kim & Becker, 2010; Nam et al., 2003; van Houwelingen, Arends, & Stijnen, 2002; Wei & Higgins, 2013b), a number of challenges have been identified in its application to practice.

Some challenges in applying multivariate meta-analysis include dealing with missing information in estimating effect sizes and their associated within-study variance–covariance matrix of multiple correlated effect sizes (Becker, 1992, 2009; Furlow & Beretvas, 2005; Ishak, Platt, Joseph, & Hanley, 2008; Riley, 2009; Riley, Thompson, & Abrams, 2008; Wei & Higgins, 2013a), an estimation of between-study variance–covariance matrix in performing a random-effects model or mixed-effects model (White, 2009), the number of primary studies exploring outcomes/constructs of researcher's interest that is sufficient enough for multivariate meta-analysis, and potential differences in the psychometric properties of outcome(s) representing the underlying construct. Likewise, multivariate meta-analysis might not be applicable for all the circumstances. Therefore, researchers are encouraged to evaluate whether to use univariate or multivariate method in advance and choose the most appropriate method for their dataset.

In this chapter, we demonstrated the steps for performing both univariate and multivariate meta-analyses using an existing dataset for answering essentially the same research questions. We do so in hopes to equip readers with the knowledge of available tools and provide information that helps to choose the most appropriate one for their own research. We believe that paying more attention to the recent advances in meta-analysis and the capacities of available computer software available to conduct meta-analysis will lead to more accurate results. In addition, we encourage researchers to adhere to the guidelines for reporting meta-analytic results. These include (i) Preferred Reporting Items for Systematic Reviews and Meta-Analyses (PRISMA), which can be found in http://www.prisma-statement.org/, and (ii) Meta-Analysis Reporting Standards (MARS), which can be found in https://www.apa.org/pubs/authors/jars.pdf.

# Acknowledgment

We appreciate Dr. Meng-jia Wu (Associate Professor at the Loyola University Chicago) for her through and helpful review of this chapter.

# References

Ahn, S., & Fedewa, A. L. (2011). A meta-analysis of the relationship between children's physical activity and mental health. *Journal of Pediatric Psychology, 36*, 385–397. doi:10.1093/jpepsy/jsq107

Becker, B. J. (1992). Using results from replicated studies to estimate linear models. *Journal of Educational and Behavioral Statistics, 17*, 341–362. doi:10.2307/1165128

Becker, B. J. (2000). Multivariate meta-analysis. In H. E. A. Tinsley & S. D. Brown (Eds.), *Handbook of applied multivariate statistics and mathematical modeling* (pp. 499–525). San Diego, CA: Academic Press.

Becker, B. J. (2009). Model-based meta-analysis. In H. Cooper, L. V. Hedges, & J. C. Valentine (Eds.), *The handbook of research synthesis and meta-analysis* (2nd ed., pp. 377–395). New York, NY: Russell Sage Foundation.

Becker, B. J., & Ahn, S. (2012). Synthesizing measurement outcomes through meta-analysis. In G. Tenenbaum, R. C. Eklund, & A. Kamata (Eds.), *Measurement in sport and exercise psychology* (pp. 153–168). Champaign, IL: Human Kinetics.

Becker, B. J., & Schram, C. M. (1994). Examining explanatory models through research synthesis. In H. Cooper & L. V. Hedges (Eds.), *The handbook of research synthesis* (pp. 357–381). New York, NY: Russell Sage Foundation.

Borenstein, M., Hedges, L. V., Higgins, J., & Rothstein, H. (2009). *Introduction to meta-analysis*. Chichester, England: John Wiley & Sons, Ltd.

Cooper, H. M. (1984). *The integrative research review: A systematic approach*. Beverly Hills, CA: Sage.

Cooper, H. (2010). *Research synthesis and meta-analysis: A step-by-step approach* (4th ed.). Thousand Oaks, CA: Sage.

Cooper, H., & Hedges, L. V. (1994). *The handbook of research synthesis*. New York, NY: Russell Sage Foundation.

Cooper, H., Hedges, L. V., & Valentine, J. C. (2009). *The handbook of research synthesis and meta-analysis* (2nd ed.). New York, NY: Russell Sage Foundation.

Craft, L. L., Magyar, T. M., Becker, B. J., & Feltz, D. L. (2003). The relationship between the competitive state anxiety inventory-2 and sport performance: A meta-analysis. *Journal of Sport & Exercise Psychology, 25*(1), 44–65.

DerSimonian, R. & Laird, N. (1986). Meta-analysis in clinical trials. *Controlled Clinical Trials, 7*(3), 177–186.

Furlow, C. F., & Beretvas, S. N. (2005). Meta-analytic methods of pooling correlation matrices for structural equation modeling under different patterns of missing data. *Psychological Methods, 10*, 227–254. doi:10.1037/1082-989X.10.2.227

Gasparrini, A., Armstrong, B., & Kenward, M. G. (2012). Multivariate meta-analysis for non-linear and other multi-parameter associations. *Statistics in Medicine, 31*, 3821–3839. doi:10.1002/sim.5471

Glass, G. V. (1976). Primary, secondary, and meta-analysis of research. *Educational Researcher, 5*(10), 3–8.

Gleser, L. J., & Olkin, I. (1994). Stochastically dependent effect sizes. In H. Cooper & L. V. Hedges (Eds.), *The handbook of research synthesis* (pp. 339–355). New York, NY: Russell Sage Foundation.

Gleser, L. J., & Olkin, I. (2009). Stochastically dependent effect sizes. In H. Cooper, L. V. Hedges, & J. C. Valentine (Eds.), *The handbook of research synthesis and meta-analysis* (2nd ed., pp. 357–376). New York, NY: Russell Sage Foundation.

Hagger, M. S. (2006). Meta-analysis in sport and exercise research: Review, recent developments, and recommendations. *European Journal of Sport Sciences, 6*, 103–115. doi:10.1080/17461390500528527

Hedges, L. V. (1983). A random effects model for effect size. *Psychological Bulletin, 93*, 388–395.

Hedges, L. V., & Olkin, I. (1985). *Statistical methods for meta-analysis*. New York, NY: Academic Press.

Hedges, L. V., & Vevea, J. L. (1998). Fixed- and random-effects models in meta-analysis. *Psychological Methods, 3*, 486–504. doi:10.1037/1082-989X.3.4.486

Hunter, J. E. & Schmidt, F. L. (1990). *Methods of meta-analysis: correcting error and bias in research findings*. Newburry Park, CA: Sage.

Ishak, K. J., Platt, R. W., Joseph, L., & Hanley, J. A. (2008). Impact of approximating or ignoring within-study covariances in multivariate meta-analyses. *Statistics in Medicine, 27*, 670–686. doi:10.1002/sim.2913

Kim, R.-S., & Becker, B. J. (2010). The degree of dependence between multiple-treatment effect sizes. *Multivariate Behavioral Research, 45*, 213–238. doi:10.1037/a0032734

Nam, I. S., Mengersen, K., & Garthwaite, P. (2003). Multivariate meta-analysis. *Statistics in Medicine, 22*, 2309–2333. doi:10.1002/sim.1410

Olkin, I., & Siotain, M. (1976). Asymptotic distribution of function of a correlation matrix. In I. S. Ikeda (Ed.), *Essays in probability and statistics* (pp. 235–251). Tokyo, Japan: Shinko Tsusho

R Development Core Team. (2014). *R: A language and environment for statistical computing*. Vienna, Austria: R Foundation for Statistical Computing. Retrieved from http://www.R-project.org

Raudenbush, S. W., & Bryk, A. S. (2002). *Hierarchical linear models: Applications and data analysis methods* (2nd ed). Thousand Oaks, CA: Sage.

Riley, R. D. (2009). Multivariate meta-analysis: The effect of ignoring within-study correlation. *Journal of the Royal Statistical Society: Series A (Statistics in Society), 172*, 789–811. doi:10.1111/j.1467-985X.2008.00593.x

Riley, R. D., Thompson, J. R., & Abrams, K. R. (2008). An alternative model for bivariate random-effects meta-analysis when the within-study correlations are unknown. *Biostatistics, 9*, 172–186. doi:10.1093/biostatistics/kxm023

Ryan, E. D., Blakeslee, T., & Furst, D. M. (1986). Mental practice and motor skill learning: An indirect test of the neuromuscular feedback hypothesis. *International Journal of Sport and Exercise Psychology, 17*(1), 60–70.

Van Houwelingen, H. C., Arends, L. R., & Stijnen, T. (2002). Advanced methods in meta-analysis: Multivariate approach and meta-regression. *Statistics in Medicine, 21,* 589–624. doi:10.1002/sim.1040

Viechtbauer, W. (2005). Bias and efficiency of meta-analytic variance estimators in the random-effects model. *Journal of Educational and Behavioral Statistics, 30,* 261–293. doi:10.3102/10769986030003261

Viechtbauer, W. (2010). Conducting meta-analyses in R with the metafor package. *Journal of Statistical Software, 36*(3), 1–48. Retrieved from http://www.jstatsoft.org/v36/i03/

Wanous, J. P., Sullivan, S. E., & Malinak, J. (1989). The role of judgment calls in meta-analysis. *Journal of Applied Psychology, 74,* 259–264. doi:10.1037/0021-9010.74.2.259

Wei, Y., & Higgins, J. P. T. (2013a). Estimating within-study covariances in multivariate meta-analysis with multiple outcomes. *Statistics in Medicine, 32,* 1191–1205. doi:10.1002/sim.5679

Wei, Y., & Higgins, J. P. T. (2013b). Bayesian multivariate meta-analysis with multiple outcomes. *Statistics in Medicine, 32,* 2911–2934. doi:10.1002/sim.5745

White, I. R. (2009). Multivariate random-effects meta-analysis. *Stata Journal, 9*(1), 40.

# 12

# Reliability and stability of variables/instruments used in sport science and sport medicine

## Alan M. Nevill[1], Andrew M. Lane[1], and Michael J. Duncan[2]

[1] Faculty of Education, Health and Wellbeing, University of Wolverhampton, Walsall, UK
[2] Faculty of Health and Life Sciences, Coventry University, Coventry, UK

## Introduction

It is the responsibility of all research scientists to ensure that minimal measurement error is present when collecting data. To minimize error, research scientists should scrutinize the decision they make when they analyze data. Scientists should be clear on the type of data (level of measurement) being used and the extent to which it describes accurate and meaningful differences. Regardless of whether data are either interval- or ratio-type data (reliability) or when asking respondents to complete discrete categorical/Likert-type data taken from psychometric questionnaires (stability), scientists must engage in determining the reliability/stability of their data. In this chapter, we will outline the most appropriate techniques to assess the test–retest agreement, that is, the extent to which two measures differ or agree when assessed

*An Introduction to Intermediate and Advanced Statistical Analyses for Sport and Exercise Scientists*, First Edition.
Edited by Nikos Ntoumanis and Nicholas D. Myers.
© 2016 John Wiley & Sons, Ltd. Published 2016 by John Wiley & Sons, Ltd.
Companion website: www.wiley.com/go/ntoumanis/sport

more than once. We will look at how data would be analyzed using (A) if the measurement tool is continuous, recorded on the interval or ratio scale, and (B) when the measurement instrument is discrete, such as the responses to Likert-type questions taken from psychometric questionnaires. A take-home message that we wish to make in our study is that traditional methods such as correlation, which researchers have been using routinely in test–retest studies, might not be appropriate. We encourage research scientists to consider what the research question and consider options that answer that question; sometimes, the traditional method is not the best one.

## A. Assessment of Test–Retest Agreement Using Interval/Ratio Data

In the past, statistical tests used to assess the agreement or reliability of interval- or ratio-type data have been (i) correlations (e.g., Pearson's product-moment correlation, intraclass correlation (ICC)) and/or (ii) the paired sample $t$-test. However, Altman and Bland (1983) and Bland and Altman (1986) have criticized the use of both these techniques, in particular the use of correlation coefficients since they are measures of **relationship** rather than **agreement** and are highly influenced by the range of participants' measurements. For example, when comparing the results of a new test to measure $VO_2$ max with an existing test, if the chosen sample contains young and old, male and female, and heavy and light participants, the correlation is likely to be high. If, on the other hand, the same two tests are to be compared using only male participants, all of approximately the same age and similar body mass, the correlation between the results of the two tests will be relatively small, **but not necessarily less valid**.

Similarly, the paired or correlated sample $t$-test and repeated measures ANOVA are equally inconclusive when assessing repeatability or agreement between two or more measurement methods. Although such tests of significance will formally examine the hypothesis that no bias exists between the repeated measurements, that is, $H_0: \mu_1 = \mu_2 = \cdots = \mu_n$ versus $H_1: \mu_1 \neq \mu_2 \neq \cdots \neq \mu_n$, if the variance within participants (the residual mean square) is **large**, the null hypothesis ($H_0$) could be accepted, but the repeated measurements will still display unacceptable random variation.

Based on these shortcomings, Bland and Altman (1986), Nevill and Atkinson (1997), and Atkinson and Nevill (1998) proposed an alternative simple method of assessing agreement, based on means, standard deviations, and simple graphs. The authors argue that in order to assess the size of the error (i.e., the agreement or the reliability of a measurement tool) recorded on the interval or ratio scale, the most appropriate statistic to report is either the test–retest standard deviation of differences or the "95% limits of agreement." The precise form that these intervals take depends on whether a positive relationship exists between the differences (errors) and the size of the measurements, that is, evidence of heteroscedastic errors. If a positive and significant relationship exists, the recommended procedure is to report either the coefficient of variation (CV%) or "the ratio limits of agreement" calculated using log-transformed measurements.

Assuming no relationship is found between the measurement differences (errors) and their means, the "95% limits of agreement" are obtained as follows:

(i) Calculate the mean ($d$) and the standard deviation ($s$) of the differences that indicate the level of bias and the random variation between the two methods, respectively.

(ii) Provided the differences are normally distributed, the 95% "limits of agreement" are given by $d \pm (1.96 \times s)$.

Bland and Altman (1986) argued that provided differences within these limits are not clinically important, the two measurement methods can be used interchangeably. Similarly, if the same measurement is being assessed for test–retest reliability, provided the differences within these limits are not clinically important, the measurement can be considered reliable.

To examine whether a positive relationship exists between the measurement errors and the means, Bland and Altman (1986) recommend a plot of the differences (errors) against the measurement mean (known as the Bland and Altman plot). This can be confirmed by calculating the correlation between the **absolute** differences and the mean. If a positive relationship is observed, the analysis described previously should be applied to the log-transformed measurements (once again provided the differences between the natural log-transformed measurements are normally distributed). [Note that the difference between two log-transformed measurements is equivalent to the log transformation of the ratio between the two measurements, i.e., $\log_e(X_1) - \log_e(X_2) = \log_e(X_1/X_2)$]. By taking antilogs of the resulting "limits of agreement," we obtain an average (the geometric mean) dimensionless ratio (obtained by dividing one measurement method by the second) that describes the measurement bias, multiplied or divided by a second ratio that indicates the level of agreement. The latter ratio is not dissimilar to the concept of a coefficient of variation except the new ratio limits should contain 95% of the observed ratios. Note that if the "agreement ratio" were equal to 1, we would have perfect agreement between the measurement methods.

# A Worked Example Using the Test–Retest Differences of the Biceps Skinfold Measurements

Table 12.1 provides the test–retest skinfold measurements of the biceps for a large sample of male participants ($n = 962$) taken for the Allied Dunbar National Fitness Survey (AHR, ADNFS, 1992):

$$\text{The 95\% "limits of agreement"} = d \pm (1.96 \times s)$$
$$= 0.042 \pm 0.760$$

Given that the mean biceps measurement was 9.5, most sport scientists specializing in kinanthropometry would regard this within subject variation $= \pm 0.760$ mm, as an acceptable level of test–rest error. As stated previously, we need to assess whether the error is associated with the size of the measurements using the Bland and Altman plots, that is, to plot the differences against the means (see Figure 12.1).

Table 12.1   The biceps raised skinfolds measured on two occasions, sample of male participants ($n = 962$) taken for the Allied Dunbar National Fitness Survey.

| | Biceps1 (mm) | Biceps2 (mm) | Differences ($d$) | Means |
|---|---|---|---|---|
| | 12.8 | 13.2 | 0.4 | 13 |
| | 12.6 | 12.2 | −0.4 | 12.4 |
| | 34.4 | 34.6 | 0.2 | 34.5 |
| | 7.8 | 8.2 | 0.4 | 8 |
| | 5.4 | 5.6 | 0.2 | 5.5 |
| | 7.2 | 7.2 | 0 | 7.2 |
| | 6.6 | 6.6 | 0 | 6.6 |
| | 5.6 | 5.6 | 0 | 5.6 |
| | 8.2 | 8.4 | 0.2 | 8.3 |
| | . | . | . | . |
| | . | . | . | . |
| | . | . | . | . |
| | 8.8 | 8.4 | −0.4 | 8.6 |
| | 7.4 | 7.6 | 0.2 | 7.5 |
| | 4.6 | 4.6 | 0 | 4.6 |
| | 6.2 | 5.8 | −0.4 | 6 |
| | 5.6 | 5.6 | 0 | 5.6 |
| **Mean** | **9.595** | **9.553** | **0.042** | **9.574** |
| $s$ | **5.486** | **5.468** | **0.388** | **5.474** |

$s$, standard deviation.

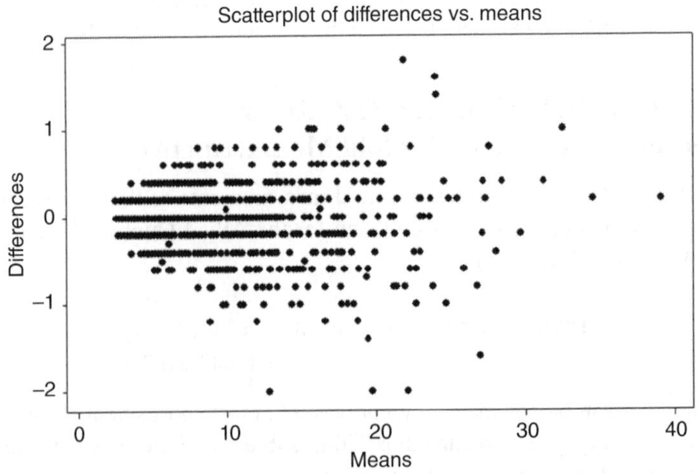

Figure 12.1   The differences (biceps 1 and biceps 2) versus their means.

Clearly, there is strong evidence of heteroscedastic errors with a wider spread of scores observed with means greater than 15 mm (sometimes referred to as the shotgun effect). This was confirmed when we calculated the correlation between the **absolute** differences and the means, found to be $r=0.409$ ($P<0.001$). As recommended previously, if such a positive relationship is observed, the analysis should be repeated but applied to the log-transformed measurements (once again provided the differences between the natural log-transformed measurements are normally distributed) (see Table 12.2).

Having taken natural logarithms of both biceps measurements, the mean difference (±standard deviation) was found to be $0.0042 \pm 0.0403$. Assuming the data are normally distributed, 95% of the differences should lie between the limits $0.0042$ ($\pm 1.96 \times 0.0403$), that is, from $-0.075$ to $0.083$. Taking antilogs of the measurements, the mean (bias) ratio was estimated as $1.004$, multiplied or divided by the agreement ratio ($*/\div 1.082$), that is, 95% of the ratios (measurement 2 divided by measurement 1) should lie between $0.928$ and $1.087$. These calculations can be summarized as follows:

$$\text{The 95% "ratio limits of agreement"} = \exp(d) * / \div \exp(1.96 \times (s))$$
$$= \exp(0.0042) * / \div \exp(1.96 \times 0.04033)$$
$$= 1.004 * / \div (1.082)$$
$$= 0.928 \text{ to } 1.087$$

Table 12.2    The log-transformed biceps raised skinfolds measured on two occasions, sample of male participants ($n=962$) taken for the Allied Dunbar National Fitness Survey.

| | ln(biceps1) | ln(biceps2) | Difference | Mean |
|---|---|---|---|---|
| | 2.549 | 2.580 | 0.0308 | 2.565 |
| | 2.534 | 2.501 | −0.0323 | 2.518 |
| | 3.538 | 3.544 | 0.0058 | 3.541 |
| | 2.054 | 2.104 | 0.0500 | 2.079 |
| | 1.686 | 1.723 | 0.0364 | 1.705 |
| | 1.974 | 1.974 | 0.0000 | 1.974 |
| | 1.887 | 1.887 | 0.0000 | 1.887 |
| | 1.723 | 1.723 | 0.0000 | 1.723 |
| | 2.104 | 2.128 | 0.0241 | 2.116 |
| | · | · | · | · |
| | 2.175 | 2.128 | −0.0465 | 2.151 |
| | 2.001 | 2.028 | 0.0267 | 2.015 |
| | 1.526 | 1.526 | 0.0000 | 1.526 |
| | 1.825 | 1.758 | −0.0667 | 1.791 |
| | 1.723 | 1.723 | 0.0000 | 1.723 |
| **Mean** | **2.1162** | **2.112** | **0.0042** | **2.1141** |
| $s$ | **0.533** | **0.5324** | **0.0403** | **0.5323** |

$s$, standard deviations.

In order to help the reader interpret these limits, if the participant's estimated biceps thickness was 10 mm on the first occasion, it is possible (worst-case scenario) that the same participant could obtain a biceps skinfold estimate as low as 9.28 mm or as high as 10.87 mm on the second occasion. Indeed, if the participants' measurement on the first occasion had been much lower at 5 mm, the second occasion measurement might have been as low as 4.64 mm or as high as 5.44 mm. These ranges are unlikely to be of serious concern to most sport scientists or clinicians involved in body-size assessment and kinanthropometry.

Bland and Altman (1986) also point out that simply by taking the antilogs of the standard deviation of differences summarized at the bottom of Table 12.2, that is, expressed as a ratio, $\exp(s) = \exp(0.04033) = 1.041$, we can obtain an estimate of the coefficient of variation, CV% $= (1.041 - 1) \times 100 = 4.1\%$. Once again, a CV% of just over 4% is normally acceptable, well within the levels of measurement error associated with skinfold assessment in most kinanthropometry laboratories.

# B. Utility of the Assessment of Test–Retest Stability Using Categorical/Likert-Type Data

The use of Likert scales to assess constructs is prevalent in sport and exercise sciences. The use of Likert-type data provides a time and labor economical means to gather data on a diverse array of topics, and the use of Likert scales is prevalent in many aspects of sport- and exercise-related research. This section will use an example from the topic of body image and, in particular, the MBSRQ to highlight the importance and utility of assessing test–retest stability when using data assessed on a Likert scale.

The argument that researchers should investigate the validity and reliability of measures is fundamental to theory testing. Interventions designed to improve any construct assessed using a pre–post design with a self-report rely on the scale that has minimal random error. In this context, it is important to distinguish reliability from stability. Stability refers to the concept that constructs retain a degree of resistance to change over time. An aspect of stability is the extent to which test–retest scores are reproducible, regardless of environment conditions. Reliability is defined as the ratio of true variance to error variance (Cohen, 1960) and is typically assessed using correlation. Although stability and reliability are closely related, there are important differences. Moreover, the prevalent approach in sport- and exercise-related research in establishing the robustness of self-report measures has been to test the test–retest reliability using Pearson's product-moment correlations. While this method is appropriate in determining association, it does not indicate anything about how stable the measure is over time. Likewise, the point-biserial correlation approach, where an individual item score is compared to total scale scores on a psychometric, has also been advocated as one means to assess stability. This approach suffers from similar limitations to the use of Pearson's product-moment correlations and is also only appropriate where there is a need to compare a dichotomous variable with a continuous variable.

It is important that researchers should be aware of the limitation of the methods they use. Methods such as the Pearson product-moment correlation, point-biserial correlation, and more recently ICC and kappa have been used to assess test–retest stability. In such cases, these measures do not assess stability. It is also common for researchers to treat reliability and stability as synonymous. Criterion values for acceptable test–retest stability using correlation suggest that the coefficient should be greater than $r=0.80$ (Kline, 1993). Research has questioned using correlational methods as a measure of test–retest stability since correlation is a measure of relationship rather than agreement (Bland & Altman, 1986; Nevill, 1996; Nevill, Lane, Kilgour, Bowes, & Whyte, 2001; Wilson & Batterham, 1999). For example, a perfect correlation ($\underline{r}=1.00$) can be found with no agreement, when measures are unstable. Consider the following example to illustrate this point. Scores taken from three participants at one point in time of 1, 2, and 3 will correlate perfectly with scores recorded at a second point in time of 3, 4, and 5. Thus, researchers should also assess the agreement between scores.

In this example, we will use scores taken from a sample of 99 young adults (aged 18–30 years) on the Multidimensional Body–Self Relations Questionnaire—Appearance Scales (MBSRQ-AS) (Cash, 2000) and will employ the nonparametric approach to assessing test–retest stability (Bland & Altman, 1999; Nevill et al., 2001).

# The Substantive Example

The MBSRQ-AS, designed for use with participants aged 15 years or older, asks participants to rate their response to 34 items on a five-point Likert scale (definitely disagree to definitely agree). It comprises five subscales related to the following appearance-related constructs of body image: Appearance Evaluation, Appearance Orientation, Overweight Preoccupation, and Body Areas Satisfaction. Acceptable internal consistency test–retest reliability values for each scale have been previously reported (Cash, 2000; Untas, Koleck, Rascle, & Borteyrou, 2009; Vossbeck-Elsebusch et al., 2014). Data relating to whether this instrument is stable over time has yet to be examined.

Scientists and researchers interested in this type of construct (or any other instrument employing Likert-type data) are interested in increases and decreases in the magnitude of scores on each scale as a result of some form of intervention (e.g., exercise training, dietary manipulation). Any instrument which pertains to be useful in this context needs to not only show validity and reliability but also needs to balance being able to be sufficiently sensitive to change while at the same time be sufficiently resistant to the effects of random error. Understanding how to calculate test–retest stability in such cases may therefore be useful and relevant to sport and exercise scientists and researchers.

## Utility of the Test–Retest Stability Using Nonparametric Data

Agreement or stability between the test–retest measurements of a psychometric questionnaire can be quantified simply by calculating for each item the differences between the responses recorded on two separate occasions. Clearly, these differences are discrete and hence will not have a normal distribution. Under such circumstances, we recommend adopting the nonparametric approach to assessing agreement proposed by Bland and Altman (1999) and Nevill et al. (2001). Systematic bias from test to retest can then be assessed using the nonparametric median sign test. It is also worthwhile to note that, unlike ratio data, self-report data from Likert scales should not be log transformed. Nevill and Lane (2007) pointed out that if you transform a 5-point scale that went from 0 to 4 (0 = not at all and 4 = very much so) and then used those numbers in subsequent analyses, then you would get completely different results than if the same scale went from 1 to 5.

The recommended procedure involves calculating the proportion of differences within some reference value, chosen to equate with no practically important difference (e.g., ±1). Nevill et al. (2001) suggested that a dispositional construct utilizing a five-point scale should show that the majority of participants (90%) should record differences within a referent value ±1. Although this reference value is arbitrary, it should be emphasized that self-report measures provide estimates of psychological constructs and cannot be relied on as objective and observable scores (see Nisbett & Ross, 1980; Nisbett & Wilson, 1977). For example, an individual might be genuinely unclear about what he/she is feeling and could only be accurate within ±1.

# The Synergy

To illustrate, the frequency distributions of two items from the MBSRQ-AS (item 1 ("Before going out in public, I always notice how I look") and item 3 ("My body is sexually appealing")) are presented in Table 12.3 and serve to illustrate the recommended assessment of agreement/stability.

Table 12.3    The frequency distribution of the test–retest differences (within participants) for items 1 and 3 of Multidimensional Body–Self Relations Questionnaire—Appearance Scale.

| Q1, Before going out in public, I always notice how I look | | | Q3, My body is sexually appealing | | |
| --- | --- | --- | --- | --- | --- |
| Difference | Freq | % | Difference | Freq | % |
| 4 | 0 | 0 | 4 | 0 | 0 |
| 3 | 0 | 0 | 3 | 3 | 3.03 |
| 2 | 1 | 1.01 | 2 | 7 | 7.07 |
| 1 | 10 | 10.10 | 1 | 7 | 7.07 |
| 0 | 55 | 55.56 | 0 | 50 | 50.51 |
| −1 | 27 | 27.27 | −1 | 20 | 20.20 |
| −2 | 5 | 5.05 | −2 | 8 | 8.08 |
| −3 | 1 | 1.01 | −3 | 2 | 2.02 |
| −4 | 0 | 0 | −4 | 2 | 2.02 |
| Total | 99 | 100 | | 99 | 100 |

Difference = test1 − test2.

Clearly, both items 1 and 3 find a similar number of participants who recorded the same response on both occasions (proportion of agreements (PAs) of 55 and 50, respectively). However, by observing Table 12.3, when responding to item 1 (Before going out in public, I always notice how I look), 92 of the participants (92.9%) differed by just ±1 point, indicating a relatively stable response to this item. In contrast, only 77 of the participants (77.8%) recorded a difference less of than or equal (±1) point for item 3 (My body is sexually appealing), suggesting a relatively unstable or transient response to item 3, that is, there appear to be quite contrasting levels of stability for these two items, an interpretation that would be missed by reporting just the PAs.

## Utility of the Item by Item Approach to Test–Retest Stability

To understand test–retest stability of any given measure that employs a Likert-type response, it is therefore important to assess whether each individual question (rather than simply the overall questionnaire scores) is stable. Using the same example as in the preceding text, the number of participants with test–retest differences within (±1), the proportion of agreement (PA = 0), and the median sign test of differences for all 34 items are given in Table 12.4. Note that items Q3 ("My body is sexually appealing"), Q9 ("Most people would consider me good-looking"), Q12 ("I like the way I look without my clothes on"), Q16 ("I don't care what people think about my appearance"), and Q28 ("How satisfied are you with your lower torso (buttocks, hips, thighs, and legs)") appear to demonstrate unstable behavior (<90% of participant differences from test to retest were ≤±1; see Nevill et al., 2001).

# The Synergy

The median sign test can then be used to identify whether bias exists in the test–retest responses for each question. In this case, the median sign test identified significant bias for 14 items (9 items where the participants recorded significantly lower responses on the retest (identified by the symbol < in Table 12.4) and 5 items where participants recorded significantly higher responses on the retest (identified by the symbol > in Table 12.4), all $P<0.05$). Note that the all five items where participants recorded significantly higher responses on the retest (Q11, "I use very few grooming products"; Q14, "I usually wear whatever is handy without caring how it looks"; Q16, "I don't care what people think about my appearance"; Q18, "I dislike my physique"; and Q20, "I never think about my appearance") are required to be "reversed" when calculating the factor scales.

Using the example of test–retest responses to the MBSRQ-AS provided here and by calculating the proportion of differences between test and retest scores that fall within ±1, the relative stability of a measure using categorical/Likert-type data can be determined. The median sign test can then be employed to determine bias in the test–retest data. In this instance, the test–retest differences of 29 of the 34 items of the MBSRQ-AS appear to indicate stable behavior (see Table 12.2), that is, items where more than 90% of participants recorded test–retest differences within (±1), see Nevill

Table 12.4    The number of participants with test–retest differences (test1 – test2) within (±1), the proportion of agreement (PA = 0), and the median sign test of differences for all 34 items.

| Item | ≤±1 | (%) | >±1 | Total | Median sign test | | | $P$ value | > vs < |
|------|-----|-----|-----|-------|-------|------|-------|-----------|--------|
|      |     |     |     |       | Below | PA = 0 | Above |           |        |
| 1  | 92 | 92.9 | 7  | 99 | 11 | 55 | 33 | 0.00 | > |
| 2  | 93 | 93.9 | 6  | 99 | 6  | 69 | 24 | 0.00 | > |
| 3  | 77 | 77.8 | 22 | 99 | 17 | 50 | 32 | 0.04 | > |
| 4  | 95 | 96.0 | 4  | 99 | 14 | 65 | 20 | 0.39 |   |
| 5  | 93 | 93.9 | 6  | 99 | 15 | 70 | 14 | 1.00 |   |
| 6  | 96 | 97.0 | 3  | 99 | 6  | 84 | 9  | 0.61 |   |
| 7  | 96 | 97.0 | 3  | 99 | 15 | 70 | 14 | 1.00 |   |
| 8  | 96 | 97.0 | 3  | 99 | 9  | 79 | 11 | 0.82 |   |
| 9  | 80 | 80.8 | 19 | 99 | 8  | 53 | 38 | 0.00 | > |
| 10 | 99 | 100.0 | 0 | 99 | 9  | 81 | 9  | 1.00 |   |
| 11 | 98 | 99.0 | 1  | 99 | 15 | 79 | 5  | 0.04 | < |
| 12 | 78 | 78.8 | 21 | 99 | 12 | 67 | 20 | 0.22 |   |
| 13 | 99 | 100.0 | 0 | 99 | 9  | 84 | 6  | 0.61 |   |
| 14 | 97 | 98.0 | 2  | 99 | 17 | 78 | 4  | 0.01 | < |
| 15 | 98 | 99.0 | 1  | 99 | 13 | 71 | 15 | 0.85 |   |
| 16 | 86 | 86.9 | 13 | 99 | 27 | 64 | 8  | 0.00 | < |
| 17 | 98 | 99.0 | 1  | 99 | 10 | 76 | 13 | 0.68 |   |
| 18 | 96 | 97.0 | 3  | 99 | 19 | 72 | 8  | 0.05 | < |
| 19 | 96 | 97.0 | 3  | 99 | 21 | 59 | 19 | 0.87 |   |
| 20 | 96 | 97.0 | 3  | 99 | 24 | 70 | 5  | 0.00 | < |
| 21 | 98 | 99.0 | 1  | 99 | 11 | 78 | 10 | 1.00 |   |
| 22 | 98 | 99.0 | 1  | 99 | 1  | 88 | 10 | 0.01 | > |
| 23 | 98 | 99.0 | 1  | 99 | 0  | 71 | 28 | 0.00 | > |
| 24 | 97 | 98.0 | 2  | 99 | 10 | 73 | 16 | 0.33 |   |
| 25 | 94 | 94.9 | 5  | 99 | 13 | 72 | 14 | 1.00 |   |
| 26 | 98 | 99.0 | 1  | 99 | 4  | 79 | 16 | 0.01 | > |
| 27 | 99 | 100.0 | 0 | 99 | 9  | 76 | 14 | 0.40 |   |
| 28 | 89 | 89.9 | 10 | 99 | 4  | 64 | 31 | 0.00 | > |
| 29 | 93 | 93.9 | 6  | 99 | 9  | 66 | 24 | 0.01 | > |
| 30 | 95 | 96.0 | 4  | 99 | 15 | 71 | 13 | 0.85 |   |
| 31 | 95 | 96.0 | 4  | 99 | 17 | 70 | 12 | 0.46 |   |
| 32 | 94 | 94.9 | 5  | 99 | 16 | 67 | 16 | 1.00 |   |
| 33 | 99 | 100.0 | 0 | 99 | 10 | 77 | 12 | 0.83 |   |
| 34 | 97 | 98.0 | 2  | 99 | 12 | 79 | 8  | 0.50 |   |

et al. (2001). In contrast, five items—Q3, "My body is sexually appealing"; Q9, "Most people would consider me good-looking"; Q12, "I like the way I look without my clothes on"; Q16, "I don't care what people think about my appearance"; and Q28,

"How satisfied are you with your lower torso (buttocks, hips, thighs, legs)"—appear to demonstrate unstable behavior. The results from the median sign test then identified 14 items with directional bias, where body image scores were lower on the second occasion in all 14 items. Understanding whether individual scale items are unstable is important in refining psychometric tests that use Likert-type data but is also essential in determining whether the whole scale is stable. If individual items lack stability, then the stability of the whole scale can be questioned.

The presence of unstable items within any self-report-type measure represents a point of theoretical and practical concern. The MBSRQ-AS, as used in this example, can be used to assess changes in a test–retest design, and given the link between body image and other negative health-related variables, it can be used in an intervention outcome targeted on improving scores. The majority of questions on the MBSRQ-AS (Cash, 2000) should be conceptualized as relatively stable as self-report perceptions can be examined in conjunction with factual information. For example, when responding to the items such as "I am on a weight-loss diet" and "I take special care with my hair grooming," we expect stable scores on items such as this, provided the individual has not made substantial changes to their lifestyle, with going on a diet being a clear example of how behavior and responses to scores on the scale should correlate.

However, unstable items could lead to a misleading interpretation, and for practitioners, this could be problematic. In the body image example here, unstable items could lead to the researcher interpreting that someone has excessive concerns over her/his appearance or that someone with excessive concerns is not identified. Identifying underlying issues that explain such changes is highly important, irrespective of the measure employed. However, we do not believe that evidence of instability is necessarily a negative quality of the scale. We suggest that items do not need to show the same degrees of stability, but researchers and practitioners need to know which ones are relatively stable and which ones are not. As normal practice involves calculating factor scores, it is important that each item in a factor shows equal stability scores and if there is instability, differences over time go in the same direction. We suggest that assessing the test–retest agreements for each item (see Nevill et al., 2001) is a user-friendly method that could be used to do this.

# Summary

The assessment of test–retest stability is useful in sport science and medicine research in better understanding agreement between repeated measures than the traditionally used Pearson's product-moment correlation. When interval or ratio data are employed, agreement may be best expressed as the standard deviation of differences X 1.96. In such cases, ratio data tends to require log transformation prior to analysis, whereas agreement for true interval data does not. When using nonparametric data calculating the proportion of differences between test and retest scores that fall within ±1, allow the relative stability of a measure to be determined. The median sign test can then be employed as a strategy to understand if there is any bias in the test–retest stability data.

# References

Activity and Health Research, Allied Dunbar National Fitness Survey. (1992). *A report on activity patterns and fitness levels: Main findings*. London, UK: Sports Council and Health Education Authority.

Altman, D. G., & Bland, J. M. (1983). Measurement in medicine: The analysis of method comparison studies. *Statistician, 32*, 307–317.

Atkinson, G., & Nevill, A. M. (1998). A review of the statistical methods employed to assess measurement error (reliability) in variables relevant in sports medicine. *Sports Medicine, 26*, 217–238.

Bland, J. M., & Altman, D. G. (1986). Statistical methods for assessing agreement between two methods of clinical measurement. *The Lancet, i*, 307–310.

Bland, J. M., & Altman, D. G. (1999). Measuring agreement in methods comparison studies. *Statistical Methods in Medical Research, 8*, 135–160.

Cash T. (2000). *The multidimensional body self relations questionnaire*. Norfolk, VA: Old Dominion University.

Cohen, J. (1960). A coefficient of agreement for nominal scales. *Educational and Psychological Measurement, 20*, 37–46.

Kline, P. (1993). *Handbook of psychological testing*. London, UK: Routledge.

Nevill, A. M. (1996). Validity and measurement agreement in sports performance. *Journal of Sports Sciences, 14*, 199.

Nevill, A. M., & Atkinson, G. (1997). Assessing agreement between measurements recorded on a ratio scale in sports medicine and sports science. *British Journal of Sports Medicine, 31*, 314–318.

Nevill, A. M., & Lane, A. M. (2007). Why self-report 'Likert' scale data should not be log-transformed. *Journal of Sports Sciences, 25*, 1–2.

Nevill, A. M., Lane, A. M., Kilgour, L. J., Bowes, N., & Whyte, G. P. (2001). Stability of psychometric questionnaires. *Journal of Sports Sciences, 19*, 273–278.

Nisbett, R., & Ross, L. (1980). *Human Inference: Strategies and Shortcomings of Social Judgment*. Englewood Cliffs, NJ: Prentice Hall.

Nisbett, R. E., & Wilson, T. D. (1977). Telling more than we know: Verbal reports of mental processes. *Psychological Review, 84*, 213–279.

Untas, A., Koleck, M., Rascle, N., & Borteyrou, X. (2009). Psychometric properties of the French adaptation of the multidimensional body self-relations questionnaire-appearance scales. *Psychological Reports, 105*(2), 461–471.

Vossbeck-Elsebusch, A. N., Waldorf, M., Legenbauer, T., Bauer, A. Cordes, M., & Vocks, S. (2014). German version of the multidimensional body-self relations questionnaire-appearance scales (MBSRQ-AS): Confirmatory factor analysis and validation. *Body Image, 11*(3), 191–200.

Wilson, K., & Batterham, A. (1999). Stability of questionnaire items in sport and exercise psychology: Bootstrap limits of agreements. *Journal of Sports Sciences, 17*, 725–734.

# 13

# Sample size determination and power estimation in structural equation modeling

## Nicholas D. Myers[1], Seniz Celimli[1], Jeffrey J. Martin[2], and Gregory R. Hancock[3]

[1] *School of Education and Human Development, University of Miami, Coral Gables, FL, USA*
[2] *Division of Kinesiology, Health and Sport Studies, Wayne State University, Detroit, MI, USA*
[3] *Department of Human Development and Quantitative Methodology, University of Maryland, College Park, MD, USA*

## General Introduction

Applications of structural equation modeling (SEM) can be found within many influential journals in sport and exercise science. For example, in *Exercise and Sport Sciences Reviews*, Duncan, Duncan, Strycker, and Chaumeton (2004) provided preliminary findings from a longitudinal study of youth physical activity. In *Medicine and Science in Sports and Exercise*, Motl, Dishman, Felton, and Pate (2003) investigated self-motivation and physical activity among black and white adolescent girls. In the *British Journal of Sports Medicine*, Smith and Hale (2004) examined the factor structure of a bodybuilding dependence scale. In the *Scandinavian Journal of Medicine and Science in Sports*, Felton and Jowett (2013) explored links between

*An Introduction to Intermediate and Advanced Statistical Analyses for Sport and Exercise Scientists*, First Edition.
Edited by Nikos Ntoumanis and Nicholas D. Myers.
© 2016 John Wiley & Sons, Ltd. Published 2016 by John Wiley & Sons, Ltd.
Companion website: www.wiley.com/go/ntoumanis/sport

coach interpersonal behaviors, coach–athlete relationships, and athletes' psychological need satisfaction and well-being. We believe that applications of SEM will continue to play an important role in sport and exercise science, in part because SEM programs can provide the user with statistical tests for (i) the entire model and (ii) specific parameters of interest within that model.

## Power

The power of a statistical test of interest is an important consideration when interpreting related results (e.g., Cohen, 1994). Statistical power can be defined as the probability of rejecting a false null hypothesis. A priori power analysis occurs prior to data collection (i.e., power is fixed and an estimate of sample size is sought) and from this point forward is referred to as *sample size determination*. Post hoc power analysis occurs after data have been collected (i.e., sample size is fixed and an estimate of power is sought) and from this point forward is referred to as *power estimation*. From this point forward, the expression *power analysis* is used when referring to sample size determination and power estimation simultaneously.

Providing information on power analysis in a published report may improve the methodological approach within a particular study and, perhaps more importantly, may positively influence the quality of related studies in the future. For example, sample size determination may encourage alterations to the research design that can lead to greater efficiency (e.g., recruit fewer participants than previously thought while achieving an acceptable level of power). Or, conversely, power estimation can provide an important context for a statistically nonsignificant result (e.g., subsequent research may need to recruit more participants than the current study in order to achieve an acceptable level of power). In either type of power analysis, effect size is a key issue that is worthy of attention in and of itself (e.g., Kelley & Preacher, 2012; Maxwell, 2004).

## Power Analysis in SEM

Within the SEM domain, a methodological literature on power analysis has emerged (e.g., MacCallum, Browne, & Sugawara, 1996; Satorra & Saris, 1985). Based on this literature, power analysis for two different purposes has materialized. The first purpose focuses on the entire model only and from this point forward is referred to as *power analysis regarding model-data fit*. The second purpose focuses on one or more specific parameters within a broader model and from this point forward is referred to as *power analysis regarding focal parameters*. Monte Carlo methods are an approach that can be used to implement a power analysis in SEM for both purposes (Muthén & Muthén, 2002). A Monte Carlo (simulation-based) approach to power analysis in SEM is not reviewed in this chapter for two reasons. The first reason is that a Monte Carlo approach to power analysis in SEM recently has been reviewed in sport and exercise science (Myers, Ahn, & Jin, 2011) and more generally (Bandalos & Leite, 2013). The second reason is that a Monte Carlo approach to power analysis in SEM can be more labor intensive, as compared to the more automated approaches that will be described in the synergy section of this chapter, for the researcher.

Power analysis in SEM relies on three core statistical concepts generally covered in a graduate-level research course. The first concept involves hypotheses, both null (which we generally wish to reject) and alternative. The second concept involves test statistics to assess null hypotheses, which differ for power analysis regarding model-data fit and focal parameters. The third concept involves central distributions (when a null hypothesis is true) and noncentral distributions (when an alternative hypothesis is true) that define the expected sampling distribution of a test statistic. The reader is referred to Hancock and French (2013) for a thorough and more technical treatment of each of these core topics.

Power analysis is typically not reported (though exceptions certainly exist) in published applications of SEM in sport and exercise science (Myers, Ahn et al., 2011). Therefore, the purpose of this chapter is to demonstrate how to implement (i) an a priori plan for sample size determination when power is fixed and (ii) a post hoc plan for power estimation when sample size is fixed. This chapter is organized within a substantive-methodological synergy format (e.g., Marsh & Hau, 2007) in an effort to make the material accessible (including minimizing the use of symbols) and relevant to the intended audience.

# Utility of the Methodology in Sport and Exercise Science

This section more formally introduces power analysis in SEM by making more explicit the three core statistical concepts referred to previously. Each introduction is intended to provide a possible (and general) starting point for future applications of SEM in sport and exercise science. The synergy section will demonstrate how to conduct power analysis for a specific example.

## Power Analysis Regarding Model-Data Fit: An Introduction

Power analysis regarding model-data fit focuses on the entire model (e.g., MacCallum et al., 1996). The root mean square error of approximation (RMSEA or $\varepsilon$; Steiger & Lind, 1980) is used to characterize model-data fit, where larger values indicate more misfit.[1] The lower boundary of unacceptable model-data fit is set to a value (e.g., 0.05; Browne & Cudeck, 1993). The researcher needs to determine the degrees of freedom for the entire model.

*Sample Size Determination.* The core task is to determine a necessary sample size for a fixed level of power for the purpose of rejecting the null hypothesis that the population model-data fit is at or exceeds a particular value (e.g., the lower boundary of unacceptable misfit).

*Hypotheses.* The null hypothesis is that the population model-data fit ($\varepsilon$) is poor, that is, greater than or equal to the lower boundary for unacceptable model-data misfit ($\varepsilon_0$). The alternative hypothesis is that the population model-data fit is acceptable, that

---

[1] It should be noted that this entire approach may be more accurately described as model-data *mis*fit.

is, less than the lower boundary for unacceptable model-data misfit. An efficient and general depiction of these hypotheses is

$$H_0 : \varepsilon \geq \varepsilon_0$$
$$H_1 : \varepsilon < \varepsilon_0 \qquad (13.1)$$

*Test Statistic.* The RMSEA is the test statistic used to test the null hypothesis. Given the form of Equation 13.1 (and assuming that $\varepsilon_0$=the lower boundary of unacceptable misfit), it is clear that rejecting the null hypothesis provides evidence for acceptable model-data fit. So the statistical question becomes: is the RMSEA estimate $\left( \hat{\varepsilon} \right)$ statistically significantly less than a particular value of $\varepsilon_0$?

*Distributions.* Under the null (and alternative) hypothesis, the central (and noncentral) sampling distribution of $\hat{\varepsilon}$ is asymptotically known due to the connection of $\varepsilon$ to a $\chi^2$ distribution (with a noncentrality parameter). While Equation 13.1 suggests a range of possible values for $\varepsilon$ under both the null and alternative condition, at this point, the researcher will select a value for both the null condition (e.g., null RMSEA=0.05) and the alternative condition (e.g., alternative RMSEA=0.00, 0.02, 0.04, ..., 0.049). Holding the null RMSEA value constant, smaller values of the alternative RMSEA will require a smaller sample size.

*Power Estimation.* The core task is to provide an estimate of power for a fixed sample size for the purpose of rejecting the null hypothesis that the population model-data fit is at or exceeds a particular value (e.g., the lower boundary of unacceptable misfit). Due to the close connection power estimation and sample size determination, only the steps that a researcher may need to take are provided below:

1. Select an α-level.

2. Determine degrees of freedom for the entire model.

3. Provide a sample size.

4. Provide an RMSEA value for the null condition.

5. Provide an RMSEA value for the alternative condition.

Note that if the researcher substitutes *desired level of power* for *sample size* in Step 3, then this list is applicable for sample size determination as well.

## Power Analysis Regarding Focal Parameters: An Introduction

Identifying that a pair of models is nested is a necessary condition for conducting a power analysis regarding focal parameters in the way that is described in this chapter.[2] For this reason, four terms commonly used to describe a pair of nested models are

---

[2] See Levy and Hancock (2007) for a framework of statistical tests for comparing a broader set of SEM models.

defined prior to dealing with power analysis in particular. The *full model* is defined by q number of parameters. The *reduced model* does not freely estimate (e.g., omit entirely) at least one parameter within the full model and does not contain any parameter excluded from the full model. Parameters common to both the full and the reduced model are considered to be *peripheral parameters*. Each parameter in the full model but not in the reduced model is considered to be a *focal parameter*.

Power analysis regarding focal parameters focuses on one or more focal parameters in the full model but not in the reduced model (e.g., MacCallum, Browne, & Cai, 2006). The full model contains the peripheral parameters plus at least one additional focal parameter and is characterized by some level of model-data misfit. The reduced model contains the peripheral parameters (but not the focal parameters) and is characterized by some level of model-data misfit. It is assumed that neither model is egregiously misspecified (Steiger, Shapiro, & Browne, 1985). The RMSEA is used to characterize model-data misfit. The researcher will need to determine degrees of freedom for both the reduced and the full model.

***Sample Size Determination.*** The core task is to determine a necessary sample size for a fixed level of power for the purpose of rejecting the null hypothesis that the difference in model-data misfit between the nested full and reduced models is a particular value (e.g., 0; MacCallum et al., 2006).

*Hypotheses.* The null hypothesis is that the population model-data misfit for the reduced model ($\varepsilon_R$) is equal to the population model-data misfit for the full model ($\varepsilon_F$), that is, that the focal parameters are unnecessary. The alternative hypothesis is that the population model-data misfit for the reduced model is greater than the population model-data misfit for the full model. An efficient and general depiction of these hypotheses is

$$H_0 : \varepsilon_R - \varepsilon_F = 0$$
$$H_1 : \varepsilon_R - \varepsilon_F > 0 \ . \tag{13.2}$$

*Test Statistic.* The difference between sample estimates of $\varepsilon_R$ and $\varepsilon_F$ can be translated to the difference between $\chi_R^2$ and $\chi_F^2$ $\left( \text{i.e.,} \chi_{\text{diff}}^2 = \chi_R^2 - \chi_F^2 \right)$, which is the test statistic (with *df* equal to $df_R - df_F$) used to test the null hypothesis (MacCallum et al., 2006). Given the form of Equation 13.2, it is clear that rejecting the null hypothesis provides evidence for the inclusion of the focal parameters. So the statistical question becomes: is the $\chi_{\text{diff}}^2$ statistically significantly greater than 0?

*Distributions.* Under the null (and alternative) hypothesis, the central (and noncentral) sampling distribution of $\chi_{\text{diff}}^2$ is known due to its at least approximate connection to a $\chi^2$ distribution. Given that the metric of $\chi_{\text{diff}}^2$ may be difficult to work with directly, and given the connection between ε and the model $\chi^2$, the researcher can return to the RMSEA metric when selecting a value for both the full and reduced model. Holding constant the RMSEA value for the full model (e.g., 0.00), larger RMSEA values for the reduced model will require a smaller sample size.

***Power Estimation.*** The core task is to provide an estimate of power for a fixed sample size for the purpose of rejecting the null hypothesis that the difference in model-data misfit between the nested full and reduced models is a particular value.

Due to the close connection between power estimation and sample size determination, only the steps that a researcher may need to take are provided below:

1. Select an α-level.

2. Determine degrees of freedom for the reduced model.

3. Determine degrees of freedom for the full model.

4. Provide a sample size.

5. Provide an RMSEA value for the reduced model.

6. Provide an RMSEA value for the full model.

Note that if the researcher substitutes *desired level of power* for *sample size* in Step 4, then this list is applicable for sample size determination as well.

# The Substantive Example

This section briefly considers the conceptual utility of the bifactor model for the Physical Education Teaching Efficacy Scale (PETES; Humphries, Hebert, Daigle, & Martin, 2012). A general case for the utility of bifactor analysis in sport and exercise science has been put forth (Myers, Martin, Ntoumanis, Celimli, & Bartholomew, 2014) and is summarized later prior to considering the PETES in particular. Two competing forms of the bifactor model for the PETES will provide a relevant substantive example for the subsequent demonstration of power analysis in SEM in the synergy section.

## Bifactor Model in Sport and Exercise Science

Theory-based scales in sport and exercise science often are developed to measure a general continuous latent construct along with several more narrowly defined continuous latent subdomains (Tenenbaum, Eklund, & Kamata, 2012). The bifactor model (Holzinger & Swineford, 1937) has a general factor (e.g., self-efficacy to produce a given attainment) and more specific group factors (e.g., self-efficacy for subdomains required to produce a given attainment) and a pattern (or "loading") matrix with a bifactor structure in which each item loads on the general factor and also may load on a group factor. In confirmatory bifactor analysis (CBFA), researchers are required to specify an explicit and complete bifactor structure a priori based on substantive measurement theory.

The exploratory form of the bifactor model was put forth because the complete a priori knowledge that is required under a CBFA often is incomplete in practice (Jennrich & Bentler, 2011). Exploratory bifactor analysis (EBFA) is an exploratory factor analysis (EFA) with a bifactor rotation criterion. Exploratory structural equation modeling (ESEM; Asparouhov & Muthén, 2009) has recently been put forth as a way to place EFA within the broader SEM framework. Thus, recent methodological developments that allow EBFA, in addition to CBFA, provide flexibility to accommodate the incomplete substantive measurement theory (e.g., when unsure if an item cross-loads on an unintended factor) that is often observed in sport and exercise science (e.g., Myers, Chase, Pierce, & Martin, 2011). EBFA and CBFA may be compared to each other statistically (as will be done in the synergy section) as well as conceptually (as will be done in the next section).

## Bifactor Model and the PETES

Investigations of self-efficacy theory (Bandura, 1997) are frequent in sport and exercise science (Feltz, Short, & Sullivan, 2008). Self-efficacy can be defined as individual's belief in her/his capability to produce given attainments. There is reason to speculate that responses to items designed to measure multifaceted efficacy beliefs may, at least in some cases, follow a bifactor structure. For example, items designed to measure multifaceted efficacy beliefs (e.g., group factors) residing within subsections of a broader conceptual space (e.g., a general self-efficacy factor) may be directly influenced by both the intended group factor and a more diffuse general self-efficacy factor that extends across, and defines the boundaries of, the entire conceptual space.

The PETES was developed to reflect the standards described for physical education (PE) teachers by the National Association of Sport and Physical Education (NASPE, 2009). Its purpose was to build upon previous research by developing "a broader, multi-dimensional teaching efficacy instrument specific to personal teaching efficacy for PE" (Humphries et al., 2012, p. 286). Personal teaching efficacy has been defined as the extent to which a teacher believes that he/she has the capacity to perform the necessary tasks to affect the learning of his/her students (Gibson & Dembo, 1984). Thus, within the previous quotation from Humphries et al., 2012, there is a reference to both a general construct (i.e., personal teaching efficacy for PE) and to more specific subdomains (i.e., group factors) residing within subsections of the broader conceptual space.

A CBFA of responses to the PETES could posit a general factor as well as seven group factors. The general factor, *PE teaching efficacy* (PETE), exerts a direct effect on responses to all 35 items and is defined as the extent to which a PE teacher believes that he/she has the capacity to perform the necessary tasks to affect the learning of his/her students. The group factors exert a direct effect on each of the items that they were designed to measure and are conceptualized as *content knowledge* (CK, 5 items), *scientific knowledge* (SK, 4 items), *accommodating skill differences* (ASD, 5 items), *teaching students with special needs* (SSN, 5 items), *instruction* (IN, 6 items), *assessment* (AS, 5 items), and *using technology* (TE, 5 items).

Figure 13.1 depicts two competing forms of the bifactor model for the PETES—from the more complex (i.e., Panel A) to the simpler (i.e., Panel B). An EBFA for the PETES is depicted in Panel A. An advantage of this model is the flexibility to accommodate unintended cross-loadings, while its potential weakness is less fidelity to the a priori measurement theory (e.g., each item is directly

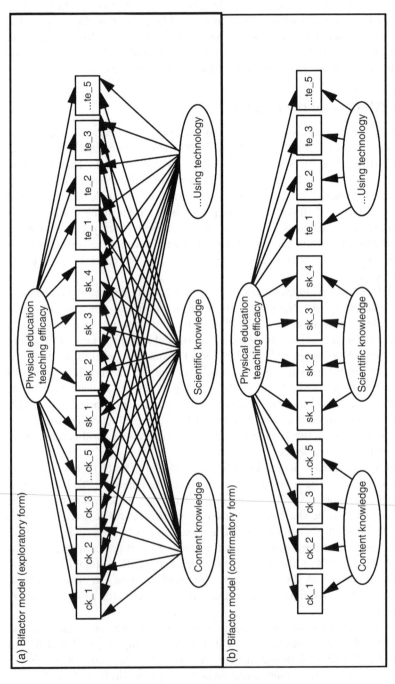

*Figure 13.1 Two competing forms of the bifactor model for the physical education teaching self-efficacy scale. Model parameters (e.g., variances), identification constraints, group factors, and items sometimes were omitted to reduce clutter. The sequence of figures follows a nested order: from Panel a (the more complex) to Panel b (the simpler).*

influenced by unintended group factors). A CBFA for the PETES is depicted in Panel B. An advantage of this is greater fidelity to the a priori measurement theory, while its potential weakness is placing too many restrictions on the data (e.g., each item is directly influenced the intended group factor only). The plausibility of, and the nested relationship between, the models depicted in Figure 13.1 provide a relevant example for demonstrating power analysis regarding both model-data fit (i.e., each model is considered separately) and focal parameters (i.e., the nested relationship between the models is emphasized). Before moving on to the synergy section, however, it should be noted the authors of this chapter are not aware of any published reports fitting real data to either form of the bifactor model for the PETES depicted in Figure 13.1. Therefore, subsequent steps in this chapter that require particular values to summarize model-data fit (e.g., $\varepsilon$) should be viewed as artificial values supplied in an effort to accomplish the pedagogical purposes of this chapter.

# The Synergy

This section demonstrates power analysis in SEM for two different purposes with regard to the two forms of the bifactor model for the PETES depicted in Figure 13.1. For each example, the reader can reproduce the result by repeating the steps and consulting relevant tables (e.g., Hancock & French, 2013) and/or an online utility (Preacher & Coffman, 2006) at http://quantpsy.org/rmsea/rmsea.htm and/or submitting code directly to R (R Core Team, 2013).[3]

Each demonstration is intended to display a reasonable (but certainly not the only) way to proceed in many applications of SEM in sport and exercise science. Some decisions are made, in part, for the sake of textual parsimony and should be altered as justified within subsequent applications in practice. Type I error rate is set to $\alpha = 0.05$. Power is set to 0.80. Assumptions, too, are made about the model(s) to be imposed (e.g., not egregiously misspecified), the data to be analyzed (e.g., conditionally multivariate normal), and the estimation method that will be used (i.e., maximum likelihood).

Degrees of freedom are determined for each model depicted in Figure 13.1 by subtracting the total number of parameters to be estimated ($q$) from the total number of observations available for the analysis ($u$). Given that the means are assumed to be in the model, $u$ can be determined by finding the value of $p(p+3)/2$, where $p$ is the number of observed variables. The value of $u$ is 665 for both models (i.e., 35(35 + 3)/2). The value of $q$ varies for the two models: for EBFA, $q = 322$, and for the CBFA, $q = 140$. Specific parameters for both models are as follows. For the EBFA, there are 35 intercepts, 252 pattern coefficients or "loadings," and 35 residual variances. For the CBFA, there are 35 intercepts, 70 pattern coefficients or "loadings," and 35 residual variances. The value of $df$ varies for the two models: for EBFA, $df = 343$ (i.e., 665–322), and for CBFA, $df = 525$ (i.e., 665–140).

---

[3] R code generated by the online utility (Preacher & Coffman, 2006) is provided in the appendices.

## Power Analysis Regarding Model-Data Fit: A Demonstration

Suppose that power analysis regarding model-data fit for each of the two competing forms of the bifactor model for the PETES depicted in Figure 13.1 is considered separately. Each measurement theory (i.e., measurement model) posits structural relationships between the latent and observed variables and allows for measurement error.[4] Each model yields some unknown level of population model-data fit.

*Sample Size Determination for the EBFA.* A necessary sample size is determined for the purpose of rejecting the null hypothesis that the population model-data fit is at or exceeds an RMSEA of 0.05. The alternative hypothesis is that the population model-data fit is an RMSEA of 0.00 or 0.02 or 0.04 which may be consistent with a range of optimism likely to be observed in practice (Hancock & French, 2013). All necessary information is now provided and is listed below:

1. α-level = 0.05

2. Degrees of freedom = 343

3. Desired level of power = 0.80

4. RMSEA value for the null condition = 0.05

5. RMSEA value for the alternative condition = 0.00 or 0.02 or 0.04

6. Necessary sample size = 85 or 104 or 322

Figure 13.2 provides a screenshot of the online utility for the first example. Appendix 13.1 provides R code for the three examples from this section.

*Sample Size Determination for the CBFA.* The null and alternative hypotheses are the same as for the EBFA in the previous paragraph. Steps with different values (as compared to the EBFA in the previous paragraph) are listed below:

2. Degrees of freedom = 525

6. Necessary sample size = 68 or 82 or 241

Notice the decrease in necessary sample size with an increase in degrees of freedom (i.e., an increase in model parsimony) while holding all other relevant values (e.g., RMSEA for the alternative condition) constant. Appendix 13.2 provides R code for the three examples from this section.

*Power Estimation for the EBFA.* An estimate of power is provided for a fixed sample size for the purpose of rejecting the null hypothesis that the population model-data fit is at or exceeds an RMSEA of 0.05. Sample size is equal to 300 or 400 or 500, which are values commonly observed in sport and exercise science (Myers, Ahn

---

[4] Clearly, there are instances when a substantive theory cannot be fully represented in a statistical model, but in this chapter, competing theories are manifest as competing statistical models, and thus, the expressions "model" and "theory" are sometimes used interchangeably.

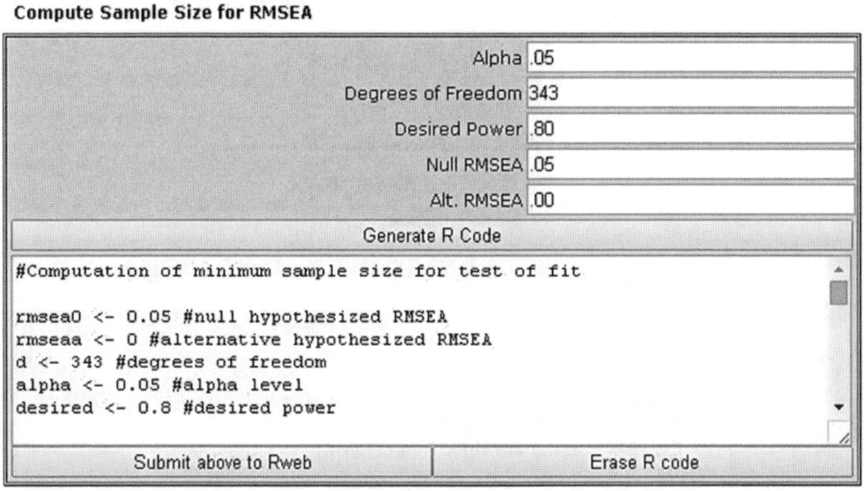

**Compute Sample Size for RMSEA**

| | |
|---|---|
| Alpha | .05 |
| Degrees of Freedom | 343 |
| Desired Power | .80 |
| Null RMSEA | .05 |
| Alt. RMSEA | .00 |

Generate R Code

```
#Computation of minimum sample size for test of fit

rmsea0 <- 0.05 #null hypothesized RMSEA
rmseaa <- 0 #alternative hypothesized RMSEA
d <- 343 #degrees of freedom
alpha <- 0.05 #alpha level
desired <- 0.8 #desired power
```

| Submit above to Rweb | Erase R code |
|---|---|

*Figure 13.2    Screenshot of the Compute Sample Size for RMSEA section within the online utility provided by Preacher and Coffman (2006). After the input is entered, the user can select Generate R Code and then Submit above to Rweb. The desired result (e.g., necessary sample size) appears near the bottom of the Results from Rweb page (i.e., for the first example: [1] 84.76). (Preacher & Coffman, 2006. Reproduced with permission from Kristopher J. Preacher.)*

et al., 2011). The alternative hypothesis is that the population model-data fit is 0.04, a value that may reflect a magnitude of misfit that is often observed in practice (Hancock & French, 2013). All necessary information is now provided and is listed below:

1. $\alpha$-level = 0.05
2. Degrees of freedom = 343
3. Sample size = 300 or 400 or 500
4. RMSEA value for the null condition = 0.05
5. RMSEA value for the alternative condition = 0.04
6. Power = 0.76 or 0.90 or 0.96

Figure 13.3 provides a screenshot of the online utility for the first example. Appendix 13.3 provides R code for the three examples from this section.

**Power Estimation for the CBFA.** The null and alternative hypotheses are the same as for the EBFA in the previous paragraph. Steps with different values (as compared to the EBFA) are listed below:

2. Degrees of freedom = 525
6. Power = 0.90 or 0.97 or 0.99

**Compute Power for RMSEA**

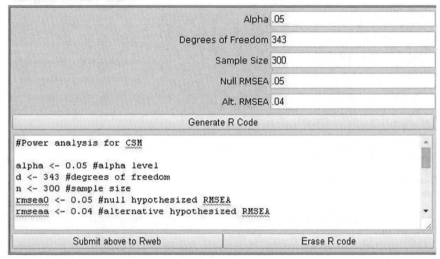

*Figure 13.3    Screenshot of the Compute Power for RMSEA section within the online utility provided by Preacher and Coffman (2006). After the input is entered, the user can select Generate R Code and then Submit above to Rweb. The desired result (e.g., power estimate) appears near the bottom of the Results from Rweb page (i.e., for the first example: [1] 0.76). (Preacher & Coffman, 2006. Reproduced with permission from Kristopher J. Preacher.)*

Notice the increase in power estimation with an increase in degrees of freedom (i.e., an increase in model parsimony) while holding all other relevant values (e.g., sample size) constant. Appendix 13.4 provides R code for the three examples from this section.

## Power Analysis Regarding Focal Parameters: A Demonstration

Suppose that the two forms of the bifactor model for the PETES depicted in Figure 13.1, which are nested models, are viewed as competing theories and power analysis regarding the focal parameters is sought. The EBFA (or the full model) contains all of the parameters of the CBFA (the reduced model). The 182 loadings estimated in the EBFA (i.e., unintended loadings on group factors) and not estimated (and forced to equal 0) in the CBFA are the focal parameters.[5] Each model yields some unknown level of population model-data fit, but due to the nesting of the CBFA within the EBFA, the CBFA cannot yield better overall fit than the EBFA.

*Sample Size Determination for the Nested Model Comparison.* A necessary sample size is determined for the purpose of rejecting the null hypothesis that the difference in population model-data misfit for the reduced model (i.e., the CBFA) as compared to the full model (i.e., the EBFA) is an RMSEA of zero. The alternative

---

[5] For identification purposes, we assume that 28 loadings (e.g., those loadings in the upper triangle of the loading matrix) in the EBFA are initially fixed to 0 (e.g., Algina, 1980).

hypothesis is that the difference in population model-data misfit for the reduced model as compared to the full model is an RMSEA of 0.02 or 0.03. The population model-data fit for the full model is an RMSEA of 0.02, while the population model-data fit for the reduced model is an RMSEA of 0.04 or 0.05 which is consistent with a similar comparison in sport and exercise science (Myers et al., 2014). All necessary information is now provided and is listed below:

1. α-level=0.05

2. Degrees of freedom for the reduced model=525

3. Degrees of freedom for the full model=343

4. Desired level of power=0.80

5. RMSEA for the reduced model=0.04 or 0.05

6. RMSEA for the full model=0.02

7. Necessary sample size=76 or 46

Figure 13.4 provides a screenshot of the online utility for the first example. Appendix 13.5 provides R code for the three examples from this section.

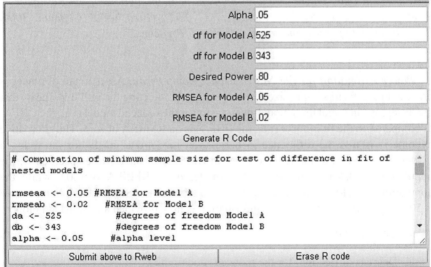

*Figure 13.4    Screenshot of the Compute Sample Size for RMSEA (nested models) section within the online utility provided by Preacher and Coffman (2006). After the input is entered, the user can select Generate R Code and then Submit above to Rweb. The desired result (e.g., necessary sample size) appears near the bottom of the Results from Rweb page (i.e., for the first example: [1] 76.17). (Preacher & Coffman, 2006. Reproduced with permission from Kristopher J. Preacher.)*

**Compute Power for RMSEA (nested models)**

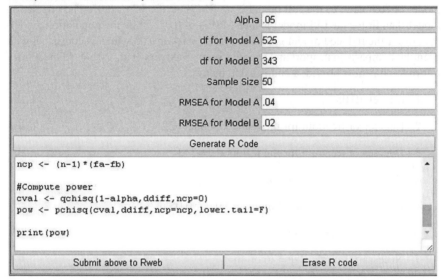

*Figure 13.5    Screenshot of the Compute Power for RMSEA (nested models) section within the online utility provided by Preacher and Coffman (2006). After the input is entered, the user can select Generate R Code and then Submit above to Rweb. The desired result (e.g., power estimate) appears near the bottom of the Results from Rweb page (i.e., for the first example: [1] 0.52). (Preacher & Coffman, 2006. Reproduced with permission from Kristopher J. Preacher.)*

**Power Estimation for the Nested Model Comparison.** An estimate of power is provided for a fixed sample size for the purpose of rejecting the null hypothesis that the difference in population model-data misfit for the reduced model (i.e., the CBFA) as compared to the full model (i.e., the EBFA) is an RMSEA of zero. The alternative hypothesis is that the difference in population model-data misfit for the reduced model as compared to the full model is an RMSEA of 0.02. More specifically, the population model-data fit for the full model is an RMSEA of 0.02, while the population model-data fit for the reduced model is an RMSEA of 0.04. Sample size is 50 or 75 or 100.[6] All necessary information is now provided and is listed below:

1. $\alpha$-level = 0.05

2. Degrees of freedom for the reduced model = 525

3. Degrees of freedom for the full model = 343

---

4. Sample size = 50 or 75 or 100

5. RMSEA for the reduced model = 0.04

6. RMSEA for the full model = 0.02

7. Power = 0.52 or 0.79 or 0.93

Figure 13.5 provides a screenshot of the online utility for the first example. Appendix 13.6 provides R code for the three examples from this section.

## Summary

Applications of SEM can be found within many influential journals in sport and exercise science. It is relatively uncommon, however, that the result of a relevant power analysis is reported within a published application of SEM in sport and exercise science. We believe that providing the result of a relevant power analysis in a published report is important because it may improve the methodological approach within a particular study and, perhaps more importantly, may positively influence the quality of related studies in the future. Therefore, the purpose of this chapter was to demonstrate power analysis (i.e., sample size determination and/or power estimation) in SEM for two different purposes (i.e., regarding model-data fit, regarding focal parameters) with a relevant example. While the PETES example allowed for illustrating how to deal with more details and in greater depth within both approaches in the synergy section, the focus of this section is more general.

Power analysis in SEM regarding model-data fit focuses on an entire model. This analysis may be appropriate when the primary purpose of a study is at the model level and not at the level of one or more focal parameters within a model. Sample size determination may be most useful at the design stage of such a study (i.e., data collection plan is being developed), whereas power estimation may be most useful at the analysis stage of such a study (i.e., data collection is closed). Some necessary conditions for performing a power analysis regarding model-data fit are that the model to be tested is well defined, a desired level of power (or sample size in the case of power estimation) can be declared, a lower boundary of model-data misfit can be specified, and a specific value of model-data misfit for the model to be tested ($\varepsilon$) can be put forth. Providing a value for $\varepsilon$ may prove to be the most difficult and the most debatable.

Power analysis in SEM regarding focal parameters focuses on one or more focal parameters that are included in the full model but not in the reduced model. This analysis may be appropriate when the primary purpose of a study is at the level of one or more focal parameters within a model. As with power analysis regarding model-data fit, sample size determination may be most useful at the design stage of such a study, whereas power estimation may be most useful at the analysis stage of such a study. Some unique necessary conditions for performing a power analysis regarding focal parameters (as compared to power analysis regarding model-data fit) are that the full model to be tested is well defined, the reduced model to be tested is well defined, a specific value of model-data misfit for the full model ($\varepsilon_F$) can be put forth, and a specific value of model-data misfit for the reduced model ($\varepsilon_R$) can be put forth. Providing a value for $\varepsilon_F$ and $\varepsilon_R$ may prove to be the most difficult and the most debatable.

Power analysis regarding focal parameters can be implemented in at least two ways although only one way was demonstrated in this chapter. The first way (e.g., Satorra & Saris, 1985) explicitly requires a value for each parameter within both the full and reduced model and was not reviewed in this chapter (see Hancock & French, 2013, for a review). An advantage (and disadvantage) of this type of implementation is that the researcher has the opportunity to (and, in fact, has to) provide a value for each parameter in the model. The second way (e.g., MacCallum et al., 1996) requires a value for model-data misfit for both the full and reduced model and was reviewed in this chapter. The first type of implementation may be of use when a priori information exists at a level to provide a plausible value for each parameter, while the second type of implementation may be of use when a priori information exists at a level to provide a plausible model-data fit value for each model only (and not a value for each parameter within a model). Readers are referred to MacCallum, Lee, and Browne (2010) for a comparison of these two implementations.

Power analysis in SEM requires the analyst to provide values for typically unknown entities (e.g., $\varepsilon, \varepsilon_R, \varepsilon_F$) that may heavily influence the result of a power analysis (e.g., estimate of sample size or power). In many cases, a range of specific values for these typically unknown entities may be put forth and therefore yield a range of values for sample size determination and/or power estimation. Providing justification for the (range of) value(s) selected for the typically unknown entities when possible to do so (e.g., previous research, pilot data, etc.) is suggested. Perhaps more important, however, is to clearly communicate all values provided by the user for a power analysis. The lists provided within the synergy section of this chapter provide a framework for a succinct paragraph (or two) where all relevant information may be summarized within a published manuscript. While the values selected for the typically unknown entities may be reasonably debated, the fact that a power analysis occurred and was thoroughly reported may provide a solid framework upon which the results of the current study can be evaluated and subsequent studies can build.

# References

Algina, J. (1980). A note on identification in the oblique and orthogonal factor-analysis models. *Psychometrika, 3,* 393–396.

Asparouhov, T., & Muthén, B. O. (2009). Exploratory structural equation modeling. *Structural Equation Modeling: A Multidisciplinary Journal, 16,* 397–438.

Bandalos, D. L., & Leite, W. (2013). Use of Monte Carlo studies in structural equation modeling. In G. R. Hancock & R. O. Mueller (Eds.), *Structural equation modeling: A second course* (2nd ed., pp. 625–666). Charlotte, NC: Information Age Publishing.

Bandura, A. (1997). *Self-efficacy: The exercise of control.* New York, NY: W. H. Freeman.

Browne, M. W., & Cudeck, R. (1993). Alternative ways of assessing model fit. In K. A. Bollen & J. S. Long (Eds.), *Testing structural equation models* (pp. 136–162). Newbury Park, CA: Sage.

Cohen, J. (1994). The earth is round ($p < .05$). *American Psychologist, 49*, 997–1003.

Duncan, S. C., Duncan, T. E., Strycker, L. A., & Chaumeton, N. R. (2004). A multilevel approach to youth physical activity research. *Exercise and Sport Sciences Reviews, 32*(3), 95–99.

Felton, L., & Jowett, S. (2013). "What do coaches do" and "how do they relate": Their effects on athletes' psychological needs and functioning. *Scandinavian Journal of Medicine & Science in Sports, 23*, e130–e139.

Feltz, D. L., Short, S. E., & Sullivan, P. J. (2008). *Self-efficacy in sport*. Champaign, IL: Human Kinetics.

Gibson, S., & Dembo, M. H. (1984). Teacher efficacy: A construct validation. *Journal of Educational Psychology, 76*, 569–582.

Hancock, G. R., & French, B. F. (2013). Power analysis in covariance structure models. In G. R. Hancock & R. O. Mueller (Eds.), *Structural equation modeling: A second course* (2nd ed., pp. 117–159). Charlotte, NC: Information Age Publishing.

Holzinger, K. J., & Swineford, S. (1937). The bi-factor method. *Psychometrika, 47*, 41–54.

Humphries, C. A., Hebert, E., Daigle, K., & Martin, J. (2012). Development of a physical education teaching efficacy scale. *Measurement in Physical Education and Exercise Science, 16*, 284–299.

Jennrich, R. I., & Bentler, P. M. (2011). Exploratory bi-factor analysis. *Psychometrika, 76*, 537–549.

Kelley, K., & Preacher, K. J. (2012). On effect size. *Psychological Methods, 17*, 137–152.

Levy, R., & Hancock, G. R. (2007). A framework of statistical tests for comparing mean and covariance structure models. *Multivariate Behavioral Research, 42*, 33–66.

MacCallum, R. C., Browne, M. W., & Cai, L. (2006). Testing differences between nested covariance structure models: Power analysis and null hypotheses. *Psychological Methods, 11*, 19–35.

MacCallum, R. C., Browne, M. W., & Sugawara, H. M. (1996). Power analysis and determination of sample size for covariance structure modeling. *Psychological Methods, 1*, 130–149.

MacCallum, R. C., Lee, T., & Browne, M. W. (2010). The issue of isopower in power analysis for tests of structural equation models. *Structural Equation Modeling: A Multidisciplinary Journal, 17*, 23–41.

Marsh, H. W., & Hau, K.-T. (2007). Application of latent variable models in educational psychology: The need for methodological-substantive synergies. *Contemporary Educational Psychology, 32*, 151–171.

Maxwell, S. E. (2004). The persistence of underpowered studies in psychological research: Causes, consequences, and remedies. *Psychological Methods, 9*, 147–163.

Motl, R. W., Dishman, R. K., Felton, G., & Pate, R. R. (2003). Self-motivation and physical activity among black and white adolescent girls. *Medicine & Science in Sports & Exercise, 35*, 128–136.

Muthén, L., & Muthén, B. (2002). How to use a Monte Carlo study to decide on sample size and determine power. *Structural Equation Modeling: A Multidisciplinary Journal, 9*, 599–620.

Myers, N. D., Ahn, S., & Jin, Y. (2011). Sample size and power estimates for a confirmatory factor analytic model in exercise and sport: A Monte Carlo approach. *Research Quarterly for Exercise and Sport, 82*, 412–423.

Myers, N. D., Chase, M. A., Pierce, S. W., & Martin, E. (2011). Coaching efficacy and exploratory structural equation modeling: A substantive-methodological synergy. *Journal of Sport &
Exercise Psychology, 33*, 779–806.

Myers, N. D., Martin, J. J., Ntoumanis, N., Celimli, S., & Bartholomew, K. J. (2014).
Exploratory bi-factor analysis in sport, exercise, and performance psychology: A substantive-methodological synergy. *Sport, Exercise, and Performance Psychology, 3*(4), 258–272.

National Association for Sport and Physical Education (NASPE). (2009). *National standards &
guidelines for physical education teacher education.* Reston, VA: Author.

Preacher, K. J., & Coffman, D. L. (2006, May). Computing power and minimum sample size
for RMSEA [Computer software]. Retrieved from http://quantpsy.org/

R Core Team. (2013). R: A language and environment for statistical computing. R Foundation
for Statistical Computing, Vienna, Austria. Retrieved from http://www.R-project.org/

Satorra, A., & Saris, W. E. (1985). Power of the likelihood ratio test in covariance structure
analysis. *Psychometrika, 50*, 83–90.

Smith, D., & Hale, B. (2004). Validity and factor structure of the bodybuilding dependence
scale. *British Journal of Sports Medicine, 38*, 177–181.

Steiger, J. H., & Lind, J. M. (1980, June). *Statistically based tests for the number of common
factors.* Paper presented at the annual meeting of the Psychometric Society, Iowa City, IA,
May 30, 1980.

Steiger, J. H., Shapiro, A., & Browne, M. W. (1985). On the multivariate asymptotic distribution of sequential chi-square statistics. *Psychometrika, 50*, 253–263.

Tenenbaum, G., Eklund, R. C., & Kamata, A. (2012). Measurement in sport and exercise
psychology: Some general thoughts about scale construction. In G. Tenenbaum, R. C.
Eklund, & A. Kamata (Eds.), *Handbook of measurement in sport and exercise psychology*
(pp. 3–7). Champaign, IL: Human Kinetics.

# Index

*An Introduction to Intermediate and Advanced Statistical Analyses for Sport and Exercise Scientists*, First Edition.
Edited by Nikos Ntoumanis and Nicholas D. Myers.
© 2016 John Wiley & Sons, Ltd. Published 2016 by John Wiley & Sons, Ltd.
Companion website: www.wiley.com/go/ntoumanis/sport